Age-Friendly Health Systems

Age-Friendly Health Systems

A Guide to Using the 4Ms While Caring for Older Adults

EDITORS

Terry Fulmer, PhD, RN, FAAN and Leslie Pelton, MPA

ASSOCIATE EDITORS

Jinghan Zhang, MPH, and Wendy Huang, MHA

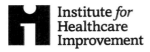

AGE-FRIENDLY HEALTH SYSTEMS
A Guide to Using the 4Ms While Caring for Older Adults

ISBN   978-1-5445-2750-5 *Hardcover*
            978-1-5445-2748-2 *Paperback*
            978-1-5445-2749-9 *Ebook*

This book is dedicated to the Age-Friendly Health System members of our movement in the United States and around the world. Your commitment to improving care for older adults is both inspiring and profoundly impactful. Because of your work, older adults can be assured they will receive equitable, reliable, quality care focused on what matters to those receiving care.

—Terry Fulmer, New York, NY, Spring 2022

Contents

Age-Friendly Health Care Contributors **ix**

Foreword *by Donald M. Berwick* **xvii**

Preface **xxiii**

Chapter 1   Care and Support With Older Adults and Their Families   **1**

Chapter 2   What Matters to Older Adults: The Basis of Age-Friendly Healthcare   **9**

Chapter 3   Conversations That Matter   **41**

Chapter 4   Medication   **63**

Chapter 5   Mentation   **93**

Chapter 6   Mobility   **109**

Chapter 7   4Ms Care   **145**

Chapter 8   4Ms Measures   **171**

Chapter 9   The Business Case for Becoming an Age-Friendly Health System *by Victor Tabbush, UCLA*   **201**

Chapter 10   Role of the Electronic Health Record in Aging   **225**

Chapter 11   Transitions of Care   **253**

Chapter 12   The Big Challenge: Spread and Scale   **267**

Chapter 13   Role of Public Health in
Age-Friendly Health Systems   309

Chapter 14   What Recognition, Credentialing, and Accreditation
Do We Need for Age-Friendly Health Systems?   325

Conclusion   333

Appendix A   Detailed Information on What Matters
Process and Outcome Measures   335

Appendix B   Resources to Support What Matters
Conversations With Older Adults   341

Appendix C   A Multicultural Tool for Getting to Know
You and What Matters to You   347

Appendix D   Examples of What Matters Conversations   351

Appendix E   Process Walkthrough   355

Appendix F   4Ms Age-Friendly Care Description Worksheets   357

Appendix G   Key Actions and Getting
Started with Age-Friendly Care   367

Appendix H   Age-Friendly Care Workflow Examples   389

Appendix I   Implementing Reliable 4Ms: Age-Friendly Care   395

Appendix J   Additional Measurement Guidance
and Recommendations   397

Appendix K   Example PDSA Cycles for Age-Friendly Care   401

Appendix L   Measuring the Impact of 4Ms Age-Friendly Care   409

Appendix M   IHI Age-Friendly Health Systems
Inpatient ROI Calculator Instructions   411

Index   425

Age-Friendly Health Care Contributors

(in formation as of Summer 2021)

Age-Friendly Health Systems Advisory Group

Don Berwick, MD, MPP (chair), President Emeritus and Senior Fellow, Institute for Healthcare Improvement; Former Administrator of the Centers for Medicare & Medicaid Services; Lecturer of Health Care Policy, Department of Health Care Policy, Harvard Medical School

Faith Mitchell, PhD (co-chair), Institute Fellow, Urban Institute

Jonathan Perlin, MD (co-chair), CMO and President, Clinical Services, Hospital Corporation of America (HCA)

Mary Tinetti, MD (founding co-chair), Gladys Phillips Crofoot Professor of Medicine (Geriatrics) and Professor, Institution for Social and Policy Studies; Section Chief, Geriatrics, Yale School of Medicine

Ann Hendrich, PhD, RN (founding co-chair), Researcher and Content Expert, Health Systems; Nursing and Safety Executive

Kyle Allen, DO, AGSF, Vice President, Enterprise Medical Director, CareSource

Kevin Biese, MD, Associate Professor, Emergency Medicine; Co-Director, Division of Geriatric Emergency Medicine; Director, Emergency Medicine Residency Program; Advisor to Gary and Mary West Health Institute

Alice Bonner, PhD, RN, Advisor, Care of Older Adults, Institute for Healthcare Improvement

Peg Bradke, RN, MA, Vice President, Post-Acute Care, UnityPoint Health— St. Luke's Hospital

Nicole Brandt, PharmD, MBA, Professor, Department of Pharmacy Practice and Science, University of Maryland School of Pharmacy; Executive Director, Peter Lamy Center on Drug Therapy and Aging

Marie Cleary-Fishman, BSN, MS, MBA, CPHQ Vice President, Clinical Quality, AHA Center for Health Innovation, American Hospital Association

Lenise Cummings-Vaughn, MD, Associate Professor of Medicine, Washington University's School of Medicine

Thomas E. Edes, MD, MS, Senior Medical Advisor, Office of Geriatrics and Extended Care, US Department of Veterans Affairs

Glyn Elwyn, MD, PhD, The Dartmouth Institute for Health Policy and Clinical Practice

Wes Ely, MD, MPH, Professor of Medicine, Vanderbilt University School of Medicine

Donna Fick, PhD, RN, Elouise Ross Eberly Professor of Nursing, Professor of Medicine, and Director of Center of Geriatric Nursing Excellence, Pennsylvania State University; Editor, Journal of Gerontological Nursing

Terry Fulmer, PhD, RN, President, The John A. Hartford Foundation

Sherry A. Greenberg, PhD, RN, GNP-BC, Associate Professor, Seton Hall University College of Nursing

Carrie Hays McElroy, MSN, RN, Gero-BC, ACM, Vice President, Clinical Operations, / Chief Nursing Officer, Chief Integrity and Compliance Officer, Trinity Health PACE

Kate Hilton, JD, MTS, Faculty, Institute for Healthcare Improvement and Atlantic Fellows for Health Equity, The George Washington University

Ann Hwang, MD, Director of the Center for Consumer Engagement in Health Innovation, Community Catalyst

Barbara Jacobs, RN, Vice President, Nursing, and Chief Nursing Officer, Anne Arundel Medical Center

Maulik Joshi, DrPH, Chief Executive Officer, Meritus Health

Doug Koekkoek, MD, Chief Executive, Providence Medical Group

Bruce Leff, MD, Professor, Johns Hopkins Medicine, and Director, The Center for Transformative Geriatric Research, Johns Hopkins University School of Medicine

Shari M. Ling, MD, Acting CMS Chief Medical Officer

Nancy Lundebjerg, MPA, Chief Executive Officer, American Geriatrics Society

Joe McCannon, Founder, Shared Nation, Formerly Founder and Chief Executive Officer, Billions Institute

Angela Patterson, DNP, FNP-BC, NEA-BC, FAANP, Chief Nurse Practitioner Officer, CVS MinuteClinic; Vice President, CVS Health

VJ Periyakoil, MD, Director, Palliative Care Education and Training, Stanford University School of Medicine; VA Palo Alto Health Care System, Division of Primary Care and Population Health

Eric Rackow, MD, Executive Chairman and Co-Founder, eFamilyCare; President Emeritus, NYU Hospital Center; Professor of Medicine, NYU School of Medicine

Stephanie Rogers, MD, MPH, Assistant Professor, Medicine, University of California, San Francisco

Ronnie Rosenthal, MD, Professor of Surgery, Yale School of Medicine; Surgeon-in-Chief, VA Connecticut Healthcare System

Nirav Shah, MD, MPH, Adjunct Professor at the School of Medicine, Stanford University

Albert Siu, MD, Professor and System Chair, Geriatrics and Palliative Medicine, Population Health Science and Policy, General Internal Medicine

Victor Tabbush, PhD, Adjunct Professor Emeritus, UCLA Anderson School of Management

Julie Trocchio, MSN, Senior Director, Community Benefit and Continuing Care, Catholic Health Association of the United States

Age-Friendly Health Systems IHI Team

Karen Baldoza, MSW, Vice President:

Matt Berry, Marketing Manager: maberry@ihi.org

Alice Bonner, PhD, RN, Advisor, Care of Older Adults: abonner@ihi.org

Chelsea Canedy, Project Manager: ccanedy@ihi.org

Shea Donie, Project Manager: sdonie@ihi.org

Luisana Henriquez Garcia, Associate Project Manager: lgarcia@ihi.org

Laura Howell, Project Manager: lhowell@ihi.org

Kevin Little, PhD, Improvement Advisor: klittle@ihi.org

Sumire Maki, Associate Project Manager: smaki@ihi.org
Kedar Mate, MD, President and CEO, Senior Sponsor: kmate@ihi.org
Leslie Pelton, MPA, Vice President: lpelton@ihi.org
KellyAnne Pepin, MPH, Project Director: kpepin@ihi.org
Christina Southey, Improvement Advisor: csouthey@ihi.org

Age-Friendly Health Systems American Hospital Association Team

Raahat Ansari, MS, Program Manager: ransari@aha.org
Kavita Bhat, MD, MPH, CPHQ, Performance Improvement Coach: kbhat@
  aha.org
Marie Cleary-Fishman, BSN, MS, MBA, CPHQ, CPPS, CHCQM, Vice
  President: mfishman@aha.org
Louella Hung, MPH, Director: lhung@aha.org
Radhika Parekh, MHA, Performance Improvement Coach: rparkeh@aha.org
Tarek Shagosh, Project Specialist: tshagosh@aha.org
Aisha Syeda, MPH, Program Manager: saisha@aha.org

Age-Friendly Health Systems Catholic Health Association of the United States Team

Julie Trocchio, MSN, Senior Director, Community Benefit and Continuing
  Care, Catholic Health Association of the United States

Age-Friendly Health Systems CVS Team

Angela Patterson, DNP, FNP-BC, NEA-BC, FAANP, Chief Nurse
  Practitioner Officer, CVS MinuteClinic; Vice President, CVS Health
Anne Pohnert, MSN, FNP-BC, Director of Clinical Quality, MinuteClinic,
  Anne.Pohnert@cvshealth.com
Sarah Ball, MSN, FNP-BC, Educator, Technology Consultant, Sarah.Ball@
  cvshealth.com
Elizabeth Evans, MSN, APRN, FNP-BC, Senior Practice Manager | Region
  57 | Area 05 | San Antonio and Corpus Christi; Champion Co-Leads,
  Age-Friendly Health Systems Ambulatory Care Continuum Grant

Mary Gattuso, Senior Manager, Corporate Communications, CVS Health MinuteClinic; Communications Consultant, Age-Friendly Health Systems Ambulatory Care Continuum Grant

Holly Kouts, MSN, APRN, Area Director, CVS Health MinuteClinic; Champion Co-Leads, Age-Friendly Health Systems Ambulatory Care Continuum Grant

Mary McCormack, MSN, FNP-BC, Educator, Professional Development Consultant, Mary.McCormack@cvshealth.com

Jennifer Nabong, FNP, Healthcare Business Partner, CVS Health MinuteClinic; Champion Co-Leads, Age-Friendly Health Systems Ambulatory Care Continuum Grant

Lilia Pino, PhD, Educator, Evaluation Consultant, Lilia.Pino@cvshealth.com

Case Western Reserve University Age-Friendly Health Systems Ambulatory Care Continuum Team

Mary A. Dolansky, PhD, RN, FAAN, Associate Professor, Case Western Reserve University; Associate Director, National VA Quality Scholars Program (VAQS); Senior Nurse Fellow VAQS, Louis Stokes Cleveland VA; Principal Investigator, Age-Friendly Health Systems Ambulatory Care Continuum Grant

Anna E. Bender, MSW, LSW, Doctoral Candidate, Jack, Joseph and Morton Mandel School of Applied Social Sciences, Case Western Reserve University; Qualitative Researcher, Age-Friendly Health Systems Ambulatory Care Continuum Grant

Brian Crick, BA, Computer Science Staff, Frances Payne Bolton School of Nursing, Case Western Reserve University; Lead, Computer Game Programmer / Software Developer, Age-Friendly Health Systems Ambulatory Care Continuum Implementation Grant

Evelyn G. Duffy, DNP, AGPCNP-BC, FAANP, Florence Cellar Professor of Gerontological Nursing, Director of the Adult-Gerontology Nurse Practitioner Program; Associate Director of the University Center on Aging and Health, Frances Payne Bolton School of Nursing, Case Western Reserve University; Professional Development Team Lead, Age-Friendly Health Systems Ambulatory Care Continuum Grant

Jackson Fielder, BA, Chemistry, Unity Developer and Educational Game Designer, Technology Team, Age-Friendly Health Systems Ambulatory Care Continuum Grant

Megan Foradori, RN, MSN, Doctoral Student, Frances Payne Bolton School of Nursing, Case Western Reserve University; Evaluation Team, Age-Friendly Health Systems Ambulatory Care Continuum Grant

Ronald L. Hickman, Jr., PhD, RN, ACNP-BC, FNAP, FAAN, The Ruth M. Anderson Endowed Chair and Associate Dean for Research, Frances Payne Bolton School of Nursing, Case Western Reserve University; Associate Editor, Applied Nursing Research; Implementation Team Lead, Age-Friendly Health Systems Ambulatory Care Continuum Grant

Robin Y. Hughes, MSN, AGNP-BC, Project Manager, Age-Friendly Health Systems Ambulatory Care Continuum Grant

Haley L. Kuhner, MN, RN, Graduate Research Assistant, Age-Friendly Health Systems Ambulatory Care Continuum Grant

Brant J. Oliver, PhD, MS, MPH, FNP-BC, PMHNP-BC, Associate Professor, Healthcare Improvement Scientist, Departments of Community & Family Medicine, Psychiatry, and The Dartmouth Institute, Geisel School of Medicine at Dartmouth College; Director, Chronic Health Improvement Research Program; Faculty Senior Scholar, Department of Veterans Affairs Health Professions Education, Evaluation, and Research Fellowship (HPEER); National Core Faculty (Methods and Analysis Curriculum Lead), Department of Veterans Affairs National Quality Scholars Fellowship (VAQS); Consultant, Age-Friendly Health Systems Ambulatory Care Continuum Grant

Glen Ona, Second-Year Nursing Student Research Assistant, Age-Friendly Health Systems Ambulatory Care Continuum Grant

Kelli Qua, PhD, Interim Director of Evaluation and CQI, Center for Medical Education; Senior Research and Evaluation Associate, Clinical and Translational Science Collaborative (CTSC) School of Medicine, Case Western Reserve University; Evaluation Team Consultant, Age-Friendly Health Systems Ambulatory Care Continuum Grant

Nicholas K. Schiltz, PhD, Assistant Professor, Frances Payne Bolton School of Nursing; Assistant Professor, Department of Population and Quantitative Health Sciences Center for Community Health Integration, Case Western Reserve University; Evaluation Team Lead, Age-Friendly Health Systems Ambulatory Care Continuum Grant

Ilona Seaman, BA, Computer Software Programmer, Lead Evaluation and Technology Analyst, Frances Payne Bolton School of Nursing, Case Western Reserve University; Age-Friendly Health Systems Ambulatory Care Continuum Grant

Barb Tassell, DNP, RN, NPD-BC, Evidence-Based Practice (CH), Frances Payne Bolton School of Nursing, Case Western Reserve University; Continuing Education Consultant, Age-Friendly Health Systems Ambulatory Care Continuum Grant

Elizabeth Zimmermann, DNP, MSN, RN, CHSE, Assistant Professor, NLN-Jonas Scholar 2013–2014, Frances Payne Bolton School of Nursing, Case Western Reserve University; Simulation Consultant, Age-Friendly Health Systems Ambulatory Care Continuum Grant

Foreword

by Donald M. Berwick, MD, MPP

President Emeritus and Senior Fellow, Institute for Healthcare Improvement

May 30, 2021

Taking a good idea to full scale should be simple, right? We have a problem, someone tests a solution, it works, we learn about the solution, and so we—all of us—adopt it too. Bingo: Problem solved for us all! What could be easier?

Sadly, no. That simple sequence is not, in fact, routine at all in human endeavor generally, nor in healthcare in particular. The clutch slips at every interface. Problems often remain undetected, unspoken, or ill-defined. Creative and practical minds do often come up with local solutions, but they tend to remain local, bottled up. Most are not published, since the inventors are too busy doing their own work to spend effort spreading their news. And even published innovations usually remain exactly where they appear; that is, in print, not in widespread practice.

Notorious exceptions do exist: Google, smartphones, pet rocks, and kale salad, for example. Some healthcare changes—good ones and bad ones—spread to large scale fast. Think of fiber-optic and robotic surgery, and, recently in the COVID-19 pandemic, virtual care, face masks, and, thankfully, vaccination. The drivers of rapid change are hard to pin down, but they appear to include vigorous commercial interests, meeting a strongly felt need, social contagion, and governmental action. But that is hardly a well-formed theory.

Reviewing the vast literature on large-scale change, even if confined to healthcare, would require far more space than this whole book, let alone the Foreword. Two research camps give just a small sample of a vast field.

The most comprehensive summary of the scientific knowledge about the diffusion of innovations is probably still the magisterial book of that name by Professor Everett Rogers, first published in 1962, and as of 2003, in its fifth edition. Trying to explain how and why changes spread, Rogers's explorations include two major branches, among others: first, properties of the innovation itself, and second, characteristics of subgroups in the potentially adopting communities. Properties of innovations favoring spread were five:

- pertinence to a felt need
- compatibility with the existing context
- simplicity
- trialability (the opportunity to taste before commitment)
- observability (the opportunity to see the change in operation elsewhere)

The strata in the adopting community, now widely known, included (a) innovators, (b) early adopters, (c) the early majority, (d) the late majority, and (e) laggards. Although Rogers's research and summaries yielding these models were nearly purely descriptive, most students of diffusion today translate them, with perhaps more enthusiasm than evidence, into prescriptions for accelerating wide-scale change.

Somewhat more recent than Rogers's original work are the insights of students of the theories of complex adaptive systems, who emphasize the inevitable non-linearities and instabilities (like the so-called butterfly effect) that render simple cause-and-effect explanations, expectations, and prescriptions inadequate or even hazardous under the conditions of complexity, which profoundly characterize healthcare. Much like Rogers, the complex adaptive systems theorists have been largely more successful in describing the phenomena than in prescribing evidence-based activity.

Though theories have blossomed, successes in large-scale healthcare improvement remain erratic and all too sparse. The problem of "spread of improvement" remains frustrating, and if a Nobel Prize in Physiology or Medicine is ever awarded in the field of improvement of healthcare, I would not be surprised if it is for solving the barriers to scaling.

Which is what makes the tale this book tells so remarkable. *Age-Friendly Health Systems: A Guide to Using the 4Ms While Caring for Older Adult* is an account of successful spread of an important improvement at a pace and scale nearly unparalleled by any other complex health system intervention. Barely five years after inception, from a standing start, over 2,000 US healthcare organizations have been recognized as Age-Friendly Health Systems.

At the simplest level, the "Age-Friendly Health Systems" movement has exactly the elements recited earlier in this Foreword: (a) a big problem recognized and spoken: the inadequacy of the healthcare system to meet the needs of a quickly aging population, many of whom are increasingly frail; (b) two decades of accumulating good ideas for improvement, tested in localities, often by disciplined clinical and health services researchers; (c) those solutions assembled and made accessible in a form (the 4Ms) easily understood; and (d) most remarkably, surging interest within less than five years in adoption of those solutions in thousands of healthcare organizations.

This progress was not accidental. It took specific stewards—in this case, a combination of The John A. Hartford Foundation and the Institute for Healthcare Improvement (which began the campaign), joined shortly afterward by the American Hospital Association and the Catholic Health Association, as well as a few pioneering organizations willing to trust and test the model in the first round of the project: Anne Arundel Medical System, Ascension, Kaiser Permanente, Providence St. Joseph, and Trinity. And it took a community of researchers, many connected as siblings by prior support from The John A. Hartford Foundation, to pool their knowledge openly and generously, and together to sculpt the 4Ms framework itself.

I suspect that Everett Rogers would have smiled to see the 4Ms (What Matters, Medication, Mentation, and Mobility). In the context of the Age-Friendly Health Systems movement, it is nearly an archetype of the five favorable characteristics of an innovation more likely than others to "diffuse." It addresses the serious problem of care for aged people; it is tested and proven in the real-world context of the early-adopting pioneers; it is a simple and memorable formulation of hundreds of research findings; it can be tried out at a small scale (as beautifully documented in this book); and its use has been made highly transparent through the collaborative mechanisms of the Age-Friendly Health Systems movement.

But, quite frankly, those explanations do not seem to me to be quite enough to account for the enormous success of age-friendly care so far. Something else is afoot, and I am not quite sure what that is, even though I have been privileged to be attached to and watch this program from the moment of its inception as a gleam in the eye of Dr. Terry Fulmer. Her enthusiasm, optimism, and sustained attention—along with those of her colleagues, like Amy Berman, Leslie Pelton, Kedar Mate, and Alice Bonner (to name just a few)—are, I am quite sure, part of the causal pathway. Credit is due also, in very large measure, to the vision and generosity of the vast community of participants who have searched out, studied, practiced, and shared in their lessons learned from the use of the 4Ms model in tough and complex settings. Attending one of their collaborative learning sessions is a vivid experience in seeing how proper improvement and joy in work are bound to each other.

This book assembles those lessons in a form easy to consume and to apply by any who wish to build on the successes to date and to sign their names to the growing roster of transformed healthcare systems much better fit to help an aging population. In so doing, they will become part of a story of spread of change whose implications and benefits will, I am totally convinced, extend far beyond the original target—excellence in care for older people—and into the vast enterprise of bringing effective innovations to all who can benefit therefrom.

Preface

In 2016, The John A. Hartford Foundation and the Institute for Healthcare Improvement (IHI) set out to improve care for older adults. We, our partners, and experts in the field all agreed that proven, evidence-based best practices were not making it to the "bedsides" of older adults. In hospitals, nursing homes, convenient care clinics, and primary care offices, the story was the same: the essential 4Ms components—described in this book—were not being reliably practiced. Five years later, along with the thousands of health system teams engaged in the Age-Friendly Health Systems movement, we have learned a great deal. We understand that any book we write today will be ready for a new edition by next year, but we believe that this is another important way to support and engage Age-Friendly Health Systems around the country and around the world. As you read it, think about how you can create a more seamless, safer, and higher-quality care encounter for your older patients in every setting of care they experience. The goal is to have excellent communication across care settings, health records, and most importantly, with the older person and their family. We refer to this as reliability. Further, as you use this book, let us know where it can be improved so we can continually make it more useful and of the highest quality possible. You will find several valuable guides as well as useful tools and charts that are yours to adopt to your own healthcare system. This is an open-source textbook, and all content is available at no cost, just like all Age-Friendly Health Systems materials on the IHI website.

This book is dedicated to those systems in appreciation for their years of stellar work. The success of the Age-Friendly Health Systems movement is due to the passion, the energy, and the wisdom that we have found in all our colleagues. Their generosity, leadership, and commitment to improving care for older adults has made this movement into what it is today: a transformational force that, every day, is improving health and well-being for older adults.

We also want to honor and express our thanks to the hundreds of thousands of older adults who have shaped our work and who have helped us create the Age-Friendly Health Systems that we all need and deserve.

Thanks so much to all who have contributed to date and to all who will contribute in the future.

Terry Fulmer, PhD, RN, FAAN
New York, NY, Summer 2021

Kedar Mate, MD
Boston, MA, Summer 2021

CHAPTER 1

Care and Support With Older Adults and Their Families

T he United States is aging; the number of adults over the age of 65 is projected to double over the next 25 years (Centers for Disease Control and Prevention, 2013). This has been well documented for decades, and yet our healthcare system seems surprisingly unprepared for the increasing proportion of older people brought on by the successful aging of the Baby Boomers. Meanwhile, US health expenditure is growing exponentially, increasing by 4.6% in 2019 and reaching $3.8 trillion (Centers for Medicare & Medicaid Services, 2019). Though people aged 55 and over make up 29% of the population, they are a high-need, high-cost population that accounts for 56% of health spending (Sawyer & Claxton, 2019).

Supporting an aging population is increasingly expensive, as clinical needs become more complex—approximately 80% of older adults have at least one chronic disease, and 77% have at least two (Centers for Disease Control and Prevention, 2013). Yet, many US health systems are ill-equipped to deal with the social complexity many older adults face, including, but not limited to, loss of loved ones, retirement, or relocation of residence (National Council on Aging, 2021). Our system of care treats people in silos defined by their disease processes. Older adults visit an endocrinologist for their diabetes, a cardiologist for their heart condition, and an orthopedic specialist or rheumatologist for their joint pain.

Providing excellent primary care in this fractured system is challenging; most people over 65 have three to five chronic diseases or disorders, and seldom do the experts have the opportunity to provide careful analysis across specialties. Older adults have higher rates of healthcare utilization compared to other age groups and experience higher healthcare-related harm, delay, and discoordination. They also visit emergency department four times as often as younger populations (Abrams & Milstein, 2016). The poor transitions in care and a failure to approach care in a person-centered manner result in potentially avoidable harms related to polypharmacy and falls, increased readmissions, and a greater risk of institutionalization, which further financially burden the US healthcare system.

Furthermore, the US is becoming more diverse, such that by 2030, the non-Hispanic white population will be the numerical minority. Though various ethnic and racial groups are living longer, socioeconomic disparities also bring about a disproportionate risk for adverse health outcomes compared with whites (Rowe et al., 2016). The COVID-19 pandemic has exposed these long-standing systemic disparities, as death rates have been disproportionately higher among African American, Native American, and Latinx communities. This stems from inequitable living and working conditions, higher rates of chronic medical conditions, and lower access to healthcare that predispose minority groups to worse COVID-19 outcomes (Tai et al., 2021). This highlights a need for effective care management by increasing collaboration between the older person, family caregivers, and clinicians to identify the older person's needs and goals and implement individualized care plans to achieve higher-quality healthcare (Rowe et al., 2016).

This book discusses care and support for older adults and utilizes the terms "people," "residents," and "patients" as appropriate to the content and setting herein.

Creating Age-Friendly Health Systems

The systems currently in place are clearly inadequate to serve an aging population's health needs. Fortunately, we now have the tools to create Age-Friendly Health Systems. Becoming an Age-Friendly Health System entails reliably providing a set of specific, evidence-based geriatric best-practice interventions to all older adults in your health system. Such systems do so primarily through redeploying existing health system resources to achieve

- better health outcomes for this population;
- reduced waste associated with low-quality services;
- increased utilization of cost-effective services for older adults; and
- improved reputation and market share with a rapidly growing population of older adults.

The development of these groundbreaking tools began in November 2016, when The John A. Hartford Foundation and the Institute for Healthcare Improvement (IHI), in partnership with the American Hospital Association (AHA) and the Catholic Health Association of the United States (CHA), set the bold aim that 20% of US hospitals and health systems would be Age-Friendly Health Systems by June 30, 2020.

The Framework: The 4Ms of Age-Friendly Care

The age-friendly care model that emerged is evidence-based and lends itself to reliable implementation in the healthcare setting. Age-friendly care can be encapsulated in the 4Ms.

The 4Ms—What Matters, Medication, Mentation, and Mobility—identify the core issues that should drive all decision-making with the care of older adults. They organize care and focus on the older adult's wellness and strengths rather than solely on disease. The 4Ms are relevant regardless of an older adult's individual disease(s). They apply regardless of the number of functional problems an older adult may have or that person's cultural, ethnic, or religious background (Mate et al., 2018).

The 4Ms

1. What *Matters*

Know and align care with each older adult's specific health outcome goals and care preferences, including, but not limited to, end-of-life care and across settings of care.

2. *Medication*

If medications are necessary, use age-friendly medications that do not interfere with What Matters, Mentation, or Mobility across settings of care.

3. *Mentation*

Prevent, identify, treat, and manage dementia, depression, and delirium across care settings.

4. *Mobility*

Ensure that older adults move safely every day to maintain function and do What Matters.

Each of the 4Ms is evidence-based. The innovation of an Age-Friendly Health System is the reliable practice of the 4Ms as a set (Mate et al., 2021).

The following chapters will describe the details of each of the 4Ms, though prototyping work shows that many health systems are already providing care aligned with one or more of the 4Ms with many of their older patients. Rather than asking providers to reinvent the wheel, the intention is that the 4Ms be incorporated into existing care. Much can be achieved primarily through redeploying existing health system resources to incorporate the remaining 4Ms and organize all 4Ms so that they are part of every encounter between an older adult and their caregivers.

The 4Ms provide a framework, not a program, designed to guide all care of older adults wherever they touch care and services. They are essential elements of providing high-quality care for older adults and, when implemented together, represent a broad shift by health systems to focus on the needs of older adults.

The Approach: Assess and Act

To successfully implement Age-Friendly Health Systems, there are two critical elements. First, assess every person/patient's unique situation through the lens of the 4Ms. Second, incorporate the 4Ms into the plan of care across all settings of care.

The 4Ms were first tested with hospital-based and ambulatory/primary care-based settings with expert faculty and advisors and five pioneering health systems—Anne Arundel Medical Center, Ascension, Kaiser Permanente, Providence, and Trinity Health. The resulting *Age-Friendly Health Systems: A Guide to Using the 4Ms While Caring for Older Adults* is designed to help care teams test and implement a specific set of evidence-based geriatric best practices across the 4Ms in their setting (Institute for Healthcare Improvement, 2020). In convenient care clinics and skilled nursing facilities, 4Ms care is now fully underway. Staff at these locations have the goal of implementing 4Ms care in every setting.

Summary

As the US population continues to age, healthcare expenditure exponentially rises due to the failure of the US healthcare system to address the complex social and clinical needs of older persons. The bold and rapidly spreading Age-Friendly Health Systems care model emerged to provide evidence-based interventions embedded in the 4Ms framework (What Matters, Medication, Mentation, Mobility), which aims to improve health outcomes for older persons, reduce waste associated with low-quality services, and increase the utilization of cost-effective, high-value services instead. This book is meant to facilitate your efforts to join the movement.

References

Abrams M., & Milstein, A. (2016). Matching patients to tailored care models: A strategy to enhance care, improving outcomes, and curb costs. National Academy of Medicine: Workshop Series on High-Need Patients. https://nam.edu/wp-content/uploads/2016/12/Taxonomy-and-care-model-presentation-FINAL.pdf

Centers for Disease Control and Prevention. (2013). The state of aging and health in America 2013. Centers for Disease Control and Prevention, US Department of Health and Human Services. https://www.cdc.gov/aging/pdf/State-Aging-Health-in-America-2013.pdf

Centers for Medicare & Medicaid Services. (2019). National Health Expenditure Data. https://www.cms.gov/newsroom/press-releases/cms-office-actuary-releases-2019-national-health-expenditures

Institute for Healthcare Improvement. (2020). *Age-friendly health systems: Guide to using the 4Ms in the care of older adults.* Institute for Healthcare Improvement. http://www.ihi.org/Engage/Initiatives/Age-Friendly-Health-Systems/Documents/IHIAgeFriendlyHealthSystems_GuidetoUsing4MsCare.pdf

Mate K. S., Berman A., Laderman, M., Kabcenell, A., & Fulmer, T. (2018). Creating age-friendly health systems: A vision for better care of older adults. *Healthcare*, 6(1), 4–6. https://doi.org/10.1016/j.hjdsi.2017.05.005

Mate, K. S., Fulmer, T., Pelton, L., Berman, A., Bonner, A., Huang, W., & Zhang, J. (2021). Evidence for the 4Ms: Interactions and outcomes across the care continuum. *Journal of Aging and Health*, 33(7–8). https://journals.sagepub.com/doi/full/10.1177/0898264321991658

National Council on Aging. (2021). *Get the facts on healthy aging.* https://www.ncoa.org/article/get-the-facts-on-healthy-aging

Rowe, J. W., Fulmer, T., & Fried, L. (2016). Preparing for better health and health care for an aging population. *JAMA*, 316(16), 1643–1644. https://jamanetwork.com/journals/jama/article-abstract/2556000.

Sawyer, B., & Claxton, G. (2019). *How do health expenditures vary across the population?* Peterson-KFF Health System Tracker. https://www.healthsystemtracker.org/chart-collection/health-expenditures-vary-across-population/#item-start

Tai, D. B. G., Shah, A., Doubeni, C. A., Sia, I. G., & Wieland, M. L. (2021). The disproportionate impact of COVID-19 on racial and ethnic minorities in the United States. *Clinical Infectious Diseases*, 72(4), 703–706. https://doi.org/10.1093/cid/ciaa815

CHAPTER 2

What Matters to Older Adults
The Basis of Age-Friendly Healthcare

Adapted from "What Matters" to Older Adults? A Toolkit for Health Systems to Design Better Care With Older Adults, *supported by The SCAN Foundation for Age-Friendly Health Systems*

> *Defining what matters means knowing and aligning care with each older adult's specific health outcome goals and care preferences including, but not limited to, end-of-life care, and across settings of care.*
> —The Age-Friendly Health Systems initiative

n March 2012, Michael Barry, MD, and Susan Edgman-Levitan, PA, introduced the concept of asking patients "What matters to you?" instead of only asking "What is the matter?" Their goal was to increase providers' awareness of critical issues in their patients' lives that could drive customized plans of care. Since then, IHI and other organizations around the world have been encouraging providers and healthcare organizations to ask patients and their caregivers about What Matters to them to inform their care (IHI, 2021b).

IHI's past work on The Conversation Project (IHI, 2021a) and *Conversation Ready* (Sokol-Hessner et al., 2019) has sought to encourage individuals, families, and health systems to have conversations about What Matters in the context of end-of-life care. The Age-Friendly Health Systems initiative builds upon IHI's previous work in shared decision-making, expanding the asking of What Matters beyond the context of end-of-life care to *all* care with older adults across their lifespan. The aim is to align care preferences—the healthcare activities (e.g., medications, self-management tasks, healthcare visits, testing, and procedures) that patients are willing and able (or not willing or able) to do or receive—keeping in mind the older adult's health outcome goals, as they relate to the values and activities that matter most to an individual, help motivate the individual to sustain and improve health, and could be impacted by a decline in health. For example, cherished activities might include babysitting a grandchild, walking with friends in the morning, or volunteering in the community. When identified in a specific, actionable, and reliable manner, patients' health outcome goals can guide decision-making.

What Matters conversations evolve over time, in the context of ongoing communication and relationship building between older adults and their caregivers. They also take place in more than one setting. Instead of one-time conversations between older adults and clinicians, What Matters conversations should take place at multiple points of care (e.g., annual visits, major life events, or changes in health status) and be coordinated among all members of the care team.

What Matters to Older Adults Toolkit

What Matters is arguably the most important of the 4Ms, the very foundation of the Age-Friendly Health Systems initiative, and yet, aligning care to each patient is still a relatively new concept, particularly for patients who are not seriously ill or near the end of life. Operationalizing a system to understand, document, and act on What Matters to older adults in healthcare organizations is challenging; it requires organizational culture change as well as clinician training and specific changes to workflows and the electronic health record. This chapter presents a tested toolkit to support the transition.

This What Matters to Older Adults Toolkit was developed by IHI with support from The SCAN Foundation to offer a starting place and extend an invitation to learn together how to better understand and act upon What Matters to older adults and measure progress in doing so by bringing together the best available evidence from health systems around the world (IHI, 2019).

The toolkit is intended to serve as a resource for multidisciplinary care teams, including, but not limited to, physicians, nurses, physician assistants, medical assistants, social workers, chaplains, nurse navigators, community health workers, and trained volunteers. This chapter provides actionable steps and guidance to ensure that every older adult's health outcome goals and care preferences are understood, documented, and integrated into their care by the entire healthcare team.

What Matters as the Basis of Age-Friendly Care

In the Age-Friendly Health Systems initiative, asking What Matters to the older adult is the basis for the relationship with the care team and shapes the care that is provided. What Matters integrates care and decision-making across care settings. What Matters is not limited to end-of-life planning. It is therefore essential to the older adult, the care team, and the health system that What Matters to each older adult is identified, understood, and documented so it can be acted upon and updated across settings of care following changes in care or life events.

Documenting What Matters Information

Reliable and timely documentation of the older adult's goals and preferences is a critical step in the What Matters process. Documentation of the conversation should be easily accessible to the older adult and all members of the care team so that it can be reviewed and referenced on a regular basis and during care planning. All documented information should be clear, concise, reflective of the older adult's stated goals, and recorded using their own words as much as possible.

High-Tech and Low-Tech Solutions

Where a care team chooses to document goals and preferences depends on available infrastructure and care context. A whiteboard or construction paper poster can be a quick and highly visible way to document and update What Matters for an older adult in an inpatient setting, but it is not easily shareable across settings and not a practical method for documenting information in a primary care or outpatient specialty care setting. Documenting What Matters in an electronic health record (EHR) allows clinicians to document conversations in more detail and allows the information to be reviewed over time and by multiple members of the care team.

Both methods may be used in tandem to document both short- and long-term preferences and care goals, depending on the care setting. Table 2.1 compares using physical versus electronic health records for documentation.

Table 2.1. Considerations for Documenting What Matters
Conversations in Physical Versus Electronic Formats (IHI, 2021b)

DOCUMENTATION	PHYSICAL RECORD	ELECTRONIC HEALTH RECORD (EHR)
Ideal for	• Inpatient/long-term care • Recording small amounts of information quickly (e.g., one or two sentences)	• Inpatient and outpatient care • Long-term recording • Recording detailed conversations • Sharing information across care settings
Pros	• Low cost • Easy and quick to document and update • Easily visible to any member of the care team who enters older adult's room • Does not require changes to hospital information technology (IT) infrastructure • Does not require significant training resources	• Readily accessible to all members of the care team who have access to the EHR, regardless of location • Can document What Matters conversations over time • Can document conversations with more detail • All health-related information is stored in one centralized location • Can link older adult's goals and preferences with key documents, such as advance care plan

Cons	• Not shareable across different care settings • Not good for documenting large quantities of or nuanced information • Not easily available to members of the care team who do not visit older adult's room • Not a viable method for long-term recording • Not effective for outpatient or primary care setting where exam rooms are used by multiple patients throughout the day • Not private, which could make some older adults uncomfortable	• Requires significant initial investment in EHR infrastructure modifications • Requires care team members to take time to enter information • Care team members must be trained on new processes for documenting What Matters in the EHR
Examples	• Asking a hospitalized older adult "What matters to you today?" during daily rounds and documenting responses on a whiteboard in the patient's room • Paper "Patient Passport" booklet that older adult is responsible for carrying to and from appointments	• Creating "tags" in the EHR for all notes that contain information on the older adult's goals and preferences • Creating "flags" to remind clinicians to update What Matters information • Documenting the older adult's goals in Plan of Care section of the EHR

Electronic Health Record. If the organization's EHR includes a patient portal, the organization may want to create a module for older adults to enter and review relevant healthcare proxy information, advance directives, and important notes on their care goals. Specific guidance for different EHR vendors is challenging given the variability between organizations and the newness of this work. While most examples are from organizations using Epic, the guidance for Epic could contain some applicable lessons for other EHRs. Some suggestions follow:

- **Creating tags**: Tags are keywords used to link notes in EHRs and can be used to indicate that a note contains What Matters information or any record of a serious illness conversation. Once a tag has been created, Epic can be configured so that notes with specific labels appear first in the record. This can be used to ensure that What Matters information is clearly available to whoever is checking the medical record.

- **Using the "Longitudinal Plan of Care" or other care planning feature**: These provide a central location for documenting What Matters conversations.

- **Using a patient-facing portal**: Many EHRs have patient-facing portals that allow patients to directly message their clinicians, attend e-visits, and complete questionnaires remotely (Epic, 2021). This tool can be used to send questionnaires about What Matters to older adults prior to visits. Clinicians can then use this information to facilitate further discussion.

- **Requesting a custom build**: Some organizations have worked with their EHR vendors to build a template that

works for their care team. A custom-built template may
include the following sections:

- self-perception of health status and trajectory
- health and healthcare concerns and fears
- values
- health goals
- care preferences

The Care Plan

Once the care team has begun the process of talking with an older
adult about What Matters to them, the next step is to incorporate
their expressed preferences and goals into their care plan. By anchoring an initial What Matters conversation around specific points in
the care process during which decisions about care are likely to be
made (e.g., first visit, new diagnosis, change in health status, or life
transition), the team may be in a better position to build a clinical
care plan that reflects the older adult's goals.

Below are some key strategies to ensure that an older adult's
expressed goals and preferences are incorporated into their plan
of care.

Patient Education as Part of Care Planning

Because most patients are not medical professionals, they may not be
as knowledgeable about the harms and benefits of various treatment
and care options. Applicable decision aids (e.g., patient education videos, flashcards) may be used to educate them and support conversations about various options and tradeoffs in some care decisions.
While such aids can be useful for relevant decisions, they are not a
substitute for a conversation to elicit the issues that are most important to older adults. Additionally, the uncertainty of benefits and

harms of treatment options for older adults makes the traditional approach of decision aids and shared decision-making less effective (Fried, 2016). It is incumbent upon the clinicians to understand each patient's goals and preferences and offer treatment options within the context of those goals and preferences.

When an Older Adult's Preferences Conflict With Clinical Advice

Generally, an older adult's goals and preferences should be respected as much as possible when planning their care with them. However, in some cases, an older adult may have preferences that are in direct conflict with their clinician's medical advice, or they may reject the advice of a clinician. If this is the case, more communication about What Matters to them may lead to more clarity about *why* they are rejecting certain options or plans. Both the older adult and the clinician may need to reevaluate their perspectives and work together to find alternatives.

Leveraging Interdisciplinary Resources to Address Older Adults' Needs

When asking older adults about What Matters to them, many of their preferences or concerns may involve social determinants of health on which a clinician is unable to have a direct impact (e.g., housing, food, access to social services). This is where having an interdisciplinary care team can be critical; a social worker or nurse navigator, for example, may be able to connect people with additional resources outside of the clinical sphere. Some teams use regular (e.g., weekly) interdisciplinary team huddles to discuss the results of that week's What Matters conversations and share resources that can be used to address older adults' concerns. Sharing these stories and problem solving together also helps build goodwill and improve satisfaction among members of the care team.

Engaging With Community Resources

In addition to the interdisciplinary care team, community-based organizations can be excellent resources for addressing needs beyond the health system. Maintaining a list of community organizations that can provide support for the social determinants of health (e.g., housing, food assistance, transportation, financial support, behavioral health) can facilitate the provision of referrals. Documenting any referrals given to an older adult during a What Matters conversation in the EHR also allows clinicians to follow up on these social determinants during subsequent visits.

Measuring What Matters

Why measure What Matters? The right measures can help improve how well the care team understands, documents, and acts on What Matters to older adults. Measurement for improvement relies on relatively frequent observations, tracked over time, to guide and maintain changes to work.

Table 2.2. What Matters Measures (IHI, 2021b)

MEASURE TYPE	MEASURE NAME
Process	Documentation of What Matters
Outcome	Care concordance with What Matters
Balancing	Impact on the care team

Process Measure: Documentation of What Matters
Why Measure Documentation of What Matters?

Documentation of What Matters signals that the care team has engaged the older adults they serve in these conversations, and this documentation will guide the team as they develop and carry out care plans aligned with What Matters for each older adult.

The process measure for What Matters documentation is the percentage of patients served by the relevant hospital unit or primary care team who have documentation of What Matters at the end of each measurement period. Appendix A gives measurement details for inpatient and primary care sites.

Tips for Getting Started With Measuring Documentation of What Matters

CREATE EXAMPLES

Have two care team members create or find at least three examples that the team leaders consider to be acceptable documentation. What features do the examples have that make them acceptable? Creating some good examples is a start to the formal development of an "operational definition" to support consistent measurement.

TEST THE MEASURE

1. Test 1: Have a care team member (a "tester") test the measure and review the examples of good documentation. Have the member look at one new instance of documentation. Can the tester decide whether the documentation is acceptably aligned with the What Matters questions and interaction proposed by the care team? If the tester cannot decide, what features of documentation are missing that would enable a decision?

2. Test 2: Repeat Test 1 for five instances of documentation.

3. Test 3: Have two members of the care team assess the same three patient records for quality of What Matters documentation. Compare their decisions. If two care

team members disagree on one or more decisions, discuss differences and propose changes to the features (or criteria) that characterize good What Matters documentation.

A TARGET GOAL FOR DOCUMENTATION OF WHAT MATTERS SHOULD BE 95% OR GREATER

This means there is documentation showing that the care team has engaged 95% or more of older adults in their care in What Matters conversations. Remember that the process should allow patients to decline to engage in What Matters conversations; an older adult who declines to answer should be included in the numerator for this process measure. The care team will have to assess whether the percentage of older adults who decline to answer is acceptable. If it is too high, this could be an area for study and improvement.

APPLY QUALITY IMPROVEMENT METHODS TO IMPROVE DOCUMENTATION

Directly observe the documentation steps and have the care team member doing the documenting talk out loud about the task, focusing on what is difficult or confusing. What can be changed to make it easier to document What Matters? Another idea is to review 10 patient records that do not meet the health system's standard for documentation to identify features of insufficient documentation. Then identify one problem that can be mitigated or prevented. Test changes to address this documentation problem.

Outcome Measure: Care Concordance With What Matters
Why Measure Care Concordance With What Matters?

While alignment between What Matters to older adults and the care they receive has been studied for care at the end of life, understanding and aligning care with What Matters for all older adults, regardless of life stage or prognosis, is critical.

There is currently no consensus or widely used approach to measure care concordance with What Matters, though there is great interest in this topic, and health systems will be actively testing and learning how to measure concordance in the future. We know enough now to get started and learn by doing.

The outcome measure tracks answers to closed-ended questions about care experience and What Matters (see the table in Appendix A for details).

If the health system already asks specific populations about the concordance of care with What Matters, then they should continue to use those tools. For example, a survey used for patients of palliative care services at Trinity Health includes some questions that touch on concordance of care with What Matters, ranked on a 1–5 scale (very poor to very good). These include

- the degree to which the care team addressed the patient's emotional needs;
- the care team's effort to include the patient in decisions about their treatment; and
- the care team's respect of the patient's wishes regarding continuing or discontinuing statements.

Getting Started With Measuring Care Concordance With What Matters

Most hospital units and primary care practices will not yet measure care concordance with What Matters. The next section introduces the **collabo**RATE tool to meet that need. **collabo**RATE questions, developed by researchers at The Dartmouth Institute for Health Policy & Clinical Practice, are appropriate after a specific clinic visit or during a hospital stay (Elwyn, n.d.).

As **collabo**RATE will be a new measurement tool for most health systems, care teams will need to figure out how to capture and summarize the question scores.

- For a clinic visit, the questions should be asked before the patient leaves the clinic.
- For a hospital stay, the questions may be asked at any time after the first day of the stay when the patient is able to communicate with the care team. Integration of **collabo**RATE into the course of care during the stay or at discharge increases the number of responses (rather than sending a post-discharge questionnaire).
- For those patients unable to communicate, there is a version designed for individuals acting on behalf of patients.

The wording of the three questions and the appearance of the scales have been tested and should not be varied, though the opening statement can be varied to make it appropriate for the setting. Note that the Hospital Consumer Assessment of Healthcare Providers and Systems (HCAHPS) guidelines may need to be reviewed prior to regular use of **collabo**RATE in hospital settings.

- Go to the **collabo**RATE Measurement Scales to find specific versions appropriate to your populations (a Creative Commons license allows for free noncommercial use).
- Consider joining the **collabo**RATE users group to learn more about practical use of the tool.
- Share the **collabo**RATE tool with relevant staff. Ask, "What should we change so that almost every patient will answer '9' to all three questions?"

Outline a method to capture answers to **collabo**RATE and summarize top-box scores. **collabo**RATE has been tested using different approaches; while response rates vary, researchers found similar clinician performance across different data collection approaches (Barr et al., 2017). Spreadsheet or paper systems can suffice for initial testing and local application. REDCap software can also be used to collect responses. Finally, health systems may want to investigate a third-party automated solution, using existing patient portals or messaging systems, that maintains anonymity and helps with clear reporting.

Learn about **collabo**RATE by testing to improve measurement. For example:

- Test **collabo**RATE with one patient. Ask, "How will the care team member introduce the questions? How will they record the answers?"
- Test **collabo**RATE with five patients. What does this test indicate about **collabo**RATE's impact on workflow? What will it take to engage with patients and document answers consistently?
- Repeat tests with older adults who prefer a language other than English.

Alternatives to Care Team Use of **collabo**RATE in a Hospital Setting

The **collabo**RATE questions and scale format, in principle, can be added to post-discharge patient surveys administered after HCAHPS. This requires discussion with the hospital's patient-experience-survey vendor to determine if the **collabo**RATE questions can be included.

If it is not possible to use **collabo**RATE, hospitals can track the HCAHPS scores that may indicate whether care of the older adult aligns with What Matters to the older adult.

HCAHPS Communication Score

Hospitals can track the HCAHPS nurse communication composite (HCAHPS questions 1, 2, 3) and physician communication composite (HCAHPS questions 5, 6, 7) for patients 65 years and older who are treated in the relevant unit. Note that this option will be of limited effectiveness if there are low counts of patients 65 years and older who are surveyed and respond to the survey.

HCAHPS Overall Experience Score

Hospitals can also track the HCAHPS overall experience scores using HCAHPS questions 21 and 22. It is recommended that for your analysis, the numerator be patients 65 years and older responding "top-box" to the specified questions and the denominator be patients 65 years and older responding to the HCAHPS survey. Then obtain 12 months of survey responses stratified by age group to determine the median number of responses. If the median monthly number of responses is more than 10 per month in each stratum, run charts of the HCAHPS scores are likely to be informative. If median monthly numbers are less than 10 per month per stratum, pool the monthly numbers into quarterly values.

Other Approaches

Additionally, hospitals can also conduct regular conversations with patients 65 years and older about the alignment of their care with What Matters. A related project carried out by National Health Service Scotland suggests five conversations a month provide a good basis to monitor performance and provoke improvement ideas (Healthcare Improvement Scotland, 2018). Some ideas for these conversations include:

- Ask two open-ended questions:
  - How well did we include What Matters to you in choosing what to do next?
  - What could we do better?

- Record the responses verbatim; don't attempt to reword or analyze.
- Review the verbatim responses with your team once a month. What ideas emerge that you can test to improve alignment of What Matters with patient experience of care? Then test the ideas.

Alternatives to Care Team Use of **collaboRATE** in an Ambulatory Practice Setting

CG-CAHPS Communication Composite

Practices can also track the Clinician and Group Consumer Assessment of Healthcare Providers and Systems Survey (CG-CAHPS) rating of communication (composite) using questions 11, 12, 14, and 15 in the basic CG-CAHPS version 3.0. It is recommended that for your analysis, the numerator be patients 65 years and older responding "top-box" to the specified questions and the denominator be patients 65 years and older responding to CG-CAHPS. Then obtain 12 months of survey responses stratified by age group to determine the median number of responses. If the median monthly number of responses is more than 10 per month in each stratum, run charts of the CG-CAHPS scores are likely to be informative. If median monthly numbers are less than 10 per month per stratum, use quarters as the time step.

Role of Family Councils

More than 40 million Americans perform the family caregiving role each year to someone of adult age. Family caregivers today support people with various conditions and do so in a variety of contexts:

- Close to one in three support someone in a rural area.
- 15% of care recipients are veterans.

- More than half (60%) are employed.
- One in five care for a person with mental health or emotional issues.

Family caregivers are key to the 4Ms of geriatric care:

- Knowing and acting on What Matters (honoring choice)
- Medication
- Mentation
- Mobility

Home Alone Findings

- 46% of caregivers performed medical/nursing tasks.
- More than 96% of medical/nursing caregivers also provided activities of daily living (ADL) or instrumental activities of daily living (IADL) assistance.
- 89% of care recipients are adults aged 50 and older.
- Many family caregivers perform these tasks with very little clinical guidance, leaving them feeling stressed and concerned about making mistakes (Reinhard et al., 2019).

Need for Patient- and Family-Centered Care and Patient and Family Advisory Councils (PFACs)

Patient- and family-centered care (PFCC) emphasizes collaborating with patients and families of all ages, at all levels of care, and in all healthcare settings. Further, it acknowledges that families, however they are defined, are essential to patients' health and well-being and are allies for quality and safety within the healthcare system (Bezold, 2005; Frampton et al., 2003; Gerteis, 1993). It recognizes that the very young, the very old, and those with chronic conditions—the individuals who are most dependent on hospital care and the broader healthcare system—are also those who are most dependent on families (Cacioppo & Hawkley, 2003; Chow, 1999; House, 2002). Family members are more than surrogates to be called on when the patient is unable to make decisions on their behalf; they are essential members of the care continuum and caregiving team. The literature confirms that social isolation is a health risk factor, and hospital and ambulatory care policies and practices should not separate patients and families in caregiving and decision-making.

Momentum for patient- and family-centered care crosses national borders. In the United Kingdom, the National Health Service (NHS) has mandated that there be structures in place in all NHS hospitals and primary care clinics that support patient and carer (family) participation in quality-improvement efforts. Patients Accelerating Change is a program in the United Kingdom bringing patients together with clinicians and managers in hospitals and primary care settings to transform healthcare services. The Picker Institute Europe and the NHS Clinical Governance Support Team are helping prepare and support people for this collaboration. Across Canada, patients and families are increasingly engaged with provincial and national efforts to improve quality, with a particular focus on access and patient safety.

Four Key Concepts of Patient- and Family-Centered Care

- **Dignity and respect**: Providers listen and honor patient and family perspectives and choices
- **Information sharing**: Providers share complete and unbiased information in ways that are affirming and useful
- **Participation**: Patients and families participate in care and decision-making.

- **Collaboration**: Patients and families collaborate on policy and program development, implementation and evaluation, as well as the delivery of care (Institute for Patient- and Family-Centered Care, n.d.)

Integrated Patient-, Family-, Public-, and Community-Centered Care

Table 2.3. Integrated Patient-, Family-, Public-, and Community-Centered Care (IHI, n.d.)

	LOCATION	EXAMPLES
Environment	Community, Region, State, Province	• Community groups • Care Coordination, ACOs, medical homes • Advance care planning, POLST, MOLST • School & church programs • Public health & other consumer campaigns
Organization	Health System, Trust, Hospital, Nursing Home	• Experience surveys • P&F councils, advisors, faculty • Resource centers, patient portals • Access to help and care 24/7 • Medication lists
Micro-system	Clinic, Ward, Unit, ED, Delivery	• Patient, advisors, & advisory councils • Open access, optimized flow • Family participation in rounding
Experience of Care	Bedside, Exam Room, Home	• Access to the chart • Shared care planning; adverse event reporting • "Smart Patients Ask Questions"

Policy

Patient and Family Advisory Councils (PFACs) became mandatory in Massachusetts hospitals, effective June 12, 2009. The regulations required each hospital to establish a PFAC by October 1, 2010, and to prepare a report outlining its plan to establish a PFAC no later than September 30, 2009 (Patient & Family Advisory Councils, 2014).

Case Studies

Blanchfield Army Community Hospital, Fort Campbell, Kentucky

Collect and Disseminate Data Regarding the Impact of Partnerships With Patients and Families in Order to Increase the Evidence Base for Change

Blanchfield Army Community Hospital (BACH) at Fort Campbell in Kentucky has been a leader among Military Treatment Facilities (MTFs) in creating partnerships with patient and family advisors. A Patient- and Family-Centered Care Council was established in 2005 at BACH. Over the last two years, over 25 patient and family advisors have been involved in various quality-improvement initiatives. Radiologists and hospital staff worked with patient and family advisors in redesigning the mammography experience. Women can now self-refer, and the experience is one of information sharing and support for women, enhancing patient and staff/physician satisfaction and meeting health promotion / disease prevention targets. BACH is the first MTF to meet the HEDIS performance measures for mammography screening (Blanchfield Army Community Hospital, n.d.).

The MCG Health System, Augusta, Georgia
Develop the Business Case for Partnerships
With Patients and Families

Incorporating patient and family advisors at all levels of an institution can contribute to efficiency, quality, safety, satisfaction, and even market share. The MCG Health System, an academic medical center in Augusta, Georgia, is nationally recognized for its commitment to patient- and family-centered care, and partnerships with patients and families at all levels of care. The process for change began in 1993. Today, 155 patient and family advisors serve on seven councils and 45 hospital committees and task forces, including the Patient Safety and Medicine Reconciliation Committees.

In 2001, MCG worked with the Walton Rehabilitation Hospital to create a Patient and Family Advisory Council for the Augusta Multiple Sclerosis Center. There are currently 15 patient and family members. Among the staff and physicians who attend the meetings regularly are the medical director, a clinical psychologist, an administrator for the clinic, the Multiple Sclerosis physician assistant, a Multiple Sclerosis certified nurse clinician, a staff nurse, and a research professional. Among the projects the Council has assisted with are the design and relocation of the clinic, parking accessibility, access to psychological care, and the development of the electronic personal health record system. The volume of patients followed by this clinic has grown substantially in the last five years. Currently, the Council is working with staff to develop a study to evaluate the clinic's approach to care and its impact on patient activation.

MCG's Family Practice Center created a Patient and Family Advisory Council in 2006. Fourteen patient and family members, the Family Medicine Center Manager, Family Medicine Nursing Coordinator, and Director of Ambulatory Patient Access Services serve on the Council. As the program evolves, residents and physicians will be asked to join. Others are involved as requested by the Council. The Manager of the Family Medicine Center serves as the staff liaison for the Council. Data is gathered from patients in the waiting areas through questionnaires and surveys and is shared with the Council to help plan changes. Customer service at the front desk area has improved. The Council's involvement in clinic meetings has been energizing and has improved overall staff attitudes.

By request of patient advisors, patient education programs have been developed or planned for the near future. These include orientation to the Family Medicine Center and integration of health education into computers in the exam room and other patient areas. Patient and family advisors are also asked to participate in projects separate from the Council, such as participation in monthly staff meetings and on the Safety Committee (Johnson et al., 2008).

Patient- and family-centered care has become the business model for the organization, as it impacts positively each of MCG's business metrics (finances, quality, safety, satisfaction, and market share). This academic medical center is the most cost-efficient hospital in the University HealthSystem Consortium (UHC) database. From 2001–2006, MCG reports a decrease in malpractice claims and litigation, while many other academic medical centers, as measured by the UHC, report annual increases in these expenditures. Patient- and family-centered care is central to the values, strategic plan, and personnel policies and practices. Partnerships with patients and families are embedded at all levels of the organization (Augusta University Health, 2021).

The Cambridge Health Alliance, Cambridge, Massachusetts
Use Community Advisors to Assist in Addressing
Linguistic and Multicultural Issues

The Cambridge Health Alliance in Cambridge, Massachusetts, serves the culturally diverse communities of Cambridge and Somerville, as well as other "immigrant gateway" communities near Boston. It is a unique model that incorporates public health, clinical care, academic programs, and research. Over 300 volunteer health advisors from these culturally diverse communities have been trained and provided with continuing education by the Alliance's Community Affairs Department since 2001. These advisors collectively speak 16 different languages and represent the local Haitian, Brazilian, Latinx, South Asian, African American, and African communities.

Currently, program staff and over 120 advisors work collaboratively with churches and community organizations to organize health fairs, educational events, and health screenings; provide basic health education in disease prevention and wellness; and educate community members about services. The Somerville Hospital has a PFAC helping staff develop a deeper understanding of the needs and perceptions of the diverse community it serves. The Cambridge Health Alliance also has a PFAC specific to the Haitian population. Hospital and clinic signs are all in four languages, and artwork in corridors and public spaces reflects the diversity of the cultures served. Patient and family informational materials and community educational programs are offered in many languages (Cambridge Health Alliance, 2021).

Vanderbilt Medical Center, Nashville, Tennessee
Assure That Leadership Walk-Arounds and Patient
Safety Rounds Include a Patient or Family Advisor

Patient and family advisors participate in leadership walking rounds for inpatient areas at Vanderbilt Medical Center in Nashville, Tennessee. The advisors have designed their own form that guides their participation and observations as part of this process. Plans are underway to extend these rounds to ambulatory care areas (Vanderbilt Health, 2019).

Dana-Farber Cancer Institute, Boston, Massachusetts
*Ensure That Patient and Family Perspectives, Including
Their Experiences of Care, Are Key Drivers in Changing
and Improving Care Processes and Structures*

Dana-Farber Cancer Institute in Boston has a commitment both to patient safety and to involving patients and families in decision-making regarding their own care. These commitments were joined in 2004, when a patient component was added to the Patient Safety Rounds at Dana-Farber. Selected members of the institution's Adult Patient-Family Advisory Council were trained as Patient/Family Safety Liaisons. The role of the liaisons is to interview current patients about their safety concerns. Dana-Farber has found that eliciting patient perspectives as part of safety rounds yields important insights into patient experiences of care, as well as useful information about potential safety problems. A toolkit developed by Dana-Farber can introduce other institutions to these safety rounds procedures.

At Dana-Farber Cancer Institute, there are PFACs for both the adult and pediatric oncology programs. Patient and family advisors have helped shape efforts to improve patient safety. After safety leaders invited patients to participate in developing a project to bring cockpit-style teamwork training skills to patients and their families, these advisors recommended a teamwork safety campaign with very clear, specific messages targeted to patients and their families. As it has developed, the "You CAN" campaign urges patients and families to Check, Ask, and Notify. The campaign emphasizes that safety is the responsibility of Dana-Farber staff and faculty; however, patients and families CAN help to ensure safe care, especially in handwashing and chemotherapy safety. Patient and family advisors, prepared for their roles in talking with patients and families about the experience of care, are the ambassadors for this campaign. Colorful posters will also be used to reinforce the messages of the campaign (Dana-Farber Cancer Institute, 2021).

The Whitby Mental Health Centre (WMHC), Whitby, Ontario
Develop and Support Partnerships Among
Administrators, Providers, Patients, and Families to
Improve Quality and Safety in Ambulatory Care

The Whitby Mental Health Centre (WMHC) in Whitby, Ontario, has long recognized the benefits of engaging patients and families as partners in care and within the organization. WMHC include clients and families on their 17-member Board of Directors. The vision and values for the Centre were determined with significant client, family, and community participation. There is an active Patient Council that brings the patient and family voice into developing and implementing Centre activities. Patients and families are involved in safety initiatives, programming and facility design, and educational and public awareness programs.

The Patient Council works with community organizations to build support for the Centre's vision of "recovering best health, nurturing hope, and inspiring discovery." WHMC has been recognized by the government of Ontario for its initiative titled Stomp Out Stigma Summits. This program offers the public the opportunity to hear different stories of people living well with mental illness. These stories promote proper diagnosis and treatment as well as instilling hope in individuals, families, and communities (Ontario Shores Centre for Mental Health Sciences, n.d.).

MinuteClinic, United States

In 2018, MinuteClinic, the retail medical clinic of CVS Health, received a planning grant from The John A. Hartford Foundation to participate in an Age-Friendly Health System Action Community and learn how to implement the 4Ms across its 1,100 locations. MinuteClinic's approach to becoming an Age-Friendly Health System focuses on the training and education of their workforce, particularly nurse practitioners (NPs) and physician assistants (PAs). This includes

- an orientation program for providers, explaining what the 4Ms are, how to assess them, how to act on them, and how to integrate them into the MinuteClinic workflow;
- monthly webinars that utilize case scenarios illustrating how to incorporate the 4Ms into various types of visits; and
- virtual training clinics for providers to practice the 4Ms.

MinuteClinic also updated its EHR to include a new tab for any patient aged 65 and older to document the patient's answers for What Matters, screenings conducted on Medication, Mentation, and Mobility, and actions taken to address the 4Ms. Additionally, MinuteClinic produced a brochure to facilitate communication and 4Ms care between providers, patients and patients' families, and primary care providers.

- **What Matters**: Providers integrate a discussion of What Matters into the beginning or conclusion of the visit. The messaging is "Share with me what matters most to you about your health so we can align your treatment plan with what's most important for you." Providers, to set the tone, also ensure patients are educated about what the 4Ms are and why they are integrated into the visit.

- **Mobility**: Providers observe their patients as they get up from the waiting area to enter the clinic, how they stand up and sit down, and how they get up on the exam table—as a simplified, modified version of Get Up and Go.

- **Mentation**: Providers conduct a quick assessment of memory and mood using the PHQ-9 and Mini-Cog.

MinuteClinic continues to leverage its EHR dashboard to monitor 4Ms uptake by each provider and has added new questions to the patient satisfaction survey to understand patients' perspectives on receiving 4Ms care. MinuteClinic NPs and PAs have quickly adapted to the 4Ms process and have seen value in empathizing with the patient and truly understanding their experience with their condition. Anne Pohnert, MSN, FNP-BY, Director of Clinical Quality at MinuteClinic, says, "Our strategy is to create unmatched human connection. That, to me, is exactly what the 4Ms do" (IHI, 2020).

Recommendations and Summary

The experience of the Age-Friendly Health Systems teams in the field underscores the value and importance of Patient and Family Advisory Council (PFAC) in order to support patient- and family-centered care. For those who already have such an Advisory Council in place, data to support your successes are valuable to the broader community learning how to do this work. Ensuring that care plans for older adults are focused on what matters to them and what matters to their families demands a systematic approach to assessing and documenting what matters on a regular basis and following that plan of care across the healthcare continuum. Changes in healthcare and life status, such as the loss of a spouse, would indicate the need for a review and potential revision of documentation of what matters. PFACs are a vital way to get guidance related to supporting what matters to older adults, their families, and communities.

References

Augusta University Health. (2021). *Patient and family information.* https://www.augustahealth.org/patient-family-info/

Barr, P. J., Forcino, R. C., Thompson, R., Ozanne, E. M., Arend, R., Castaldo, M. G., O'Malley, A. J., & Elwyn, G. (2017). Evaluating collaboRATE in a clinical setting: Analysis of mode effects on scores, response rates and costs of data collection, *BMJ Open*, 7(3), 1–9. https://bmjopen.bmj.com/content/7/3/e014681.

Bezold, C. (2005). The future of patient-centered care: Scenarios, visions, and audacious goals. *Journal of Alternative & Complementary Medicine*, 11(Suppl. 1), 77–84. https://doi.org/10.1089/acm.2005.11.s-77

Blanchfield Army Community Hospital. (n.d.). *Family centered care clinics: Patient-centered medical homes*. https://blanchfield.tricare.mil/Health-Services/Primary-Care/Family-Centered-Care-Clinics

Cacioppo, J. T., & Hawkley, L. C. (2003). Social isolation and health, with an emphasis on underlying mechanisms. *Perspectives in Biology and Medicine*, 46(3), S39–S52. https://muse.jhu.edu/article/168969#:~:text=10.1353/pbm.2003.0049.

Cambridge Health Alliance. (2021). *Volunteer Health Advisor Program*. https://www.challiance.org/community-health/volunteer-health-advisor-program

Chow, S. (1999). Challenging restricted visiting policies in critical care. *Official Journal of the Canadian Association of Critical Care Nurses*, 10(2), 24–27.

Dana-Farber Cancer Institute. (2021). *For patients and families: Comprehensive care for patients and their families*. https://www.dana-farber.org/for-patients-and-families/

Elwyn, G. (n.d.). *collaboRATE 5-point anchor scale*. http://www.glynelwyn.com/uploads/2/4/0/4/24040341/collaborate_for_patients_5_anchor_point_scale.pdf

Epic. (2021). *Patient experience*. https://www.epic.com/software#PatientEngagement

Frampton, S. B., Gilpin, L., & Charmel, P. A. (2003). *Putting patients first: Designing and practicing patient-centered care*. Jossey-Bass.

Fried, T. R. (2016). Shared decision-making: Finding the sweet spot. *The New England Journal of Medicine*, 374, 104–106. https://www.nejm.org/doi/full/10.1056/NEJMp1510020

Gerteis, M. (1993). *Through the patient's eyes: Understanding and promoting patient-centered care*. Wiley.

Healthcare Improvement Scotland. (2018). *Real-time and right-time care experience improvement models*. Person-Centred Health and Care

Programme. https://ihub.scot/media/6417/rtrt-evaluation-report-final-may-2018-web.pdf

House, J. S. (2002). Understanding social factors and inequalities in health: 20th-century progress and 21st-century prospects. *Journal of Health and Social Behavior, 43*(2), 125–142.

Institute for Healthcare Improvement. (n.d.). *Integrated Patient-, Family-, Public-, and Community-Centered Care* [Unpublished internal document].

Institute for Healthcare Improvement. (2019). *"What Matters" to older adults? A toolkit for health systems to design better care with older adults.* http:/.www.ihi.org/Engage/Initiatives/Age-Friendly-Health-Systems Documents/IHI_Age_Friendly_What_Matters_to_Older_Adults_Toolkit.pdf

Institute for Healthcare Improvement. (2020). *MinuteClinic.* http://www.ihi.org/Engage/Initiatives/Age-Friendly-Health-Systems/Documents/Age-Friendly-Health-Systems_MinuteClinic_Case.pdf

Institute for Healthcare Improvement. (2021a). *The Conversation Project.* https://theconversationproject.org

Institute for Healthcare Improvement. (2021b). *What matters.* http://www.ihi.org/Topics/WhatMatters/Pages/default.aspx

Institute for Patient- and Family-Centered Care. (n.d.). *Patient- and family-centered care.* https://www.ipfcc.org/about/pfcc.html

Johnson, B., Conway, J., Edgman-Levitan, S., Sodomka, P., Schlucter, K., & Ford, D. (2008). *Partnering with patients and families to design a patient- and family-centered health care system: Recommendations and promising practices.* Institute for Patient- and Family-Centered Care. https://www.ipfcc.org/resources/PartneringwithPatientsandFamilies.pdf

Ontario Shores Centre for Mental Health Sciences. (n.d.). *Patients & families.* https://www.ontarioshores.ca/patients___families

Patient & Family Advisory Councils. (2014). *A review of 2013 Massachusetts patient & family advisory council reports.* https://www.ipfcc.org/bestpractices/Review-of-PFAC-2013-Reports.pdf

Reinhard, S. C., Young, H. M., Ryan, E., & Choula, R. B. (2019). *The CARE Act implementation: Progress and promise.* AARP Public Policy Institute. https://www.aarp.org/content/dam/aarp/ppi/2019/03/the-care-act-implementation-progress-and-promise.pdf

Sokol-Hessner, L., Zambeaux, A., Little, K., Macy, L., Lally, K. M., & McCutcheon Adams, K. (2019). *"Conversation ready": A framework for improving end-of-life care* [White paper, 2nd ed.]. Institute for Healthcare Improvement. http://www.ihi.org/resources/Pages/IHIWhitePapers/ConversationReadyEndofLifeCare.aspx

Vanderbilt Health. (2019). *Patient relations.* https://www.vanderbilthealth.com/information/patient-relations

CHAPTER 3

Conversations That Matter

U nderstanding What Matters is an ongoing process built on strong relationships between care team members and older adults. While there are some critical moments when an older adult's health and care goals and preferences may need to be elicited or redefined, understanding What Matters requires a series of conversations over time that become the guide for how care is delivered. There are two considerations for What Matters conversations, as described below.

What Matters Conversations at Certain Care Touchpoints

Care touchpoints for older adults—such as regular visits, Annual Wellness Visits, a new diagnosis, a life-stage change, ongoing chronic disease management, and inpatient visits—present opportunities for What Matters conversations (see Figure 3.1). These types of care interactions tend to be time limited and specific to a clinical interaction. What Matters conversations can and should take place in various settings, including inpatient hospital, primary care, cancer care, skilled nursing facility or nursing home, home-based care, and specialty services such as rehabilitation.

Figure 3.1. *Care Touchpoints When What Matters Conversations Might Occur (IHI, 2019.)*

Regular and Annual Wellness Visits

A longer annual wellness visit can be conducive to an initial "What Matters" conversation. Regular wellness visits are also an excellent opportunity to continue "What Matters" conversations over time.

New Diagnosis or Change in Health Status

Schedule an initial "What Matters" conversation one week after the older adult has received a new diagnosis of change in health status, and use this information when planning a course of care.

Life-Stage Change

Initiate a "What Matters" conversation during a primary care appointment with an older adult who has just entered retirement or enrolled in Medicare. Review "What Matters" information at each visit following the life-stage change for any updates on the older adult's care.

Chronic Disease Management

Discuss "What Matters" during primary care visits, revisiting past conversations and discussing any changes or updated to the older adult's goals and preferences.

Inpatient Visits (Hospital, Nursing Home, Skilled Nursing Faciility)

Ask older adults what is important to them at every hospitalization and document any new information.

Note that asking older adults about What Matters can be difficult in the emergency department (ED), when decisions need to be made quickly to address the urgent issue at hand. Rather than initiating What Matters conversations in the ED setting, ED care teams are more likely interpreters of this information, using it to guide care decisions, particularly as patients in the ED may not be able to communicate their goals and preferences during an emergency encounter. Documenting What Matters information consistently and making it easily and clearly accessible to clinicians in all settings are the most important factors in ensuring patients' What Matters preferences are known and respected in the ED.

What Matters Conversations as Part of Routine and Recurring Care

Consistently incorporating What Matters as part of discussions between older adults and clinicians is a key part of relationship-based care. These conversations might be broad (e.g., "My grandchildren and knitting are important to me") or specific (e.g., "I am worried I will be too weak to attend a family reunion I've been looking forward to next month").

What Matters conversations may be more effective and actionable if anchored to something the older adult cares about by connecting their goals and preferences to the impacts of care and care decisions.

Considerations for What Matters Conversations

What Matters conversations are never the same twice. Each interaction must take into consideration the patient's cognition, health status, and identity.

Cognition
The care team must consider how older adults' cognitive status does, and does not, impact their ability to engage in meaningful

conversations about their goals and preferences. Some clinicians may think an older adult with cognitive impairment is not capable of a What Matters conversation and thus will not introduce the opportunity or will only speak with the family or caregiver.

Older adults living with cognitive impairment and dementia are often capable of expressing their goals and preferences and should participate in What Matters conversations to the degree possible. It is the care team's responsibility to get to know each older adult and engage with them directly. Careful consideration should be given to the timing of What Matters conversations. There may be times of the day when the older adult is more lucid (e.g., earlier in the day). If there is significant cognitive impairment, the most important aspect of What Matters may be finding out who the older adult relies on most to help make decisions. The guiding principle is to maximize autonomy of cognitively impaired older adults and not diminish their self-image (e.g., "changes in cognition" versus "cognitive impairment"; Fazio et al., 2018).

Health Status

Older adults' goals and preferences will likely change over time as health status changes. What matters most to someone who is functionally independent and has few health problems will differ from someone with functional disabilities and a heavy disease burden. Accordingly, the What Matters conversations to understand older adults' goals and preferences may need to vary based on health status.

Identity

It is critical to consider the impact of race, ethnicity, language, religion, culture, and other identities on how older adults view health and illness, and their preferences and willingness to engage in conversations about What Matters. Issues of trust between some populations (e.g., communities of color, the LGBTQ+ community) and the healthcare system, born of past experiences and historic mistreatment, can affect What Matters conversations.

Clinicians are also at risk of expressing their own unconscious biases, which may manifest in subtle verbal and nonverbal ways that can alienate patients. Without trust, it is challenging to truly understand What Matters to inform a treatment plan that incorporates the older adult's goals and care preferences.

What Matters conversations can open the door to more culturally competent, affirming, and humble care, as clinicians become better informed about the life and cultural contexts of each older adult. It is recommended that all clinicians undergo training on implicit bias as part of their preparation for having What Matters conversations, using tools like the Project Implicit assessments (Harvard University, 2011) and the National Standards for Culturally and Linguistically Appropriate Services (CLAS) in Health and Health Care (US Department of Health and Human Services, n.d.). Guidelines from cross-cultural care can help the care team have more-successful conversations with older adults from different cultural backgrounds (American Geriatrics Society Ethnogeriatrics Committee, 2004).

CHECKLIST FOR CULTURALLY APPROPRIATE WHAT MATTERS CONVERSATIONS

- Learn the older adult's preferred term for their cultural identity.

- Determine the appropriate degree of formality. Learn the older adult's preference for how they would like to be addressed, and use this title and the surname (e.g., Mrs. Smith), unless a less-formal address is requested.

- Determine the older adult's preferred language. If the older adult has basic or below-basic literacy or English language proficiency, seek permission from the person to have a medical interpreter assist in the What Matters conversation, or determine if a trusted individual who is literate can be present during the What Matters conversation.

- Be respectful of nonverbal communication. Watch for body language cues that might be linked to cultural norms. Adopt conservative body language, use a calm demeanor, and avoid expressive gestures.

- Address issues linked to culture, such as a lack of trust, fear of medical experimentation, fear of side effects, and unfamiliarity with Western biomedical belief systems.

- Review the medical records to determine if there has been a history of trauma, including refugee status, survivors of violence, genocide, and torture. These are very sensitive issues and must be approached with caution. Reassure the older adult of the confidentiality of the clinician-patient relationship.

- Determine the level of acculturation and recognize that this is a factor for individuals who are recent immigrants as well as for those who are not recent immigrants.

- Recognize health beliefs that include the use of alternative therapies.

- Consider how gender or gender identity might affect decision-making.

- Consider an approach to decision-making that recognizes family and community decisions and does not automatically exclude them in favor of individual autonomy.

CONVERSATIONS THAT MATTER • 47

Who Should Initiate a What Matters Conversation

Because What Matters conversations should be part of an ongoing dialogue, several members of the interdisciplinary care team may have conversations with the older adult about their goals and preferences at different times (e.g., an older adult's general values preferences may remain relatively static over time, but specific goals may change from visit to visit). It is recommended that all members of the care team undergo training on motivational interviewing and shared decision-making prior to engaging in What Matters conversations (see Appendix B: Resources to Support What Matters Conversations With Older Adults for additional resources).

Any member of the care team can initiate and document a conversation with an older adult about their goals and preferences:

- While physicians may be the default care team member guiding care decisions based on an older adult's goals and preferences, they may not have the time or the communication skills necessary to engage in these conversations during a visit.

- Nurses, physician assistants, social workers, and medical assistants may have a close relationship with the older adult and have more time for What Matters conversations. Chaplains, nurse navigators, community health workers, or trained volunteers may also be able to have meaningful conversations about goals and preferences and record that information for clinicians to access.

- What Matters can also be elicited by self-report (e.g., a form sent to an older adult prior to the Annual Wellness Visit or filled out while in the waiting room).

Regardless of who on the care team conducts the What Matters conversation, there should be a clear process for documenting and sharing this information. It is important to document and communicate the older adult's exact words, as these can be the most impactful. The documentation process might include a write-in template (see Appendix C for one example), detailed notes in the electronic health record (EHR) with information on health goals and care preferences, or (for inpatients) a whiteboard in an older adult's room that is updated with What Matters to them daily. Whichever method is used, every care team member needs to be trained on where to record their What Matters conversations and where to find documentation of previous What Matters conversations.

What to Discuss in a What Matters Conversation

What Matters conversations are more effective and actionable if they

- explore the older adult's life context, priorities, and preferences and connect them to the impacts of care, self-management, and care decisions; and
- are anchored to tangible health or care events in an older adult's life.

It may be appropriate to have an initial conversation in an outpatient setting that is focused on understanding an individual older adult's life context, then follow up with treatment-specific questions or start a conversation from a diagnosis and specific treatment decisions, and then broaden the discussion to the older adult's life preferences (Naik et al., 2018).

Understanding Life Context and Priorities

These broad conversations explore what is important to older adults in their lives outside of their health (e.g., children, family, pets, hobbies), both overall and on the day of the conversation. Questions should ideally be asked by a variety of healthcare clinicians in their everyday interactions with older adults in different settings.

GUIDING QUESTIONS: UNDERSTANDING
LIFE CONTEXT AND PRIORITIES

- What is important to you today?
- What brings you joy? What makes you happy? What makes life worth living?
- What do you worry about?
- What are some goals you hope to achieve in the next 6 months or before your next birthday?
- What would make tomorrow a really great day for you?
- What else would you like us to know about you?
- How do you learn best? For example, listening to someone, reading materials, watching a video (IHI, 2019).

Anchoring Treatment in Goals and Preferences

What Matters conversations are anchored to an older adult's health status and care needs and may be most appropriate when there is a new diagnosis, treatment decision, or change in health status. Questions need to focus on how treatment could facilitate or impede their ability to do the things they enjoy (e.g., walking, cooking, everyday activities) or attain certain life goals (e.g., attending a meaningful event). Questions also should focus on a specific time frame, such as 6 months or by the next birthday.

GUIDING QUESTIONS: ANCHORING
TREATMENT IN GOALS AND PREFERENCES

- What is the one thing about your healthcare you most want to focus on so that you can do [fill in desired activity] more often or more easily?

- What are your most important goals about your health now and as you think about the future?
- What concerns you most when you think about your health and healthcare in the future?
- What are your fears or concerns for your family?
- What are your most important goals if your health situation worsens?
- What things about your healthcare do you think aren't helping you and you find too bothersome or difficult?
- Is there anyone who should be part of this conversation with us? (IHI, 2019)

How to Prepare Older Adults and Caregivers for a What Matters Conversation

Not all older adults are ready to engage in What Matters conversations. Most have never been part of a discussion with a care team member beyond specific medical problems. Some older adults and caregivers may be concerned that the questions, which are often associated with end-of-life care, indicate a dire prognosis and spark concern that they may be terminally ill. Some may find the questions intrusive or are reluctant, unprepared, or embarrassed to share details about their lives that they deem unrelated to their healthcare, or they are looking for more didactic instructions. Others are willing and eager to guide clinical conversations with their nonclinical goals. The success of being able to understand What Matters to each older adult will depend on their (and their clinician's) comfort, readiness, and expectation for incorporating their expressed goals and preferences into care planning.

One way to prepare for What Matters conversations is to present the idea of identifying health goals and care preferences prior to a face-to-face interaction with the healthcare system. Conversations are likely to be more fruitful when older adults reflect in advance of a visit and have a chance to prepare themselves to talk about their goals and priorities. Additionally, how older adults respond to being asked depends on the framing, and the care team must be able to explain why they are asking. Thus, setting the context for the conversation, before it happens, is critical.

Some ideas for how care team members can prepare older adults and their caregivers to have What Matters conversations follow:

- Use a pre-visit survey, either on paper or through a patient-facing EHR portal, to obtain information about What Matters that is reviewed by clinicians prior to a visit.
- Meet with groups of older adults to encourage them to talk with each other about goals, preferences, and common experiences.
- Utilize existing relationships with community-based organizations, such as faith communities, to encourage more conversations about What Matters.
- Provide older adults with resources to prepare them to talk with their clinician, such as PREPARE for Your Care, the Stanford Medicine Bucket List Planner, or The Conversation Project Starter Kits (see Appendix B for more resources).
- Include a What Matters brochure in waiting areas, similar to existing brochures on healthcare proxies and advance care planning.
- Suggest that the older adult bring a family member, caregiver, or trusted friend to a conversation about their goals and preferences.

How to Conduct an Effective What Matters Conversation

Below is a list of tasks to complete before, during, and after a What Matters conversation. The guidance generally follows the framework described in the *Serious Illness Conversation Guide* from Ariadne Labs: set up the conversation, assess understanding and preferences, share prognosis, explore key topics, and close the conversation (Ariadne Labs, 2017). See Appendix D for examples of What Matters conversations.

Before the Conversation

Prepare the Older Adult for the Conversation in Advance

Introduce the idea of talking about What Matters and ask the older adult to do some reflection prior to the visit, including with their family or caregiver, if appropriate. Let the person know that they will be asked about their goals and preferences. The care team member should explain why this information is being sought, namely to identify what matters most to the individual so that care can be better aligned with What Matters. This preparation could take place during a prior visit or as part of pre-visit paperwork.

Determine Who on the Care Team Will Have the Conversation

The most appropriate person to conduct the conversation may depend on the care setting and the relationship a given care team member has with the older adult. For example, if a physician will be working closely with the older adult to design a care plan and they have the time and skills to have the discussion, it is beneficial for the physician to facilitate the What Matters conversation. Alternatively, if a nurse, care manager, or other care team member spends a significant amount of time with the older adult, then one of these people may be better positioned to facilitate the conversation and communicate the older adult's needs to the rest of the team. Time and availability are also factors, which is why training all members of the care team to facilitate What Matters conversations is important to sustaining this work.

Decide on a Setting for the Conversation

Having a What Matters conversation in a meeting room, sitting around a table as equals, may be more effective than having the discussion in an exam room, since the meeting room setting can help reduce the perceived power dynamics between the older adult and the clinician. If the conversation must take place in an exam room, the older adult and care team member should sit in chairs facing one another, with the older adult dressed in their own clothes rather than in a patient gown, if possible. If the older adult uses a hearing aid, be sure it is turned on. Home is a good location for the discussion, if feasible. For example, it can be done by a case manager, social worker, or home care nurse who already visits the older adult's home.

Review the Records of Previous What Matters Conversations

Look over notes of previous conversations about the older adult's goals and preferences, whether documented in the EHR or elsewhere, as they may provide a good starting point for the current conversation, and the information may need updating.

Conduct a Screen for Cognitive Impairment to Inform Approach for a What Matters Conversation

This screening (which should occur routinely in an Age-Friendly Health System) is critical when preparing for a What Matters conversation, given the burden of cognitive impairment among many older adults. Some potential screening tools include Ultra-Brief 2-Item Screener (Fick et al., 2015); naming four-legged animals in 1 minute (Howe, 2007); drawing a clock face, either in isolation or as part of the Mini-Cog (Borson et al., 2000); and the Short Blessed Test and Months

Backward Test (Katzman et al., 1983). It is important to bear in mind that memory deficits do not preclude capacity to make decisions about what matters. If there is cognitive impairment, consider how the older adult's cognitive status does, and does not, impact their ability to engage in a meaningful conversation about goals and preferences. Ask the person whom they rely on most to help them make decisions and consider windows of lucidity and timing of these conversations.

Prepare for the Conversation
If you will be using any handouts, prompt cards, or education tools, prepare them ahead of the conversation. If the conversation will require an interpreter, include the interpreter in any pre-meeting team conversations to ensure that they can translate questions in a way that will be understood by the older adult. Translate the materials into writing whenever possible.

During the Conversation
Invite the Older Adult to Have a Conversation
The success of a What Matters conversation depends on having a strong relationship between the older adult and their care team and both parties having similar expectations for incorporating nonclinical goals into care planning. Begin by asking the older adult if they would like to talk about their goals and preferences, and (if applicable) how involved they want others to be in the conversation. If they are not comfortable or wish for additional people to attend the conversation (e.g., family member, caregiver), ask what would make them more comfortable, and offer the option to have the conversation at a different time.

Start by Asking One or More What Matters Questions
See the section What to Discuss in a What Matters Conversation for guiding questions on how to start a conversation. Choosing an approach depends on the purpose of the conversation and the level

of comfort the care team member and the older adult have with talking about What Matters. While scripts can be helpful, many trained staff report not needing a script and prefer tailoring a conversation based on the older adult and the context. Rather than following a script, think about the older adult's health status (e.g., advanced illness, single condition, multiple chronic conditions, or generally well) and life context. See Appendix B for additional tools and resources.

Listen Carefully and Ask Questions
Give the older adult time to think and provide answers. Ask follow-up questions as needed, but do not ask an overwhelming number of questions. Try to ask the fewest number of questions to obtain the information.

Use Training and Health Literacy Tools to Facilitate
the Conversation and Provide Clarification
Being able to successfully communicate health or clinical information is a critical component of a successful What Matters conversation. Once the care team member identifies the communication method that is most comfortable for the older adult, it may be helpful to use health literacy tools such as education videos, flashcards, or pamphlets to communicate clinical information. Asking the older adult to explain the clinical information in their own words (the "Teach-Back" approach) will also help confirm that the information has been effectively communicated. Note that "Teach-Back" may not be effective for those with executive dysfunction.

Affirm the Conversation for the Older Adult
Throughout the conversation, the care team member should take time to

- acknowledge the older adult's thoughts and feelings;

- confirm the older adult's understanding of what they are communicating; and
- ask for clarification of anything that is unclear.

If the older adult has chosen to include other people in the conversation, this can also be a time to ask whether they need any clarification from either the clinician or the older adult.

After the Conversation

Incorporate What Matters Information Into the Care Plan

Once the care team has had the What Matters conversation with the older adult, the next step is to incorporate their expressed goals and preferences into their care plan. By anchoring an initial What Matters conversation around specific points in the care process during which decisions about care are likely to be made (e.g., first visit, new diagnosis, change in health status, or life transition), the team may be in a better position to build a clinical care plan that reflects the older adult's goals.

If the conversation involves clinical decision-making, the following steps are recommended:

1. Present personalized evidence, considering all steps above, to help the older adult reflect on and assess the impact of care decisions regarding their goals, preferences, and lifestyle.
2. Identify choices the older adult can make, and evaluate the clinical research in the context of their life.
3. Help the older adult reflect on the impact of different options on themselves and their family.
4. Come to a decision point with the older adult and family (when appropriate).
5. Agree on next steps and plan for follow-up.

Document the What Matters Conversation

Document the conversation, ideally in the EHR, immediately following the conversation's conclusion or within 24 hours. Use the person's own words as much as possible (e.g., "Leslie would like to be able to walk around the block" rather than "Patient wants to mobilize") and use tags to make preferences and goals readily searchable in the medical record (see section on Documenting What Matters Information for more guidance on incorporating What Matters into the EHR).

Share Information With the Care Team

If appropriate, discuss conversation outcomes with the care team during regular team huddles. If the team does not currently conduct regular team huddles, the Better Care Playbook provides strategies for care teams to use huddles ("Play," 2021). If any information requires immediate action, share it with appropriate care team members as soon as possible.

Continue the Conversation

During the next encounter with the older adult, revisit the previous What Matters conversation, discuss any new or changing topics, and update the conversation documentation in the EHR or the agreed-upon location for storing documentation.

Case Study

Providence St. Joseph Health, Oregon Region

Providence St. Joseph Health, Oregon Region, began developing a process for operationalizing What Matters conversations with older adults in February 2017. They initially formed an exploratory workgroup comprising a clinic medical director, chaplain, physician, nurse, care manager, and social worker. This workgroup shared their knowledge and experiences of having conversations with patients about What Matters and discussed what was needed to make these discussions valuable to patients and the organization. The workgroup then used their shared knowledge, along with resources from the literature, What Matters work at NHS Scotland, and the *Serious Illness Conversation Guide* to develop guidelines for successful What Matters conversations.

After reviewing the first draft of the guidelines, frontline care team staff reported that the guidelines did not provide specific-enough guidance for structuring and conducting What Matters conversations. The workgroup gathered comments and feedback from care teams and created a list of suggested questions to guide What Matters conversations. The questions were introduced with the phrase "You can consider using the following..." so an individual practitioner could select what made sense for a specific conversation. A second draft was developed and disseminated to frontline staff to begin testing with older adults in two service lines: one primary care clinic setting and one program that provided care to elders in their homes.

Following a first round of testing with five patients, the frontline care teams debriefed their experiences with the workgroup, who then used their feedback to revise the guidelines. The What Matters discussion guidelines have now been in use for several years across the continuum of care.

To date, the workgroup has noted the following learnings:

- Including an opening statement for clinicians to invite patients to participate in What Matters conversations helps make clinicians and patients feel more comfortable with having a conversation.
- What Matters conversations have typically been shorter than clinicians anticipated.

- The guidelines have been modified to indicate that a family member or surrogate is strongly encouraged to be present during conversations with patients with dementia.
- Stories about rewarding experiences of What Matters conversations and how the information from them is integrated into care planning is particularly motivating for frontline team members.

Providence St. Joseph Health has also integrated What Matters information into its Epic Electronic Health Record. The goal is to have all What Matters-type information in one place in the chart for easy access to all caregivers (IHI, 2019).

Recommendations and Summary

Preparing for conversations related to what matters is extremely important in order to ensure positive outcomes and the effectiveness of such conversations. Cultural sensitivity is essential, and in its absence, there can be a loss of trust and cohesion in the care plan. There are many examples of conversation starters that are referenced both here and in the broader literature. An Age-Friendly Health System approach commits to a learning community where all staff have knowledge about conducting or referring older adults and their families to members of the Age-Friendly Health Systems who can help navigate and document a conversation about what matters.

There is a great deal of evidence related to the positive impact of documenting what matters to an older adult and their family as well as ensuring that appropriate conversations continue to refine the understanding of goals of care on an ongoing basis. This chapter has provided several tools and references to help get this work started. There is no requirement for which clinician should be leading this work. Social workers, nurses, physicians, and clergy can all commit to learn the process and provide leadership for the interdisciplinary team to benefit older adults and their families.

References

American Geriatrics Society Ethnogeriatrics Committee. (2004). *Doorway thoughts: Cross-cultural health care for older adults.* Jones & Bartlett Learning.

Ariadne Labs. (2017). *Serious illness conversation guide.* https://www.ariadnelabs.org/areas-of-work/serious-illness-care/resources/#Downloads&%20Tools

Borson, S., Scanlan, J., Brush, M., Vitaliano, P., & Dokmak A. (2000). The mini-cog: A cognitive "vital signs" measure for dementia screening in multi-lingual elderly. *International Journal of Geriatric Psychiatry, 15*(11), 1021–1027. https://doi.org/10.1002/1099-1166(200011)15:11<1021::AID-GPS234>3.0.CO;2-6

Fazio, S., Pace, D., Flinner, J., & Kallmyer, B. (2018). The fundamentals of person-centered care for individuals with dementia. *The Gerontologist, 58*(Suppl. 1), S10–S19. https://doi.org/10.1093/geront/gnx122

Fick, D. M., Inouye, S. K., Guess J., Ngo, L. H., Jones, R. N., Saczynski, J. S., & Marcantonio, E. R. (2015). Preliminary development of an ultrabrief two-item bedside test for delirium. *Journal of Hospital Medicine, 10*(10), 645–650. https://www.journalofhospitalmedicine.com/jhospmed/article/127331/two-item-bedside-test-delirium

Harvard University. (2011). *Project Implicit.* https://implicit.harvard.edu/implicit/

Howe, E. (2007). Initial screening of patients for Alzheimer's disease and minimal cognitive impairment. *Psychiatry, 4*(7), 24.

Institute for Healthcare Improvement. (2019). *"What matters" to older adults? A toolkit for health systems to design better care with older adults.* http://www.ihi.org/Engage/Initiatives/Age-Friendly-Health-Systems/Documents/IHI_Age_Friendly_What_Matters_to_Older_Adults_Toolkit.pdf

Institute for Healthcare Improvement. (2021). *What matters.* http://www.ihi.org/Topics/WhatMatters/Pages/default.aspx

Katzman, R., Brown, T., Fuld, P., Peck, A., Schechter, R., & Schimmel, H. (1983). Validation of a short orientation-memory-concentration test of cognitive impairment. *The American Journal of Psychiatry*, 140(6), 734–739. https://doi.org/10.1176/ajp.140.6.734

Naik, A. D., Dindo, L. N., Van Liew, J. R., Hundt, N. E., Vo, L., Hernandez-Bigos, K., Esterson, J., Geda, M., Rosen, J., Blaum, C. S., & Tinetti, M. E. (2018). Development of a clinically feasible process for identifying individual health priorities. *Journal of the American Geriatrics Society*, 66(10), 1872–1879. https://doi.org/10.1111/jgs.15437

Play: Manage quality with daily huddles. (2021). Better Care Playbook. https://www.bettercareplaybook.org/plays/manage-quality-daily-huddles

US Department of Health and Human Services. (n.d.). *National Standards for Culturally and Linguistically Appropriate Services (CLAS) in health and health care*. https://thinkculturalhealth.hhs.gov/clas

CHAPTER 4

Medication

If medication is necessary, use age-friendly medication
that does not interfere with What Matters to the older
adult, Mobility, or Mentation across settings of care.
—The Age-Friendly Health Systems initiative

Older adults are particularly vulnerable to polypharmacy, as they are more likely to be living with various chronic conditions. Polypharmacy increases the risk of drug-drug interactions, adverse drug events, and nonadherence, which puts the older adult at greater risk of harm (Maher et al., 2014). Prescribing cascade is a type of polypharmacy in which a new drug is prescribed to counter the adverse reaction of a current drug that has been mistaken as a new medical condition, thereby introducing the older adult to unnecessary harm without having addressed the root of the problem (Rochon & Gurwitz, 1997). Unfortunately, problematic prescribing has increased significantly since 2005–2006, such that the concurrent use of five or more prescription medications increased from 30.6% to 35.8%. By 2010–2011, 15.1% of older adults were potentially at risk for major drug-drug interactions (Qato et al., 2016).

There is a vast body of literature that describes the effects of medications on older adults. For instance, within a national estimate that there are four emergency department visits for adverse drug events per 1,000 individuals annually, older adults account for 34.5% of these visits, while 43.6% of these visits resulted in hospitalization (Shehab et al., 2016). Meanwhile, cost-related medication nonadherence poses another challenge and is increasingly common as drugs become more unaffordable: 6.8% of older adults reported cost-related medication nonadherence. Risk factors include younger age, female sex, lower socioeconomic levels, mental distress, functional limitations, multimorbidities, and obesity (Chung et al., 2019). Thus, clinicians must manage medications to ensure that medication is only prescribed when necessary and is safely adhered to. Medication in the 4Ms framework emphasizes the utilization of age-friendly medications that do not interfere with What Matters to an older person, Mobility, or Mentation across settings of care. This requires an alertness to inappropriate medications and polypharmacy and limiting the over-prescription of high-risk medications and dose-adjusting or deprescribing when clinically appropriate.

Prescription Risks for Older Adults

There are seven categories of medications that clinicians must regularly screen for to prevent adverse effects: benzodiazepines, opioids, highly anticholinergic medications (e.g., diphenhydramine), all prescription and over-the-counter sedatives and sleep medications, muscle relaxants, tricyclic antidepressants, and antipsychotics.

Antipsychotics

Shared with permission from Dr. Cara Tannenbaum (2014a). For more information, go to deprescribingnetwork.ca.

Antipsychotic drugs are sometimes prescribed to treat disruptive behaviors in people with dementia or insomnia. However, new research shows that people who take antipsychotic drugs are putting themselves at

- a higher risk of memory and concentration problems;
- an increased risk of falls and fractures (hip, wrist);
- an increased risk of having a stroke; and
- a higher risk of dizziness, confusion, diabetes, weight gain, and high cholesterol.

The dose of the drug is related to the occurrence of side effects. Even at small doses, all antipsychotic drugs slow your brain performance and reflexes. Antipsychotic medication was developed primarily to treat schizophrenia and bipolar disease. These medications were never intended to treat insomnia or disruptive behaviors in people with dementia. Antipsychotic medication masks the symptoms of agitation in patients with dementia without addressing the underlying cause. The risks associated with these drugs are serious. They should not be taken except under very special circumstances. These drugs remain longer and longer in the person's body as the person ages. This means they can remain in the body for up to several days and can make a person tired, sleepy, and confused. They can impair one's balance and cause a stroke, or even death. They also make the person gain weight and may cause or exacerbate diabetes, high cholesterol, and memory problems. An antipsychotic's sedative properties can cause drowsiness during the day, which can lead to car accidents. Even if these symptoms are not apparent, it is imperative that older adults speak to a doctor or pharmacist for pre-vention in the future (Ralph & Espinet, 2018).

Alternate therapies are available to relieve anxiety or improve sleep with fewer side effects on quality of life. There are lifestyle changes that can help:

- Exercise. Physical activity helps people sleep better. However, avoid vigorous activity for several hours before bedtime.
- Keep a routine. Try to go to bed and wake up at about the same time every day, even on weekends.
- Try not to eat right before bedtime. Eat three hours or more before going to bed.
- Avoid caffeine after 3:00 p.m. Some people need to avoid caffeine even earlier. Avoid consuming nicotine, as it is a stimulant and may keep you awake.
- Limit alcohol. Alcohol causes sleepiness at first, followed by wakefulness.
- Create the right environment. Keep the bedroom peaceful and quiet. Avoid mental excitement before bedtime. Do not read or watch TV in bed; do so in a chair or on a couch.

If an antipsychotic drug is being used to treat disruptive behaviors in people with dementia, try these alternative solutions:

- Keep a daily routine. People with dementia often become restless or irritable around dinnertime.
  - Do activities that use more energy earlier in the day, such as bathing.
  - Eat the biggest meal at midday.
  - Set a quiet mood in the evening, with soft lighting, less noise, and soothing music.

- Help the person exercise every day. Physical activity helps use nervous energy. It improves mood and sleep.
- Do not argue with a person who is distressed.
  - Distract the person with music, singing, dancing, soft blankets, or other comforts.
  - Ask the person to help with a simple task, such as setting the table or folding clothes.
  - Take the person to another room or for a short walk.
- Plan simple activities and social time. Boredom and loneliness can increase anxiety. Adult daycare programs can provide activities for older people. They also give caretakers a break.

A tapering schedule should be carefully reviewed with the older person and their family to ensure they comprehend the process.

Encourage the older person to ask the following questions:

1. Do I need to continue my medication?
2. How do I reduce my dose?
3. Is there an alternative treatment?
4. What symptoms should I look out for when I stop my medication?
5. Whom do I follow up with and when?

Sedative-Hypnotic Drugs

Shared with permission from Dr. Cara Tannenbaum (2014b). For more information, go to deprescribingnetwork.ca.

These medications are in a family of drugs that bind to the receptors in the brain that cause sedation. It is no longer recommended to take a sedative-hypnotic drug to treat insomnia or anxiety. People who take one are putting themselves at a

- fivefold higher risk of memory and concentration problems;
- fourfold increased risk of daytime fatigue;
- twofold increased risk of falls and fractures (hip, wrist);
- twofold increased risk of having a motor vehicle accident (Hansen et al., 2015); and
- risk of problems with urine loss.

Even if the older person thinks the drugs have no side effects, even a small dose of a sedative-hypnotic drug can worsen brain performance and slow reflexes. They can stay in the body for up to several days and can cause the older person to be tired and weak, impair one's balance, and reduce the other senses. Taking these drugs can cause a physical addiction to the medication. Stopping it abruptly can result in trouble sleeping and greater anxiety. Millions of people have succeeded in slowly cutting these drugs out of their lives and finding alternatives to help their problems. Although they are effective over the short term, studies show that sedative-hypnotic drugs are not the best long-term treatment for anxiety or insomnia. Sedative-hypnotic medication covers up the symptoms without actually solving the problem. Please keep on reading to learn more about how to help an older person develop healthier sleep patterns and diminish stress (Glass et al., 2005).

If the older person is taking a sedative-hypnotic drug to aid sleep, review the following lifestyle changes with that person and their family:

- Do not read or watch TV in bed; do so in a chair or on your couch.
- Try to get up in the morning and go to bed at night at the same time every day.
- Practice deep breathing or relaxation exercises before going to bed.
- Exercise during the day, but not during the last three hours before you go to bed.

- Avoid consuming nicotine, caffeine, and alcohol, as they are stimulants and might keep you awake.
- Ask your doctor for the use of a sleep diary, which can help you understand disruptive sleep patterns.

If the older person is taking a sedative-hypnotic drug to help reduce anxiety, review the following solutions with that person and their family to deal with stress and anxiety:

- Talking to a therapist is a good way to help work out stressful situations and talk about the causes of anxiety.
- Support groups can help to relieve stress and loneliness.
- Relaxation techniques like stretching, yoga, massage, meditation, or tai chi can help relieve everyday stress and help work through anxiety.
- Talking to your doctor about other anti-anxiety medications that have less-serious side effects can be helpful.

Prescribing for Older Adults

The Beers Criteria, first described in 1991 by a renowned group of geriatricians, changed the way a prescriber thought about medications for older adults and has been regularly updated since that time. More recently, the American Geriatrics Society (AGS) made it a practice to keep the revised list updated to help ensure its likely adoption (American Geriatrics Society Beers Criteria Update Expert Panel et al., 2019).

The goal of the Beers Criteria is to improve care of older adults by reducing their exposure to potentially inappropriate medications (PIMs).

- This should be viewed as a guide for identifying medications for which the risks of use in older adults outweigh the benefits.
- These criteria are not meant to be applied in a punitive manner.
- This list is not meant to supersede clinical judgment or an individual's values and needs. Prescribing and managing disease conditions should be individualized and involve shared decision-making.
- These criteria also underscore the importance of using a team approach to prescribing and the use of nonpharmacological approaches and of having economic and organizational incentives for this type of model.

Implicit criteria, such as the Screening Tool of Older Persons' Prescriptions and Screening Tool to Alert to Right Treatment (STOPP/START) criteria and Medication Appropriateness Index, should be used in a complementary manner with the 2019 AGS Beers Criteria to guide clinicians in making decisions about safe medication use in older adults.

Table 4.1. 2019 American Geriatrics Society Beers Criteria for Potentially Inappropriate Medication Use in Older Adults

ORGAN SYSTEM, THERAPEUTIC CATEGORY, DRUG(S)	RATIONALE	RECOMMENDATION	QUALITY OF EVIDENCE	STRENGTH OF RECOMMENDATION
Anticholinergics[a]				
First-generation antihistamines Brompheniramine Carbinoxamine Chlorpheniramine Clemastine Cyproheptadine Dexbrompheniramine Dexchlorpheniramine Dimenhydrinate Diphenhydramine (oral) Doxylamine Hydroxyzine Meclizine Promethazine Pyrilamine Triprolidine	Highly anticholinergic; clearance reduced with advanced age, and tolerance develops when used as hypnotic; risk of confusion, dry mouth, consipation, and other anticholinergic effects of toxicity. Use of diphenhydramine in situations such as acute treatment of severe allergic reaction may be appropriate.	Avoid	Moderate	Strong
Antiparkinsonian agents Benztropine (oral) Trihexyphenidyl	Not recommended for prevention of treatment of extrapyramidal symptoms with antipsychotics; more effective agents available for treatment of Parkinson's disease	Avoid	Moderate	Strong

ORGAN SYSTEM, THERAPEUTIC CATEGORY, DRUG(S)	RATIONALE	RECOMMENDATION	QUALITY OF EVIDENCE	STRENGTH OF RECOMMENDATION
Antispasmodics Atropine (excludes ophthalmic) Belladonna alkaloids Clidinium-chlordiazepoxide Dicyclomine Homatropine (excludes ophthalmic) Hyoscyamine Methscopolamine Propantheline Scopolamine	Highly anticholinergic, uncertain effectiveness	Avoid	Moderate	Strong
Antithrombotics				
Dipyridamole, oral short acting (does not apply to the extended-release combination with aspirin)	May cause orthostatic hypotension; more effective alternatives available; IV form acceptable for use in cardiac stress testing	Avoid	Moderate	Strong
Anti-Infective				
Nitrofurantoin	Potential for pulmonary toxicity, hepatoxicity, and peripheral neuropathy, especially with long-term use; safer alternatives available	Avoid in individuals with creatinine clearance <30 mL/min or for long-term suppression	Low	Strong

ORGAN SYSTEM, THERAPEUTIC CATEGORY, DRUG(S)	RATIONALE	RECOMMENDATION	QUALITY OF EVIDENCE	STRENGTH OF RECOMMENDATION
Cardiovascular				
Peripheral alpha-1 blockers for treatment of hypertension Doxazosin Prazosin Terazosin	High risk of orthostatic hypotension and associated harms, especially in older adults; not recommended as routine treatment for hypertension; alternative agents have superior risk/benefit profile	Avoid use as an antihypertensive	Moderate	Strong
Central alpha-agonists		Avoid as first-line antihypertensive	Low	Strong
Clonidine for first-line treatment of hypertension Other CNS alpha-agonists Guanabenz Guanfacine Methyldopa Reserpine (>0.1mg/day)	High risk of adverse CNS effects; may cause bradycardia and orthostatic hypotension; not recommended as routine treatment for hypertension	Avoid other CNS alpha-agonists as listed	Low	Strong
Disopyramide	May induce heart failure in older adults because of potent negative intropic action; strongly anticholinergic; other antiarrhythmic drugs preferred	Avoid	Low	Strong
Digoxin for first-line treatment of atrial fibrillation or heart failure	*Use in atrial fibrillation:* should not be used as a first-line agent in atrial fibrillation, because there are safe and more effective alternatives for rate control supported by high-quality evidence	Avoid this rate control agent as first-line therapy for atrial fibrillation	*Atrial fibrillation:* low	*Atrial fibrillation:* strong

ORGAN SYSTEM, THERAPEUTIC CATEGORY, DRUG(S)	RATIONALE	RECOMMENDATION	QUALITY OF EVIDENCE	STRENGTH OF RECOMMENDATION
Digoxin for first-line treatment of atrial fibrillation or heart failure *(continued)*	*Use in heart failure:* evidence for benefits and harms of digoxin is conflicting and of lower quality; most but not all of the evidence concerns use in HFrEF. There is strong evidence for other agents as first-line therapy to reduce hospitalizations and mortality in adults with HFrEF. In heart failure, higher dosages are not associated with additional benefit and may increase risk of toxicity. Decreased renal clearance of digoxin may lead to increased risk of toxic effects; further dose reduction may be necessary in those with stage 4 or 5 chronic kidney disease.	Avoid as first-line therapy for heart failure If used for atrial fibrillation or heart failure, avoid dosages >0.125mg/day	*Heart failure:* low *Dosage >0.125 mg/day:* moderate	*Atrial fibrillation:* strong *Dosage >0.125 mg/day:* strong
Nifedipine, immediate release	Potential for hypotension; risk of precipitating myocardial ischemia	Avoid	High	Strong
Amiodarone	Effective for maintaining sinus rhythm but has greater toxicities than other antiarrhythmics used in atrial fibrillation; may be reasonable first-line therapy in patients with concomitant heart failure or substantial left ventricular hypertrophy if rhythm control is preferred over rate control	Avoid as first-line therapy for atrial fibrillation unless patient has heart failure or substantial left ventricular hypertrophy	High	Strong

ORGAN SYSTEM, THERAPEUTIC CATEGORY, DRUG(S)	RATIONALE	RECOMMENDATION	QUALITY OF EVIDENCE	STRENGTH OF RECOMMENDATION
Central Nervous System				
Antidepressants, alone or in combination Amitriptyline Amoxapine Clomipramine Desipramine Doxepin >6 mg/day Imipramine Nortriptyline Paroxetine Protriptyline Trimipramine	Highly anticholinergic, sedating, and cause orthostatic hypotension; safety profile of low-dose doxepin (≤6 mg/day) comparable to that of placebo	Avoid	High	Strong
Antipsychotics, first (conventional) and second (atypical) generation	Increase risk of cerebrovascular accident (stroke) and greater rate of cognitive decline and mortality in persons with dementia Avoid antipsychotics for behavioral problems or dementia or delirium unless nonpharmacological options (eg, behavioral interventions) have failed or are not possible *and* the older adult is threatening substantial harm to self or others	Avoid, expect in schizophrenia or bipolar disorder, or for short-term use as antiemetic during chemotherapy	Moderate	Strong

ORGAN SYSTEM, THERAPEUTIC CATEGORY, DRUG(S)	RATIONALE	RECOMMENDATION	QUALITY OF EVIDENCE	STRENGTH OF RECOMMENDATION
Barbiturates Amobarbital Butabarbital Butalbital Mephobarbital Pentobarbital Phenobarbital Secobarbital	High risk of physical dependence, tolerance to sleep benefits, greater risk of overdose at low dosages	Avoid	High	Strong
Benzodiazepines *Short and immediate acting:* Alprazolam Estazolam Lorazepam Oxazepam Temazepam Triazolam *Long acting:* Chlordiazepoxide (alone or in combination with amitriptyline or clidinium) Clonazepam Clorazepate Diazepam Flurazepam Quazepam	Older adults have increased sensitivity to benzodiazepines and decreased metabolism of long-acting agents; in general, all benziodiazepines increase risk of cognitive impairment, delirium, falls, fractures, and motor vehicle crashes in older adults May be appropriate for seizure disorders, rapid eye movement sleep behavior disorder, benzodiazepine withdrawal, ethanol withdrawal, severe generalized anxiety disorder, and periprocedural anesthesia	Avoid	Moderate	Strong

ORGAN SYSTEM, THERAPEUTIC CATEGORY, DRUG(S)	RATIONALE	RECOMMENDATION	QUALITY OF EVIDENCE	STRENGTH OF RECOMMENDATION
Meprobamate	High rate of physical dependence; sedating	Avoid	Moderate	Strong
Nonbenzodiazepine, benzodiazepine receptor agonist hypnotics (ie, Z-drugs) Eszopiclone Zaleplon Zolpidem	Nonbenzodiazepine benzodiazepine receptor agonist hypnotics (ie, Z-drugs) have adverse events similar to those of benzodiazepines in older adults (eg, delirium, falls, fractures); increased emergency room visits/ hospitalizations; motor vehicle crashes; minimal improvement in sleep latency and duration	Avoid	Moderate	Strong
Ergoloid mesylates (dehydrogenated ergot alkaloids) Isoxsuprine	Lack of efficacy	Avoid	High	Strong
Endocrine				
Androgens Methyltestosterone Testosterone	Potential for cardiac problems; contraindicated in men with prostate cancer	Avoid unless indicated for confirmed hypogonadism with clinical symptoms	Moderate	Weak
Dessicated thyroid	Concerns about cardiac effects; safer alternatives available	Avoid	Low	Strong

ORGAN SYSTEM, THERAPEUTIC CATEGORY, DRUG(S)	RATIONALE	RECOMMENDATION	QUALITY OF EVIDENCE	STRENGTH OF RECOMMENDATION
Estrogens with or without progestins	Evidence of carcinogenic potential (breast and endometrium); lack of cardioprotective effect and cognitive protection in older women	Avoid systemic estrogen (eg, oral and topical patch)	*Oral and patch:* high	*Oral and patch:* strong
	Evidence indicates that vaginal estrogens for the treatment of vaginal dryness are safe and effective; women with a history of breast cancer who do not respond to nonhormonal therapies are advised to discuss the risks and benefits of low-dose vaginal estrogen (dosages of estradiol <25 μG twice weekly) with their healthcare provider	*Vaginal cream or vaginal tablets:* acceptable to use low-dose intravaginal estrogen for management of dyspareunia, recurrent lower urinary tract infections, and other vaginal symptoms	*Vaginal cream or vaginal tablets:* moderate	*Vaginal cream or vaginal tablets:* weak
Growth hormone	Impact on body composition is small and associated with edema, arthralgia, carpal tunnel syndrome, gynecomastia, impaired fasting glucose	Avoid, except for patients rigorously diagnosed by evidence-based criteria with growth hormone deficiency due to an established etiology	High	Strong

ORGAN SYSTEM, THERAPEUTIC CATEGORY, DRUG(S)	RATIONALE	RECOMMENDATION	QUALITY OF EVIDENCE	STRENGTH OF RECOMMENDATION
Insulin, sliding scale (insulin regimens containing only short- or rapid-acting insulin dosed according to current blood glucose levels without concurrent use of basal or long-acting insulin)	Higher risk of hypoglycemia without improvement in hyperglycemia management regardless of care setting. Avoid insulin regimens that include only short- or rapid-acting insulin dosed according to current blood glucose levels with concurrent use of basal or long-acting insulin. This recommendation does not apply to regimens that contain basal insulin or long-acting insulin.	Avoid	Moderate	Strong
Megestrol	Minimal effect on weight; increases risk of thrombotic events and possibly death in older adults	Avoid	Moderate	Strong
Sulfonylureas, long-acting Chlorpropamide Glimepiride Glyburide (also known as glibenclamide)	*Chlorpropamide:* prolonged half-life in older adults; can cause prolonged hypoglycemia; causes SIADH *Glimepiride and glyburide:* higher risk of severe prolonged hypoglycemia in older adults	Avoid	High	Strong
Gastrointenstinal				
Metoclopramide	Can cause extrapyramidal effects, including tardive dyskinesia; risk may be greater in frail older adults and with prolonged exposure	Avoid, unless for gastroparesis with duration of use not to exceed 12 weeks except in rare cases	Moderate	Strong
Mineral oil, given orally	Potential for aspiration and adverse effects; safer alternative available	Avoid	Moderate	Strong

ORGAN SYSTEM, THERAPEUTIC CATEGORY, DRUG(S)	RATIONALE	RECOMMENDATION	QUALITY OF EVIDENCE	STRENGTH OF RECOMMENDATION
Proton-pump inhibitors	Risk of Clostridium difficile infection and bone loss and fractures	Avoid scheduled use for >8 weeks unless for high-risk patients (eg, oral corticosteroids or chronic NSAID use), erosive esophagitis, Barrett's esophagus, pathological hypersecretory condition, or demonstrated need for maintenance treatment (eg, because of failure of drug discontinuation trial or H2-receptor antagonists)	High	Strong
Pain Medication				
Meperidine	Oral analgesic not effective in dosages commonly used; may have higher risk of neurotoxicity, including delirium, than other opiods; safer alternatives available	Avoid	Moderate	Strong

ORGAN SYSTEM, THERAPEUTIC CATEGORY, DRUG(S)	RATIONALE	RECOMMENDATION	QUALITY OF EVIDENCE	STRENGTH OF RECOMMENDATION
Non-cyclooxygenase-selective NSAIDs, oral: Aspirin >325 mg/day Diclofenac Diflunisal Etodolac Fenoprofen Ibuprofen Ketoprofen Meclofenamate Mefenamic acid Meloxicam Nabumetone Naproxen Oxaprozin Piroxicam Sulindac Tolmetin	Increased risk of gastrointestinal bleeding or peptic ulcer disease in high-risk groups, including those >75 years or taking oral or parenteral corticosteroids, anticoagulants or antiplatelet agents; use of proton-pump inhibitor or misoprostol reduces but does not eliminate risk. Upper gastrointestinal ulcers, gross bleeding, or perforation caused by NSAIDs occur in ~1% of patients treated for 3–6 months and in ~2%–4% of patients treated for 1 year; these trends continue with longer duration of use. Also can increase blood pressure and induce kidney injury. Risks are dose related.	Avoid chronic use, unless other alternatives are not effective and patient can take gastroprotective agent (proton-pump inhibitor or misoprostol)	Moderate	Strong
Indomethacine Ketorolac, includes parenteral	Increased risk of gastrointestinal bleeding/peptic ulcer disease and acute kidney injury in older adults Indomethacin is more likely than other NSAIDs to have adverse CNS effects. Of all the NSAIDs, indomethacin has the most adverse effects.	Avoid	Moderate	Strong

ORGAN SYSTEM, THERAPEUTIC CATEGORY, DRUG(S)	RATIONALE	RECOMMENDATION	QUALITY OF EVIDENCE	STRENGTH OF RECOMMENDATION
Skeletal muscle relaxants Carisoprodol Chlorzoxazone Cyclobenzaprine Metaxalone Methocarbamol Orphenadrine	Most muscle relaxants poorly tolerated by older adults because some have anticholinergic adverse effects, sedation, increased risk of fractures; effectiveness at dosages tolerated by older adults questionable	Avoid	Moderate	Strong
Genitourinary				
Desmopressin	High risk of hyponatremia; safer alternatives available	Avoid for treatment of nocturia or nocturnal polyuria	Moderate	Strong

Abbreviations: CNS, central nervous system; HFrEF, heart failure with reduced ejection fraction; NSAID, nonsteroidal anti-inflammatory drug; SIADH, syndrome of inappropriate antidiuretic hormone secretion.

[a] See also criterion on highly anticholinergic antidepressants.

Table 4.2. 2019 American Geriatrics Society Beers Criteria for Potentially Inappropriate Medication Use in Older Adults Due to Drug–Disease or Drug-Syndrome Interaction that May Exacerbate the Disease or Syndrome

DISEASE OR SYNDROME	DRUG(S)	RATIONALE	RECOMMENDATION	QUALITY OF EVIDENCE	STRENGTH OF RECOMMENDATION
Cardiovascular					
Heart failure	*Avoid:* Cilostazol	Potential to promote fluid retention and/or exacerbate heart failure (NSAIDs and COX-2 inhibitors, nondihydropyridine CCBs, thiazolidinediones); potential to increase mortality in older adults with heart failure (cilostazol and dronedarone)	As noted, avoid or use with caution	*Cilostazol:* low	*Cilostazol:* strong
	Avoid in heart failre with reduced ejection fraction: Nondihydropyridine CCBs (diltiazem, verapamil)			*Nondihydropyridine CCDs:* moderate	*Nondihydropyridine CCDs:* strong
				NSAIDs: moderate	*NSAIDs:* strong
	Use with caution in patients with heart failure who are asymptomatic; avoid in patients with symptomatic heart failure: NSAIDs and COX-2 inhibitors			*COX-2 inhibitors:* low	*COX-2 inhibitors:* strong
				Thiazolidinediones: high	*Thiazolidinediones:* strong
	Thiazolidinediones (pioglitazone, rosiglitazone)			*Dronedarone:* high	*Dronedarone:* strong
	Dronedarone				

DISEASE OR SYNDROME	DRUG(S)	RECOMMENDATION	RATIONALE	QUALITY OF EVIDENCE	STRENGTH OF RECOMMENDATION
Syncope	AChEIs Nonselective peripheral alpha-1 blockers (ie, doxazosin, prazosin, terazosin) Tertiary TCAs Antipsychotics: Chlorpromazine, Thioridazine, Olanzapine	Avoid	AChEIs cause bradycardia and should be avoided in older adults whose syncope may be due to bradycardia. Nonselective peripheral alpha-1 blockers cause orthostatic blood pressue changes and should be avoided in older adults whose syncope may be due to orthostatic hypotension. Tertiary TCAs and the antipsychotics listed increase the risk of orthostatic hypotension or bradycardia.	AChEIs, TCAs, and antipsychotics: high Nonselective peripheral alpha-1 blockers: high	AChEIs, TCAs: strong Nonselective peripheral alpha-1 blockers and antipsychotics: weak
Nervous System					
Delirium	Anticholinergics (see Table 7 and full criteria available on www.geriatricscareonline.org) Antipsychotics[a] Benzodiazepines Corticosteroids (oral and parenteral)[b] H2-receptor antagonists: Cimetidine, Famotidine, Nizatidine, Ranitidine Meperidine Nonbenzodiazepine, benzodiazepine receptor against hypnotics: eszopiclone, zaleplon, zolpidem	Avoid	Avoid in older adults with or at high risk of delirium because of potential of inducing or worsening delirium Avoid antipsychotics for behavioral problems of dementia and/or delirium unless nonpharmacological options (eg, behavioral interventions) have failed or are not possible and the older adult is threatening substantial harm to self or others. Antipsychotics are associated with greater risk of cerebrovascular accident (stroke) and mortality in persons with dementia.	H2-receptor antagonists: low All others: moderate	Strong

DISEASE OR SYNDROME	DRUG(S)	RATIONALE	RECOMMENDATION	QUALITY OF EVIDENCE	STRENGTH OF RECOMMENDATION
Dementia or cognitive impairment	Anticholinergics (see Table 7 and full criteria available on www.geriatricscareonline.org) Benzodiazepines Nonbenzodiazepine, benzodiazepine receptor against hypnotics: eszopiclone, zaleplon, zolpidem Antipsychotics, chronic and as-needed use[a]	Avoid because of adverse CNS effects Avoid antipsychotics for behavioral problems of dementia and/or delirium unless nonpharmacological options (eg, behavioral interventions) have failed or are not possible and the older adult is threatening substantial harm to self or others. Antipsychotics are associated with greater risk of cerebrovascular accident (stroke) and mortality in persons with dementia.	Avoid	Moderate	Strong
History of falls or fractures	Antiepileptics Antipsychotics[a] Benzodiazepines Nonbenzodiazepine, benzodiazepine receptor against hypnotics: eszopiclone, zaleplon, zolpidem Antidepressants: TCAs, SSRIs, SNRIs Opiods	May cause ataxia, impaired psychomotor function, syncope, additional falls; shorter-acting benzodiazepines are not safer than long-acting ones. If one of the drugs must be used, consider reducing use of other CNS-active medications that increase risk of falls and fractures (ie, antiepileptics, opiod-receptor agonists, antipsychotics, antidepressants, nonbenzodiazepine and benzodiazepine receptor against hypnotics, other sedatives/hypnotics) and implement other strategies to reduce fall risk. Data for antidepressants are mixed but no compelling evidence that certain antidepressants confer less fall risk than others.	Avoid unless safer alternatives are not available; avoid antiepileptics except for seizure and mood disorders Opiods: avoid except for pain management in the setting of severe acute pain (eg, recent fractures or joint replacement	*Opiods:* moderate *All others:* high	Strong

DISEASE OR SYNDROME	DRUG(S)	RATIONALE	RECOMMENDATION	QUALITY OF EVIDENCE	STRENGTH OF RECOMMENDATION
Parkinson's disease	Antiemetics: Metoclopramide, Prochlorperazine, Promethazine All antipsychotics (except quetiapine, clozapine, pimavanserin)	Dopamine-receptor antagonists with potential to worsen parkinsonian symptoms Exceptions: Pimavanserin and clozapine appear to be less likely to precipitate worsening of Parkinson disease. Quetiapine has only been studied in low-quality clinical trials with efficacy comparable to that of placebo in five trials and to that of clozapine in two others.	Avoid	Moderate	Strong
Gastrointestinal					
History of gastric or duodenal ulcers	Aspirin >325mg/day Non–COX-2–selective NSAIDs	May exacerbate existing ulcers or cause new/additional ulcers	Avoid unless other alternatives are not effective and patient can take gastroprotective agent (ie, proton-pump inhibitor or misoprostol)	Moderate	Strong
Kidney/Urinary Tract					
Chronic kidney disease stage 4 or higher (creatinine clearance <30mL/min)	NSAIDs (non-COX and COX selective, oral and parenteral, nonacetylated salicylates)	May increase risk of acute kidney injury and further decline of renal function	Avoid	Moderate	Strong

Deprescribing

Deprescribing is the planned and supervised process of dose reduction or stopping of medication that might be causing harm or no longer be of benefit. Clinicians should consider deprescribing to reduce the negative effects of polypharmacy and to improve medication management for older persons. Data shows that patients favor deprescribing (Major et al., 2019; Reeve et al., 2018; Reeve et al., 2019).

- 20–92% are willing to stop one or more medications.
- 15–25% wish to decrease their dose of a medication.
- 67% want to decrease their number of medications.
  - People taking six or more medications are more willing to stop a medication or reduce their medications.
  - Remember, taking six or more medications may lead to a hospital admission due to an adverse drug reaction from a PIM.

Figure 4.1. Usual Approach Versus Proposed Approach
of Medication Management (Zullo et al., 2018)

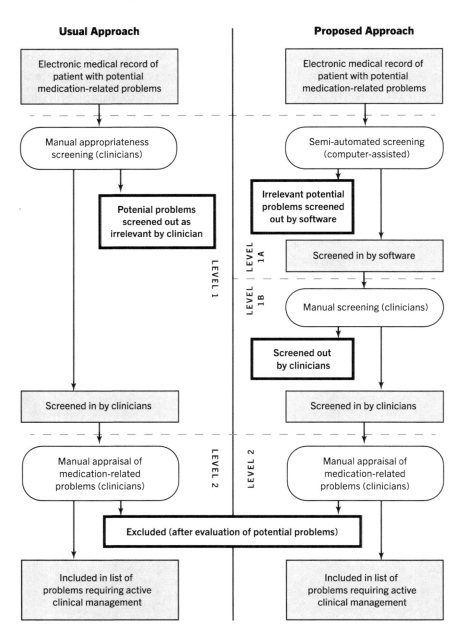

Personal Action Plans

The following is a sample action plan to distribute to older adults and families (Centers for Disease Control and Prevention, 2021).

- Ask your primary care provider or pharmacist the following questions about each of your medicines:
  - What is this medicine used for?
  - Does this medicine interact with others I am taking?
  - Could this medicine have side effects that might change my ability to drive safely or increase my risk of falling?
  - Is there another medicine or dose I should try?
  - If I stop or change this medicine, what side effects should I expect?
- Include prescription medicines, over-the-counter medicines, dietary supplements, and herbal products.
- Use this information to complete your Personal Action Plan, which consists of the provider's answers and your plan of action.

Recommendations and Summary

Gaps in the care continuum within the US continue to impede progress in achieving the goal of delivering optimal care to patients. This fragmentation is a root cause of polypharmacy, as patients with multiple chronic diseases are seen by numerous primary care providers, many of whom are not aware of the older adult's medical history. Judicious use of medication, following the Beers Criteria for regular assessment of medication, is a key strategy of an Age-Friendly Health System. Pharmacists are increasingly accelerating the delivery of patient-centered care in healthcare systems across the nation.

Recommendations for reducing unnecessary treatment, preventing adverse events, and enhancing the safe use of medications for older adults are as follows:

- Do not initiate medications to treat symptoms, adverse events, or adverse effects without determining the cause.
- Do not prescribe medications for patients taking five or more medications, or continue medications indefinitely, without a comprehensive review, including nonprescription medications and dietary supplements.
- Do not continue medications based solely on past use unless a reason for use is verified.
- Do not prescribe medications at discharge that the patient was taking prior to admission without verifying the need.
- Use only metric units when prescribing liquid medications.

The Age-Friendly Health Systems regular review of medication effectiveness and safety as one of the 4Ms is an excellent way to help older adults communicate any concerns, side effects, or benefits they are achieving with their medication plan.

References

American Geriatrics Society Beers Criteria Update Expert Panel. (2019). American Geriatrics Society 2019 updated AGS Beers Criteria for potentially inappropriate medication use in older adults. *Journal of the American Geriatrics Society, 67*(4), 674–694. https://doi.org/10.1111/jgs.15767

Centers for Disease Control and Prevention. (2021). *Personal action plan.* https://www.cdc.gov/motorvehiclesafety/pdf/older_adult_drivers/Personal-Action-Plan_FINAL_508.pdf

Chung, G. C., Marottoli, R. A., Cooney, L. M., Jr., & Rhee, T. G. (2019). Cost-related medication nonadherence among older adults: Findings from a nationally representative sample. *Journal of the American Geriatrics Society*, 67(12), 2463–2473. https://doi.org/10.1111/jgs.16141

Glass, J., Lanctôt, K. L., Herrmann, N., Sproule, B. A., & Busto, U. E. (2005). Sedative hypnotics in older people with insomnia: Meta-analysis of risks and benefits. *BMJ*, 331(7526), 1169. https://doi.org/10.1136/bmj.38623.768588.47

Hansen, R. N., Boudreau, D. M., Ebel, B. E., Grossman, D. C., & Sullivan, S. D. (2015). Sedative hypnotic medication use and the risk of motor vehicle crash. *American Journal of Public Health*, 105(8), 64–69. https://doi.org/10.2105/AJPH.2015.302723

Maher, R. L., Hanlon, J., & Hajjar, E. R. (2014). Clinical consequences of polypharmacy in elderly, *Expert Opinion Drug Safety*, 13(1), 57–65. https://doi.org/10.1517/14740338.2013.827660

Major, G. L., Mills, A., & Lowthian, J. A. (2019). Deprescribing attitudes of older adults receiving medication management support from home-based nurses. *Journal of the American Geriatrics Society*, 67(8), 1756–1757. https://doi.org/10.1111/jgs.16015

Qato, D. M., Wilder, J., Schumm, L. P., Gillet, V., & Alexander, G. C. (2016). Changes in prescription and over-the-counter medication and dietary supplement use among older adults in the United States, 2005–2011. *JAMA Internal Medicine*, 176(4), 473–482. https://doi.org/10.1001/jamainternmed.2015.8581

Ralph, S. J., & Espinet, A. J. (2018). Increased all-cause mortality by antipsychotic drugs: Updated review and meta-analysis in dementia and general mental health care. *Journal of Alzheimer's Disease Reports*, 2(1), 1–26. https://doi.org/10.3233/ADR-170042

Reeve, E., Low, L. F., & Hilmer S. N. (2019). Attitudes of older adults and caregivers in Australia toward deprescribing. *Journal of American Geriatrics Society*, 67(6), 1204–1210. https://doi.org/10.1111/jgs.15804

Reeve, E., Wolff, J. L., Skehan, M., Bayliss, E. A., Hilmer, S. N., & Boyd, C. M. (2018). Assessment of attitudes toward deprescribing in older medicare beneficiaries in the United States. *JAMA Internal Medicine*, 178(12), 1673–1680. https://doi.org/10.1001/jamainternmed.2018.4720

Rochon, P. A., & Gurwitz, J. H. (1997). Optimising drug treatment for elderly people: The prescribing cascade. *BMJ*, 315(7115), 1096–1099. https://doi.org/10.1136/bmj.315.7115.1096

Shehab, N., Lovegrove, M. C., Geller, A. I., Rose, K. O., Weidle, N. J., & Budnitz, D. S. (2016). US emergency department visits for outpatient adverse drug events, 2013–2014. *JAMA*, 316(20), 2115–2125. https://doi.org/10.1001/jama.2016.16201

Tannenbaum, C. (2014a). *Antipsychotics*. Institut universitaire gériatrie de Montréal. https://static1.squarespace.com/static/5836f01fe6f2e1fa62c11f08/t/5e14ae8d0d946d7e1fa6c36e/1578413714789/Empower_antipsych_EN_fillable.pdf

Tannenbaum, C. (2014b). *Sedative-hypnotics*. Institut universitaire gériatrie de Montréal. http://www.criugm.qc.ca/fichier/pdf/BENZOeng.pdf

Zullo, A. R., Gray, S. L, Holmes, H. M., & Marcum, Z. A. (2018). Screening for medication appropriateness in older adults. *Clinics in Geriatric Medicine*, 34(1), 39–54. https://doi.org/10.1016/j.cger.2017.09.003

CHAPTER 5

Mentation

Prevent, identify, treat, and manage dementia,
depression, and delirium across settings of care.
—The Age-Friendly Health Systems initiative

Mental Health and Older Adults

Dementia, delirium, and depression, which will be discussed in further detail, are common mental disorders among older persons that have contributed to billions of dollars in healthcare spending. Approximately 5.8 million Americans aged 65 and older are living with Alzheimer's dementia in 2020, costing the US $305 billion, including $206 billion in Medicare and Medicaid payments. The number of older people living with dementia is projected to grow to 13.8 million by 2050 ("2020 Alzheimer's Disease Facts and Figures," 2020). Meanwhile, delirium costs US hospitals more than $8 billion annually and contributes to $100 billion in post-hospital costs (e.g., skilled nursing facilities and home care). The costs are comparable to diabetes and congestive heart failure, at $152 billion (Leslie et al., 2005).

Depression exacerbates cognitive impairment and adversely impacts physical functioning as well, which significantly increases hospital admission and healthcare spending. All three disorders result in negative health outcomes, higher hospital admission and readmission, and added burden to family caregivers. Older persons are often stuck in a vicious cycle in which increased hospitalization can worsen symptoms of delirium and depression, which then requires a longer length of stay, and ultimately institutionalization if symptoms worsen. It is imperative for interdisciplinary teams of clinicians, social workers, and therapists to implement person-centered approaches to prevent, diagnose, and manage symptoms.

Dementia

Common behavioral and psychological symptoms of dementia—such as agitation, depression, apathy, repetitive questioning, psychosis, aggression, sleep problems, and wandering—are some of the most complex, stressful, and costly aspects of care. They result in poor patient health outcomes, income loss, and increased risk of depression for family caregivers, and higher hospital admission and institutionalization. The causes include neurobiologically related disease factors; unmet needs; caregiver factors; environmental triggers; and interactions of individual, caregiver, and environmental factors. Figure 5.1 is a conceptual model that depicts how degeneration caused by dementia changes the ability of people with dementia to interact with others (especially their caregivers) and the environment. The complexity of these symptoms requires patient-centered approaches tailored to the patient and involving the family and caregiver. Clinicians strongly encourage the use of nonpharmacological treatments as a first strategy, which include behavioral, environmental, and caregiver supportive interventions (see Table 5.1). However, drugs are often preferred, as providers lack training in the use of nonpharmacological strategies and a lack of general understanding and reimbursement for such approaches. If nonpharmacological treatments alone are ineffective, pharmacological treatments such as antipsychotics can reduce symptoms, but the risk-to-benefit ratio is a concern (Kales et al., 2015).

Figure 5.1. Factors Associated With Behavioral and Psychological Symptoms of Dementia (Kales et al., 2015)

Factors Associated with BPSD

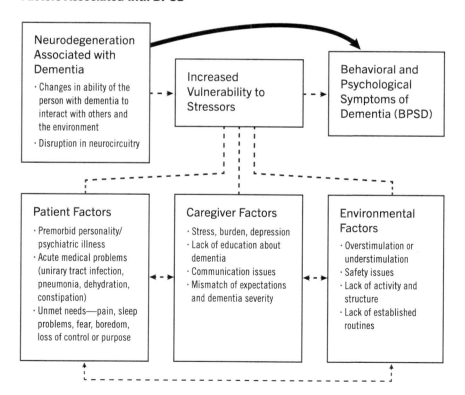

Table 5.1. *Nonpharmacological Strategies for Reducing Symptoms of Dementia (Kales et al., 2015)*

TARGETING PERSON WITH DEMENTIA	TARGETING CAREGIVER	TARGETING ENVIRONMENT
Reminiscence therapy (discussion of past experiences)	Resources for Enhancing Alzheimer's Caregiver Health (REACH II)	Tackling overstimulation (for example, excess noise, people, or clutter in the home) or understimulation (for example, lack of anything of interest to look at)
Validation therapy (working through unresolved conflicts)	REACH-VA	Tackling lack of activity and structure (for example, no regular exercise or activities that match interests and capabilities)
Simulated presence therapy (use of audiotaped recordings of family members' voices)	Tailored Activity Program (TAP)	Tackling lack of established routines (for example, frequent changes in the time, location, or sequence of daily activities)
Aromatherapy (use of fragrant plant oils)	Advancing Caregiver Training (ACT)	
Snoezelen (placing the person with dementia in a soothing and stimulating environment, known as a "Snoezelen room")		
Cognitive training and rehabilitation		
Acupuncture		
Light therapy		

Delirium

Delirium is a transient mental disorder, characterized by globally impaired cognitive functions and reduced ability to sustain or shift attention, that develops over a short period of time and fluctuates during the course of the day. Though delirium normally only lasts for a few days, symptoms may persist for weeks or even months. Over half of hospitalized older adults with dementia will develop delirium, or delirium superimposed on dementia (DSD), but it is reversible and preventable (Fick et al., 2007). Delirium increases rates of long-term cognitive impairment, rehospitalization within 30 days, and risk of permanent admission to long-term-care (LTC) facilities. Common causes of delirium include medications, infections, dehydration, electrolyte imbalance, impaired oxygenation, severe pain, and sleep deprivation. Delirium is costly, deadly, and distressing for the patient, family, clinician, and system but is often overlooked or ignored across settings of care. It is essential to develop new ways to quickly access delirium, especially in acute care but also in other care settings.

Table 5.2. Assessment of Delirium (Fick et al., 2015; Han et al., 2013; Marcantonio et al., 2014; Wei et al., 2008)

TOOL	SENSITIVITY	COMMENTS
CAM	90–98%	Has strongest evidence-based sensitivity and specificity
3D-CAM	95%	Operationalizes CAM and only 3 minutes
UB-2	93–95%	Part of a two-step approach, lower specificity but takes only 36 seconds
B-CAM	78–82%	Lower sensitivity

Confusion Assessment Method

The Confusion Assessment Method (CAM) is a five-minute evidence-based diagnostic tool that detects delirium in older persons with normal mental status or those with dementia and/or depression. It requires structured assessment to complete, including mental-status questions, interview observations, and time, training, and resources. CAM measures four key features of delirium:

- acute onset and/or fluctuating course
- inattention
- disorganized thinking
- altered level of consciousness

It has the highest sensitivity with DSD (Inouye et al., 1990).

Delirium Superimposed on Dementia Algorithm

While the CAM is a useful tool, the Delirium Superimposed on Dementia Algorithm recognizes that the patient's baseline mental status is a critical parameter for assessing and treating delirium. It recommends review of the patient's medical record for indications of preexisting dementia and checking with the patient's family, if any, as to whether the patient has a diagnosis of dementia or signs and symptoms of possible dementia. If a patient is admitted from an assisted living or LTC facility, the nurse should question the staff at the facility about the patient's baseline mental and functional status. The algorithm presents practical ways for bedside nurses to assess delirium and CAM features such as poor attention and fluctuation.

The algorithm can be used with patients with dementia who present to the hospital without previous medical evaluation or who are at increased risk for undetected delirium, and/or with family members who cannot describe the patient's mental status prehospitalization. The algorithm helps address ageism, a significant barrier to detecting the presence of delirium, wherein clinicians attribute further cognitive loss or lethargy in a person with dementia as an inevitable fact of life for older adults (Fick & Mion, 2008).

Ultra-Brief 2-Item Screener

The Ultra-Brief 2-Item Screener (UB-2) is a brief delirium screen that can be conducted in under 1 minute. While it offers a combination of tasks for the older person, the combination with the highest sensitivity (93% to detect delirium and 96% to detect DSD) consists of the following items:

1. Please tell me the day of the week.
2. Please tell me the months of the year backward (Fick et al., 2015).

ASSESSMENT TOOLS' KEY COMPONENTS

The key components of the aforementioned assessment tools comprise:

- cognitive testing
  - including formal testing of attention
- observations of symptoms
  - altered level of consciousness
  - psychomotor agitation/retardation
- presence/acuity of mental status change
  - fluctuations during assessment
  - ask patient, proxies (nurses, family)

Prevention and Treatment of Delirium

Delirium is an acute and dangerous event and is at the heart of what matters to older adults, in that losing control of one's cognitive ability to control behavior is frightening and potentially life-threatening. First, assess what matters to the older adult and their family in the event of delirium. Ensure that any medications that might be causing

Figure 5.2. *2-Item Ultra-Brief (UB-2)*
Delirium Screen Quick Guide (Fick et al., 2015)

2-Item Ultra-Brief (UB-2) Delirium Screen — Quick Guide©

Position: Try to sit at eye level
Sensory: Be sure sensory aids (glasses, hearing) are in place
Wording: Please read the script exactly as written

---

1. Please tell me the day of the week.

The participant can check anywhere (e.g., white board, newspaper, etc.), but cannot ask anyone else in the room.

---

2. Please tell me the months of the year backward; say December as your first month.

Missed Month: If participant finished reciting months but missed one or more, it is incorrect and no prompting is allowed.

Stuck: Prompt only with: *"What month comes before _____ (last month they said)?"*

Prompt up to two times; if after 2 prompts participant is frustrated, confused, or taking a long time, mark it incorrect and offer them an exit, such as, *"That's a tough one, you're doing well...let's try the next question."*

Wrong Type of Answer: If the participant begins at November, starts forward, or begins spelling, assume they don't understand the question and re-read the instructions *once*. If the participant is incorrect again, mark it as incorrect but let them finish.

If incorrect on either question, use an additional screening tool
to further assess, such as the CAM or 3D-CAM
www.hospitalyelderlifeprogram.org/request-access/delirium-instruments

Remember to avoid correcting or cuing the older adult; it's okay if they're incorrect.
Inquiries to Donna Fick: dmf21@psu.edu (Please cite Fick et al, Journal of Hospital Medicine, 2015)

delirium are discontinued, and ensure that the older person is not restrained but is kept safe during the delirium event. Then proceed with the following steps for proper care:

1. Remove or treat underlying cause(s).
2. Manage delirium behaviors.
3. Prevent or remediate complications.
4. Restore cognitive and physical function.

In addition to Age-Friendly Health Systems, two other initiatives include the Nonpharmacologic Delirium Prevention: Hospital Elder Life Program (HELP), which targets delirium risk factors for hospitalized older persons, and Nurses Improving Care for Healthsystem Elders (NICHE), which aims to deliver patient-centered nursing care for older persons across healthcare facilities (Reuben et al., 2000; Mezey et al., 2004).

Table 5.3. *Multicomponent Intervention Strategy Targeted at Six Delirium Risk Factors (Inouye et al., 1999)*

RISK FACTOR	INTERVENTION
Cognitive impairment	Reality orientation, therapeutic activities protocol
Sleep deprivation	Nonpharmacological sleep protocol, sleep enhancement protocol
Immobilization	Early mobilization protocol, minimizing immobilizing equipment
Vision impairment	Vision aids, adaptive equipment
Hearing impairment	Amplifying devices, adaptive equipment and techniques
Dehydration	Early recognition and volume repletion

Understanding Delirium and Dementia Behaviors

A person-centered approach focuses on delirium causes and unmet needs. It is important to understand these needs and their corresponding response-based behaviors, which may include agitation. Clinicians must know the person and understand their goals and emotion. Non-drug strategies are recommended, along with family participation.

Screening/Assessment Controversies

Accuracy of screening goes down at the bedside (Yanamadala et al., 2013). Universal screening should not be done if best practices for treatment and prevention are not in place, as this can hurt care. Another controversy is that screening takes too much time and training. Clinicians are often unsure which population to screen (e.g., 70 and older, 65 and older, high risk). Furthermore, screening for delirium alone—without ongoing system-wide education for trained staff who are implementing nonpharmacological preventive and treatment strategies and changes—will lead to marked increases in use of antipsychotic and sedative drugs. This will result in worsened outcomes, particularly for older adults. This would not happen with the 4Ms approach, where assessment is linked to action strategies.

Depression

Depression is a prevalent yet serious mood disorder that negatively interferes with how an individual feels, thinks, and responds to activities of daily living—such as working, eating, or sleeping—for at least 2 weeks (National Institute of Mental Health, 2021). While depression is more common than dementia among older people and affects almost seven million people aged 65 and older living in the US, it is underdiagnosed and therefore often left untreated (Allan et al., 2014; Steinman et al., 2007). Depression is more challenging to recognize among older people because symptoms often manifest differently and can be indicative of common physical illnesses in this population. Physical symptoms can include insomnia, slowed movement, weight loss, vague pain, confusion, and memory problems. It is not uncommon for older people to deny changes in mood, which further complicates diagnosis and prevents them from receiving the necessary treatment (Cahoon, 2012). Older people are also at a greater risk of becoming depressed, as risk factors—such as dementia, chronic medical conditions, poor physical and cognitive function, polypharmacy, experiencing multiple losses, retirement, and social isolation—are all more common in old age (Allan et al., 2014; Cahoon, 2012). However, depression is highly treatable once diagnosed (Cahoon, 2012).

To assess depression using the 4Ms approach, it is recommended that clinicians routinely use one of the following tools: Patient Health Questionnaire-2 (PHQ-2), Patient Health Questionnaire-9 (PHQ-9), Geriatric Depression Scale (GDS), or Geriatric Depression Scale: Short Form (GDS-15). Each tool is highly valid and reliable for culturally and linguistically diverse populations. GDS and GDS-15 are also effective in assessing depression in older adults with varying levels of education. However, cognitive function may interfere with the validity of these tools, so it is important for clinicians to test for dementia as well as to develop a comprehensive understanding of an older person's mentation (Mate et al., 2021).

Based on the severity of symptoms, treatments for depression include psychotherapy, pharmacology, electroconvulsive therapy (ECT), or a combination. Psychotherapy, such as problem-solving therapy, cognitive behavioral therapy, and interpersonal psychotherapy, is generally recommended for patients with mild to moderate symptoms and is comparable to the efficacy of antidepressants. However, it is unclear whether the influence of frailty, cognitive impairment, and physical diseases impacts the effectiveness or feasibility of psychotherapy (Kok & Reynolds, 2017). Pharmacological treatment relies on the use of antidepressants—such as selective serotonin reuptake inhibitors (SSRIs), tricyclic antidepressants (TCAs), monoamine oxidase inhibitors (MAOIs), and atypical antidepressants—and is effective for the treatment of more severe depression (Cahoon, 2012; Kok & Reynolds, 2017). It is recommended to first use SSRIs, as they do not typically cause anticholinergic effects, cardiotoxicity, hypotension, or sedation. However, medication can cause nausea and discomfort, which may lead to nonadherence and a relapse in depressive symptoms (Kales et al., 2015). Furthermore, since adverse effects are common with antidepressants, clinicians must carefully consider their patients' sensitivity to medication and the potential for drug-drug interaction. For instance, it is not recommended to use medication to treat depression in patients with dementia. Clinicians can use the STOPP/START criteria to avoid prescribing inappropriate medications or undertreatment (Kok & Reynolds, 2017). For older patients with severe depression who have been unresponsive to psychotherapy and have concerns surrounding the adverse effects of antidepressants, ECT is an effective alternative. Along with standard treatments, it is also beneficial for patients to exercise, improve sleep hygiene, and leverage community-based resources to increase social interactions and support (Kok & Reynolds, 2017; Mezey et al., 2004).

Recommendations and Summary

Previously underappreciated and referred to broadly as confusion, we now know that cognitive change in older adults is a serious and high-risk event that is often undetected with untoward outcomes. In Age-Friendly Health Systems, there is a systematic approach to screening for and detection of cognitive changes regardless of care setting. Further, there are approaches to teach families about the potential of cognitive changes and what they might look for at home. There are tools to accurately and feasibly assess for cognitive change that are

Table 5.4. *Mentation Measures: Getting the Right Baseline and Change Score (IHI, n.d.)*

Percentage of patients who have depressive symptoms	*Numerator:* Calculated by using data from Item DO3OO, the total self-reported depression severity score on PHQ-9
	Denominator: Count of patients or residents who have received an MDS assessment
Percentage of patients or residents screened positive for depression with reduction in depressive symptoms	*Numerator:* Count of patients in the denominator with a 6-month PHQ-9 score of less than 5
	Denominator: Count of non-acute patients with a diagnosis of major depression and an initial PHQ-9 score greater than 9 discharged in the measurement period
Percentage of patients screened positive for dementia with behavior management plan	*Numerator:* Count of patients in the denominator with a documented behavior management plan
	Denominator: Count of patients who screen positive for dementia among inpatient discharges or facility resident census in the measurement period
Percentage of patients meeting diagnostic criteria on the Confusion Assessment Method (CAM)	*Numerator:* Count of patients in the denominator meeting diagnostic criteria on the CAM
	Denominator: Count of inpatient discharges or facility resident census in the measurement period
Percentage of patients identified with delirium treated according to local protocol	*Numerator:* Count of patients in the denominator treated according to local protocol
	Denominator: Count of inpatient discharges or facility resident census in the measurement period meeting diagnostic criteria on the CAM

readily available. When older adults demonstrate changes in mood and memory, it can be both alarming and frightening to family, friends, and the older person. There are excellent strategies and supports from numerous resources and organizations that should be made readily available when doing a mentation assessment and care plan.

Assessing mentation for any cognitive change requires training, education, and leadership with an understanding that the 4Ms are interactive and that any of them may be advancing or harming progress. Teaching staff how to develop early mobility programs with a reduction of low-mobility activity, such as sitting in a chair, and the elimination of physical restraints supports positive mentation in older adults.

Assessing and documenting the mentation of older persons in care settings with a plan for needed support that is in line with the older person's goals and preferences is a vital component of 4Ms care.

References

2020 Alzheimer's disease facts and figures. (2020). *Alzheimer's & Dementia: The Journal of the Alzheimer's Association*, 16(3), 391–460. https://doi. org/10.1002/alz.12068

Allan, C. E., Valkanova, V., & Ebmeier, K. P. (2014). Depression in older people is underdiagnosed. *The Practitioner*, 258(1771), 19–22. https:// www.thepractitioner.co.uk//Symposium/Psychiatry/5596-/Depression-in-older-people-is-underdiagnosed

Cahoon, C. G. (2012). Depression in older adults. *American Journal of Nursing*, 112(11), 22–30. https://doi.org/10.1097/01.NAJ.0000422251.65212.4b

Fick, D. M., Hodo, D. M., Lawrence, F., & Inouye, S. K. (2007). Recognizing delirium superimposed on dementia: Assessing nurses' knowledge using case vignettes. *Journal of Gerontological Nursing*, 33(2), 40–49. https:// doi.org/10.3928/00989134-20070201-09

Fick, D. M., Inouye, S. K., Guess J., Ngo, L. H., Jones, R. N., Saczynski, J. S., & Marcantonio, E. R. (2015). Preliminary development of an ultrabrief two-item bedside test for delirium. *Journal of Hospital Medicine*, 10(10), 645–650. https://doi.org/10.1002/jhm.2418

Fick, D. M., & Mion L. C. (2008). Delirium superimposed on dementia. *American Journal of Nursing*, 108(1), 52–60. https://doi.org/10.1097/01. NAJ.0000304476.80530.7d

Han, J. H., Wilson, A., Vasilevskis, E. E., Shintani, A., Schnelle, J. F., Robert, S. D., Graves, A. J., Storrow, A. B., Shuster, J., & Ely, E. W. (2013). Diagnosing delirium in older emergency department patients: validity and reliability of the delirium triage screen and the brief confusion assessment method. *Annals of Emergency Medicine*, 62(5), 457–465. https://doi.org/10.1016/j.annemergmed.2013.05.003

Inouye, S. K., Bogardus, S. T., Jr., Charpentier, P. A., Leo-Summers, L., Acampora, D., Holford, T. R., & Cooney, L. M., Jr. (1999). A multicomponent intervention to prevent delirium in hospitalized older patients. *New England Journal of Medicine*, 340(9), 669–676. https://doi.org/10.1056/ NEJM199903043400901

Inouye, S. K., van Dyck, C. H., Alessi, C. A., Balkin, S., Siegal, A. P., & Horwitz, R. I. (1990). Clarifying confusion: The confusion assessment method. A new method for detection of delirium. *Annals of Internal Medicine*, 113(12), 941–948. https://doi.org/10.7326/0003-4819-113-12-941

Institute for Healthcare Improvement. (n.d.). *Mentation Measures: Getting the Right Baseline and Change Score* [Unpublished internal document].

Kales, H. C., Gitlin, L. N., & Lyketsos, C. G. (2015). Assessment and management of behavioral and psychological symptoms of dementia. *BMJ*, 350, h369. https://doi.org/10.1136/bmj.h369

Kok, R. M., & Reynolds III, C. F. (2017). Management of depression in older adults: A review. *JAMA*, 317(20), 2114–2122. https://doi.org/10.1001/ jama.2017.5706

Leslie, D. L, Zhang, Y., Bogardus, S. T, Holford, T. R, Leo-Summers, L. S, & Inouye, S. K. (2005). Consequences of preventing delirium in hospitalized older adults on nursing home costs. *Journal of the American Geriatrics Society*, 53(3), 405–409. https://doi.org/10.1111/j.1532-5415.2005.53156.x

Marcantonio, E. R., Ngo, L. H, O'Connor, M., Jones, R. N., Crane, P. K., Metzger, E. D., & Inouye, S. K. (2014). 3D-CAM: Derivation and validation of a 3-minute diagnostic interview for CAM-defined delirium:

A cross-sectional diagnostic test study. *Annals of Internal Medicine*, 161(8), 554–561. https://doi.org/10.7326/M14-0865

Mate, K. S., Fulmer, T., Pelton, L., Berman, A., Bonner, A., Huang, W., & Zhang, J. (2021). Evidence for the 4Ms: Interactions and outcomes across the care continuum. *Journal of Aging and Health*, 33(7–8),469–481. https://doi.org/10.1177/0898264321991658

Mezey, M., Kobayashi, M., Grossman, S., Firpo, A., Fulmer, T., & Mitty, E. (2004). Nurses Improving Care to Health System Elders (NICHE): Implementation of best practice models. *The Journal of Nursing Administration*, 34(10), 451–457. https://doi.org/10.1097/00005110-200410000-00005

National Institue of Mental Health. (2021). *Depression*. https://www.nimh.nih.gov/health/topics/depression/

Reuben, D. B., Inouye, S. K., Bogardus, S. T., Jr., Baker, D. I., Leo-Summers, L., & Cooney, L. M., Jr. (2000). Models of Geriatric Practice; The Hospital Elder Life Program: A model of care to prevent cognitive and functional decline in older hospitalized patients. Hospital Elder Life Program. *Journal of the American Geriatrics Society*, 48(12), 1697–1706. https://doi.org/10.1111/j.1532-5415.2000.tb03885.x

Steinman, L. E., Frederick, J. T., Prohaska, T., Satariano, W. A., Dornberg-Lee, S., Fisher, R., Graub, P. B., Leith, K., Presby, K., Sharkey, J., Snyder, S., Turner, D., Wilson, N., Yagoda, L., Unutzer, J., & Snowden, M. (2007). Recommendations for treating depression in community-based older adults. *American Journal of Preventive Medicine*, 33(3), 175–181. https://doi.org/10.1016/j.amepre.2007.04.034

Wei, L. A., Fearing, M. A., Sternberg, E. J., & Inouye S. K. (2008). The Confusion Assessment Method: A systematic review of current usage. *Journal of American Geriatriacs Society*, 56(5), 823–830. https://doi.org/10.1111/j.1532-5415.2008.01674.x

Yanamadala, M., Wieland, D., & Heflin, M. T. (2013). Educational interventions to improve recognition of delirium: A systematic review. *Journal of the American Geriatrics Society*, 61(11), 1983–1993. https://doi.org/10.1111/jgs.12522

CHAPTER 6

Mobility

Contributors: *Ann Hendrich, PhD, RN, FAAN, Age-Friendly Health Systems Advisor; Maryjo Phillips, MSN, RN-BC, CMSRN, Clinical Program Manager, Geriatrics, Ann May Center for Nursing and Allied Health, Hackensack Meridian Health; Brenda Belbot, MHA, MSN, RN-BC, NICHE (Nurses Improving Care for Healthsystem Elders) Consultant*

> *Ensure that older adults move safely every day in order to maintain function to do What Matters.*
> —The Age-Friendly Health Systems initiative

To promote safe mobility in older adults, it is essential to transform how individuals think about fall prevention. Despite years of effort to reduce injurious falls, falls continue to be a major health concern for older adults. In 2018, 27.5% of adults aged 65 and older in the US said that they fell at least once in the prior year. In the same year, falls were the leading cause of injury in older adults: 10.2% reported that they had a fall with an injury, and about 32,000 older adults died as a result of fall injuries. These injuries resulted in more than 950,000 hospitalizations or transfers to another facility and almost 3 million visits to the emergency department (Moreland et al., 2020). According to the Agency for Healthcare Research and Quality, 227,000 falls happened in hospitals in 2017 (Agency for Healthcare Research and Quality, 2019). In 2015, medical costs for fatal falls were estimated to be $754 million, and for nonfatal falls, $49.6 billion (Florence et al., 2018).

The current practice of fall prevention is limited all too often by the underlying assumption that the way to keep a person from falling is to keep them from moving. This assumption is most prevalent in the hospital setting and may flow in part from the pressure to achieve "zero falls" in response to the national patient safety movement and the Centers for Medicare & Medicaid Services' Hospital-Acquired Conditions Initiative, which began in 2008 and changed reimbursement practices to deny payment for injuries related to inpatient falls. In many acute-care facilities, nursing effort around fall prevention focuses on a checklist approach that emphasizes uniform environmental modifications and restrictions on mobility for all patients considered at risk for falls. Many of these interventions, such as bed alarms and nonskid socks, are not supported by the evidence (Jazayeri et al., 2021; Shorr et al., 2012). Despite the widespread implementation of fall prevention programs in the "zero falls" era, progress in reducing falls has been slow and rarely sustainable (Porter et al., 2018; Shorr et al., 2019). It is time for a more person-centered and clinically relevant approach.

The 4Ms approach of the Age-Friendly Health Systems initiative presents an exciting opportunity to reframe the way people think about fall prevention. For one thing, it encourages individuals to look beyond ageism—in which it is assumed that people fall because they are older—and instead look at the underlying risk factors that lead to falls. In other words, it is not age that makes people fall; it is the root causes correlated with aging, such as Medication (potentially inappropriate medications, polypharmacy), Mentation (delirium, dementia, depression), Mobility (gait, strength, balance; primary or secondary related to morbidities), and the failure to engage patients and caregivers in care plans designed around What Matters. A "history of falls" reveals when someone has fallen, but not *why* they are falling. Rather than a one-size-fits-all approach to fall prevention and mobility promotion, it is crucial to tailor interventions to address each person's modifiable fall risk factors, engaging the expertise of interprofessional teams across the care continuum. At the heart of this shift is how to reimagine fall risk factors as part of a larger approach to preventive care, where underlying conditions that come to light as part of the fall risk assessment are elevated to the medical problem list and addressed in both inpatient and outpatient settings and as part of transitions in care and the continuum of care.

This chapter will describe this new approach and show how it aligns with 4Ms care, promoting healthy aging and independence. The acronym ERA is utilized to designate the fundamental principles of this new era in fall prevention and safe mobility: Electronic health record integration, Risk factors that matter, and Assessment and care plans.

Why Safe Mobility Rather Than Fall Prevention?

First, it is important to emphasize a paradigm shift of the new era: the way to reduce injurious falls is to *keep* people moving rather than to keep them *from* moving. The evidence is exceedingly strong that immobility leads to adverse effects and negative outcomes (Wald et al., 2019), making a compelling case for promoting mobility among older adults, even during a short hospital stay. Hospitalized adults spend 87–100% of their time sitting or lying in bed (Fazio et al., 2020; Wald et al., 2019). Immobility during a hospital stay leads to various negative health outcomes, including pressure ulcers, venous stasis, the loss of muscle mass, frailty, and falls, that correlate with higher rates of readmission, length of stay, long-term-care placement, and even death (Barnes et al., 2013; Greysen et al., 2015; Smart et al., 2018; Wald et al., 2019). Ten days of bed rest results in a 12% decline in aerobic capacity and a 16% decline in knee extensor strength in healthy older adults (Kortebein et al., 2008). During a hospital stay, 30–60% of older patients lose their ADL function, increasing risk of ADL disability 60-fold (Boyd et al., 2008; Gill et al., 2012). In fact, one-third do not recover their ADL function within one year, resulting in a higher reliance on post-acute care and long-term institutionalization (Boyd et al., 2008).

Hospitalized older adults with low physical mobility are six times more likely to be institutionalized in nursing homes and 34 times more likely to die than those who ambulate at least twice per day (Brown et al., 2004). Implementation of mobility programs improves the health outcomes of hospitalized older adults and reduces hospital length of stay as well as costs associated with healthcare utilization (Smart et al., 2018). Furthermore, by improving the older person's ability to perform ADL, mobility assessment and action also uplift the older person's dignity through a patient-centered approach.

The Transformative Potential of the ERA Approach

Table 6.1 provides an overview of how the ERA approach can transform fall prevention and safe mobility programs. The sections that follow will provide more detail about how each of the components of ERA contributes to better patient outcomes and better use of care team time and skills.

Table 6.1. The Transformative Potential of the ERA Approach

	Current State	Desired State	Impact
E Electronic Health Record Integration	Nursing typically takes charge of fall risk assessment, and the medical problem list does not include fall risk scores or integrate modifiable risk factors into the plan.	• An interprofessional care model approach with the electronic record available across the continuum. • Modifiable risk factors are prioritized and followed across the continuum of care. • Confusion is assessed and diagnosed. Delirium is treated as a medical emergency and links to a sepsis protocol.	• Intrinsic risk factors are managed along with environmental risks to avoid injuries and decline in health if possible. • Early identification of delirium can prevent worsening and long-term effects. It can also lead to detection of unrecognized sepsis, reducing mortality. • Cognition baseline is established for preventative careand ongoing evaluations.
	Duplication and rework by all providers.	• Electronic record is auto-populated from ongoing, regular assessments and history and physical on admission.	• Saves provider time and utilizes current data feeds that can improve reliability.
	Formulary triggers (informed by Beers Criteria)	• High-risk drugs eliminated from routine prescribing. • Appropriate use informed by "what matters most" to the person and side effects of treatment with trade-offs.	• Avoidance of drug side effects and polypharmacy. • Deprescribing is a standard of care. • Pharmacists can take a lead role to collaborate with the provider in calibrating a therapy plan that is safe and meets the person's goals when possible.
	Standardized tools for modifiable risk factors not linked automatically in record.	• Standardized tools for depression screening (e.g., PHQ-9), delirium screening (e.g., CAM), etc. are automatically linked to fall risk factors for positive scores in the assessment.[1]	• Environmental safety precautions become the global standard in all environments. • Safe mobility becomes a goal that is balanced with avoidance of injurious falls.
	Gait, balance, and mobility baseline not assessed and captured as a minimum standard of care. Standardized tools not used for baseline functionality.	• Standardized activity tool(s) used for promotion and maintenance of gait and balance for all levels of care (e.g., BMAT).[1]	• Environmental safety precautions become the global standard in all environments. • Safe mobility becomes a goal that is balanced with avoidance of injurious falls.
	Documenting "what matters most" is not a minimum standard of care with frequent updates in history of record.	• Documenting "what matters most" is a standard within the record, using the words of the person.	• Person-centered, holistic care informed by the values and goals of the person, when possible.

	Current State	Desired State	Impact
R Risk Factors That Matter ⚠	Interventions are not informed by evidence-based risk factors. Assessments are based on small studies with methodological limitations or "home-grown" tools. Unintended bias forms false assumptions based on correlation versus causation (e.g., the assumption that age causes falls).	• Evidence-based risk factors, supported by reliable studies, subject matter experts, and/or quality improvement efforts known to positively impact populations, inform interventions to reduce injurious fall risk.	• Modifiable risk factors and the 4Ms become the standard of care to promote mobility, healthy aging, and independence.
A Assessment and Care Plans	The 4Ms are not used to inform and guide clinical care for older adult populations.	• Continuum of care plan is informed by integrated, coordinated care for all levels (home, acute care, long-term acute care, rehabilitation, behavioral health, etc.) with a focus on independence and healthy aging.	• Coordinated, safe, high-quality care at less cost, based on "what matters most" to the person.
	Care and information gaps in holistic assessment and coordination between primary care and special needs, referrals, and specialists.	• Risk factors are integrated into the EHR plan of care and available to all providers for continuous monitoring and follow-up.	• Reduction in needless injurious falls from attention to modifiable risk factors and preventative care to promote independence and healthy aging.
	Polypharmacy and side effects prevalent, and deprescribing not a standard of care with provider buy-in and agreement.	• Education and support for the 4Ms and Beer Criteria available to all providers with interdisciplinary approaches.	• Prescription of potentially high-risk medications and polypharmacy are greatly reduced when the focus shifts to prevention and underlying causes versus prescribing and when the care model follows the person regardless of location (community, acute care, or chronic care).

Abbreviations: BMAT: Bedside Mobility Assessment Tool; CAM: Confusion Assessment Method; PHQ-9: Patient Health Questionnaire-9.

1 For extensive lists or standardized tools, see the Institute for Healthcare Improvement's Age-Friendly Health Systems: Guide to Using the 4Ms in the Care of Older Adults, July 2020. Accessed Sept 17, 2020. http://www.ihi.org/Engage/Initiatives/Age-Friendly-Health-Systems/Documents/IHIAgeFriendlyHealthSystems_GuidetoUsing4MsCare.pdf.

Use the Electronic Health Record to Create More Efficient, More Effective Fall Prevention / Mobility Programs

One fundamental principle of the new ERA in fall prevention and safe mobility is to optimize use of the electronic health record (EHR) to improve outcomes for patients and make better use of the time of care teams. Chapter 10 provides guidance on how to use the EHR to support age-friendly care, but it is important to emphasize here the advantages of using the EHR to enhance fall prevention programs. The aim is to incorporate a valid and reliable fall risk assessment tool into the EHR so that it continuously automates and auto-populates the patient's fall risk factors into the nursing assessment form (Moskowitz et al., 2020). Auto-population from concurrent medical record data can improve frequency of fall risk assessments (which change often in acute care) and eliminates duplication in documentation. More frequent assessment leads to better patient outcomes. Environmental precautions can become a minimum standard of care in the design for all patients, eliminating redundant work by the nurse. EHR functionality can also save nursing time and enhance patient safety by using an alert system built into the record rather than relying on visual identification methods.

Most importantly, the patient's fall risk factors can link to customizable, evidence-based care plans and interventions. The nurse, in collaboration with the interprofessional team, can develop a care plan by choosing interventions based on the patient's risk factors and condition. As risk factors change, so can the care plan. For example, the Hendrich II Fall Risk Model, a fall risk assessment tool that has been validated in large, diverse study populations (Hendrich et al., 2003; Hendrich et al., 2020), has been built into the Epic™ App Orchard™[1] to enable the care team to personalize the selection of interventions and

---

1   Epic and App Orchard are trademarks or registered trademarks of Epic Systems Corporation.

Figure 6.1. Step 1—Risk Factors That Matter

	1009	**1202**	1300
Hendrich II Fall Risk Model (If new, add to Problem List for automatic scoring)			
Unable to assess any fall risk factors			
Universal fall risk interventions			
Flowsheet reviewed?	Yes		
Confusion			
Confusion/disorientation/impulsivity	4		
Behavioral health	0		
Dehydration	0		
Delirium	1		
Dementia	0		
Sepsis	0		
Medication side effects including polypharmacy	0		
Metabolic/liver failure	0		
Substance abuse/misuse (alcohol or drugs)	0		
Sleep loss/sensory deprivation	0		
Hyponatremia	0		
Symptomatic Depression			
Symptomatic depression	0		
Depression/suicide screening tool			
Altered Elimination			
Altered elimination	1		
Urinary tract or bladder infection	0		
Medication side effects or overuse of cathartics			
Postoperative surgery and anesthesia			
Removal of urinary catheter within 24 hours	1		
Undiagnosed diabetes			
Prolapsed bladder			
Bowel pattern documentation	0		
Enlarged prostate	0		
Dizziness			
Dizziness or vertigo			

care plans based on individual risk factors identified by the fall risk assessment. To walk through what this looks like in practice: Risk Factor 1 of the Hendrich II Fall Risk Model is Confusion. Confusion is not a diagnosis, so the cause of the confusion and a baseline need to be established. Figure 6.1 shows the most common causes of confusion.

In the example, the person's confusion is caused by delirium. If the hospital has standardized a tool for confusion/delirium, the form will automatically link to the tool for further assessment. Then the caregiver can choose the appropriate intervention(s) for delirium to populate the care plan (see Step 2 below). The interventions list can also be customized further to incorporate site-specific interventions that may already be in place. This gives the site maximum flexibility in adoption or editing.

Figure 6.2. *Step 2—Interventions*
Confusion/Disorientation/Impulsivity

Delirium
Problem Interventions — Frequency

- Ensure sufficient oral hydration (see dehydration interventions) ×
- Reorient patient/resident to person, place, time, and situation ×
- Ensure person has their personal adaptive equipment (e.g., glasses, hearing aids, dentures, walkers) ×
- Prevent sleep interruptions by avoiding overnight vital checks and blood draws unless necessary ×
- Use nonpharmacological interventions to support sleep (e.g., earplugs, sleeping masks, muscle relaxation such as hand massage, posture and relaxation training, white noise and music, and educational strategies) ×
- Consult with team to avoid or minimize high-risk medications ×
- Provide a consistent routine ×

As this example illustrates, integration of the fall risk assessment tool into the EHR can facilitate a holistic, person-centered approach to fall prevention that enables the care team to use their critical thinking skills and efficiently address the root causes of the person's fall risk.

Figure 6.3. Step 3—Care Plan

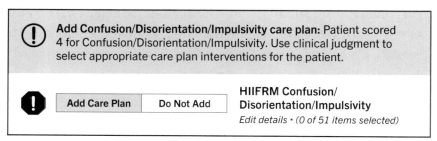

Keep the Focus on Risk Factors That Matter

The foundation of fall prevention is the assessment of fall risk using a tool that is based on risk factors that have been scientifically validated. Most falls are based on multiple factors intrinsic to the person, so it is important to look at how the factors interact. "Reluctance to simplify" is central to providing highly reliable care (Weick & Sutcliffe, 2015).

To build on the example used to illustrate EHR integration, the Hendrich II Fall Risk Model (HIIFRM), a validated tool used across the United States and internationally (https://hendrichfallriskmodel. com/fall-risk-model-validation/), assesses eight fall risk factors that were scientifically identified as necessary to predict falls:

- mental status (confusion, disorientation, impulsivity)
- symptomatic depression

- altered elimination
- dizziness/vertigo
- two categories of medications (antiepileptics and benzodiazepines)
    - Note that statistical analyses found that only these two drug categories increased fall risk within the model. The most common side effects of other medications—such as effects on orthostatic hypotension, mobility, gait, cognition, mood, or elimination—are already assessed as part of other HIIFRM risk factors.
- gender (male)
- functional status (the "Rising from a Chair" item from the Get Up and Go Test)

The Hendrich research team published a large electronic health-validation study of the HIIFRM, based on a sample of 214,358 adult inpatients (625 falls) admitted consecutively over a three-year period to nine varied acute-care sites and across all departments (Hendrich et al., 2020). The study sites had patient populations that were diverse in terms of race, gender, age, ethnicity, case-mix, and length of stay and included hospitals of various sizes, in both urban and rural locations, and academic and nonacademic settings. The results confirmed the validity and accuracy of the model to predict falls in practice and in the EHR.

Figure 6.4 shows how the eight risk factors of the HIIFRM align with the 4Ms framework.

No matter what fall risk assessment tool a facility uses, it is imperative that it is scientifically validated to identify the risk factors that matter in preventing falls. Other validated fall risk assessment tools include the Johns Hopkins Fall Risk Assessment Tool (JHFRAT), a risk stratification tool that is highly effective when combined with a comprehensive protocol and fall prevention products and technologies.

The Johns Hopkins Hospital used the JHFRAT to reduce its fall rate by 21% and fall injury rate by 51% (Poe et al., 2005). The JHFRAT is reliable, with high sensitivity and negative predictive validity. However, specificity and positive predictive validity were lower than expected (Poe et al., 2018).

Figure 6.4. *Alignment of the 4Ms Framework With the Eight Fall Risk Factors of the Hendrich II Fall Risk Model®*

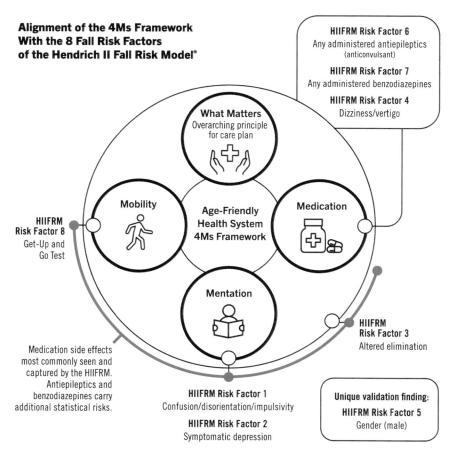

The Stopping Elderly Accidents, Deaths & Injuries (STEADI) initiative is a fall prevention approach developed by the Centers for Disease Control and Prevention's Injury Center. It consists of three core elements:

1. Screen patients for fall risk.
2. Assess modifiable risk factors.
3. Intervene to reduce risk by using effective clinical and community strategies.

STEADI includes various tools and resources, which consist of basic information about falls, screening options, information on medications linked to falls, standardized gait and balance assessment tests, and online trainings that offer continuing education. Systematic implementation of STEADI can help clinical teams reduce older-patient fall risks, improve health outcomes, and reduce healthcare expenditures (Eckstrom et al., 2017).

Create Care Plans to Manage Fall Risk Factors, in Alignment With the 4Ms

The older adult's intrinsic fall risk factors are closely aligned with the 4Ms. Once these factors are identified for an individual patient, it is time to take action to select and implement individualized interventions. A crucial shift in perspective is to think of fall risk assessment not only as a way to identify patients at risk of falling but as an opportunity to diagnose and address underlying conditions. For example, if a person is admitted to the hospital for a heart condition and the fall risk assessment identifies depression as a fall risk factor, depression should be added to the medical problem list and become part of both the inpatient and transitional care plan.

One way in which What Matters conversations can support fall prevention and safe mobility for patients is that they provide an occasion to weigh the risks and benefits of various physical activities in consultation with the care provider. The person, with their family / care proxy, can clarify their values and goals and provide input on a mobility plan that works for them. In the context of a hospital stay, it is important to establish the person's baseline for mobility and build a mobility plan to sustain at least their current capabilities. In the hospital, as well as at home and in their community, a person who values maintaining personal independence may prefer to take on some level of personal risk to stay mobile, even if it means their risk of falling is greater than zero. It is important to avoid injurious falls whenever possible, but a realistic mobility plan may provide more support to their overall physical and mental health than avoiding all risk of falls. As emphasized, healthy aging is all about keeping moving rather than stopping moving, and What Matters conversations can facilitate ongoing adaptation of the mobility plan to reflect the patient's current condition.

Issues related to Mentation and Medication increase the risk of falling. Chapter 5 details how preventing, identifying, treating, and managing dementia, depression, and delirium across settings of care is central to age-friendly care. It should also be borne in mind that each of these issues of mentation is also a fall risk factor, interfering with safe mobility. Similarly, the use of potentially inappropriate medications, as detailed in Chapter 4, and polypharmacy can cause side effects such as cognition changes, dehydration, mobility and gait disturbances, mood changes, hypotension, and altered elimination—side effects that heighten vulnerability to falls and poor mobility. Thus, when a patient's fall risk assessment identifies mentation- or medication-related risk factors, these risk factors should be evaluated as part of the comprehensive assessment and integrated into the overall plan of care.

The Mobility Care Plan

The mobility care plan should be grounded in regular assessment of the person's capability for movement, using a validated tool—ideally, a tool that has been integrated into the EHR workflow. In the inpatient setting, a good choice is the Bedside Mobility Assessment Tool (BMAT), which uses a simple functional assessment and guides selection of appropriate equipment to safely mobilize the patient (Boynton et al., 2020).

The mobility care plan should get the same attention as any other written order. The EHR can facilitate this attention with prompts and by ensuring that an order of "bed rest" is either not an option or must be justified for any hospitalized patient. A study implementing a hospital mobility program that assisted older hospitalized patients with ambulation up to twice daily and incorporated a behavioral strategy to encourage mobility found that participants were able to maintain prehospitalization community mobility (Brown et al., 2016). Some critical care units are creating mobility plans even for ventilated patients, reducing complications and lengths of stay (Escalon et al., 2020). Technological advances should enable EHRs to connect to inexpensive wearable devices that can track steps and distance against weekly, daily, or shift goals in the hospital or at home.

Case Study

Implementing the ERA Approach at Hackensack Meridian Health

Hackensack Meridian Health is a leading not-for-profit healthcare organization that is the largest, most comprehensive, and truly integrated healthcare network in New Jersey, offering a complete range of medical services, innovative research, and life-enhancing care. The network includes 17 hospitals from Bergen to Ocean counties, three academic medical centers, a behavioral health hospital, two rehabilitation hospitals, and more than 500 other patient care locations throughout New Jersey, including 16 long-term-care facilities. The nursing strategic vision focuses on strengthening the nursing workforce; inspiring, generating, and implementing new knowledge and innovation; advancing a culture of nursing excellence; developing transformational nurse leaders for the future; supporting a culture of continuous improvement; and humanizing care for patients, communities, and each other.

To begin the journey to transform fall prevention efforts and strengthen early mobility programs, leaders at Hackensack Meridian Health knew they needed to kickstart the necessary culture change. They created an interdisciplinary team with a shared vision, including nursing executives, nurse educators, nurse scientists, physicians, pharmacists, physical therapists, frontline nurses, policy experts, risk managers, and nurse information technology, among others. Historically, nurses had been responsible for completing fall risk assessments and for implementing fall prevention interventions such as nonskid socks, bed position, access to the call bell, and adequate lighting, but there was a growing realization that nurses cannot and should not be solely responsible for fall prevention (Porter et al., 2018). In addition, relying only on environmental modifications was not enabling nurses and other members of the care team to capture the entire picture and address the true root cause of the fall risk. The interdisciplinary team was charged with creating a new culture around fall prevention in which nurses would collaborate with the interprofessional care team via the EHR to create a comprehensive fall risk plan that places appropriate emphasis on both environmental and inherent risk factors to develop patient-centered interventions (Hendrich et al., 2020; Phelan et al., 2016).

A priority for the team was building the Hendrich II Fall Risk Model (HIIFRM) into the EHR. The core team, comprising an Epic analyst, nurse informaticist, fall prevention advisor, policy administrator, and frontline nurse, worked closely with the interdisciplinary team to understand their current workflow, with the goal of transforming their processes so that there is less redundancy, more support for interdisciplinary collaboration, and enhanced critical thinking (Chin-Yee & Upshur, 2020). Another overarching goal was to give valuable time back to nurses to focus on human interaction, which is vital to establish What Matters to the patient and family, and to create an individualized and meaningful fall prevention plan.

The HIIFRM automated build pulls data from discrete fields across the disciplines, such as diagnoses entered upon admission by the physician and gender data entered by registration. This data are then quantified using the HIIFRM and used to strengthen, not replace, clinical judgment. The build also includes an evidence-based care pathway for each fall risk factor and links to evidence-based tools, such as the Confusion Assessment Method (CAM), to assist the care team in diagnosing underlying conditions and developing care plans. Automating a manual tool allows the clinician to expertly collaborate with all members of the care team electronically. Additionally, in some instances, up-to-the-minute documentation updates in the EHR can reflect real-time risk status updates and allow for enhanced caregiver communication and patient safety, unlike a static door sign or armband. Figure 6.5 shows the logic within the EHR for the automated scoring of Risk Factor 1, Confusion, on the HIIFRM.

Figure 6.5. Automated Scoring of Confusion on the HIIFRM

CONFUSION

The system performs the below checks, in order, assigning the specified number of points based on the first check that evaluates to true.

1. If the patient has an active diagnosis (excludes resolved diagnoses) on the problem list that has an ICD-10-CM code matching one of the specific ICD-10-CM codes.
    *   R41.0
    *   F44.9

- R41.82
- R45.87
- F03.91
- G31.84
- F01.50
- R41.9
- F05

If the above is true, 4 points are assigned.

2. If the last filed value in the Level of Consciousness flowsheet row (single select) is more recent than the last filed value in the Neuro (WDL) flowsheet row where WDL was documented, check if the last filed value in the past 24 hours in the Level of Consciousness flowsheet row is Lethargic, Obtunded, Stuporous, Semi-Comatose, or Comatose. In the event that the last filed value in the Level of Consciousness flowsheet row and the last filed in the Neuro (WDL) flowsheet row where WDL was documented in the same time column, this check is performed.

If the above is true, 4 points are assigned.

3. If the last filed value in the Orientation Level flowsheet row (multi-select) is more recent than the last filed value in the Neuro (WDL) flowsheet row where WDL was documented, check if the last filed value in the past 24 hours in the Orientation Level flowsheet row contains a response of Disoriented X3. In the event that the last filed value in the Orientation Level flowsheet row and the last filed in the Neuro (WDL) flowsheet row where WDL was documented were documented in the same time column, this check is performed.

If the above is true, 4 points are assigned.

4. If the last filed value in the Cognition flowsheet row (multi-select) is more recent than the last filed value in the Neuro (WDL) flowsheet row where WDL was documented, check if the last filed value in the past 24 hours in the Cognition flowsheet row contains a response of Confusion, Impulsive, Poor judgement, Poor safety awareness, Poor attention/concentration, Short term memory loss, or Unable to follow commands. In the event that the last filed value in the Cognition flowsheet row and the last filed in the Neuro (WDL) flowsheet row where WDL was documented were documented in the same time column, this check is performed.

If the above is true, 4 points are assigned.

5. Check if the last filed value in the CAM Delirium Present/Absent flowsheet row in Present.

If the above is true, 4 points are assigned. Note: There is no check against WDL documentation and no lookback time frame, so this will continue to give the patient 4 points until Present is no longer the last filed value.

6. Check if the last filed value in the Overall CAM-ICU flowsheet row in Positive.

If the above is true, 4 points are assigned. Note: There is no check against WDL documentation and no lookback time frame, so this will continue to give the patient 4 points until Present is no longer the last filed value.

7. Check if the last filed value in the Mini Cog Score flowsheet row in Positive.

   If the above is true, 4 points are assigned. Note: *There is no check against WDL documentation and no lookback time frame, so this will continue to give the patient 4 points until Present is no longer the last filed value.*

Fall prevention does not occur in a silo and does not stop with the use of an evidence-based fall risk assessment. For example, success of the mobility program at Hackensack Meridian Health includes drawing a connection between the automated HIIFRM and evidence-based mobility assessments, together providing support for patients and clinicians to safely and quickly mobilize patients to mitigate risk. Nurses use the BMAT (Boynton et al., 2020) to determine the patient's mobility status and the assistive devices required to mobilize their patients, independent of a provider order or physical therapy evaluation. The BMAT provides the underpinnings of a successful nurse-led early mobility program and, when used with the automated HIIFRM, increases the confidence of the clinicians as they advocate for safe mobility to decrease injurious falls.

The COVID-19 pandemic slowed the momentum of the transformation efforts at Hackensack Meridian Health. However, this historic event also fueled the need for immediate action, as many healthcare organizations continue to see alarmingly high fall rates with devastating consequences and expect to see increased falls as a result of immobility for months to come (De La Cámara et al., 2020). Reengaging the care team in 2021—with this new and exciting innovation, an approach that produces tangible results they can truly be proud of—will allow the team to be reenergized and demonstrate their continued commitment to excellence and patient safety, following the extraordinarily difficult challenges created by the pandemic. Figure 6.6 shows the 2021 rollout plan.

Figure 6.6. Network RISE Meeting 2021 Hendrich Rollout Plan

Network R.I.S.E. Meeting
(Reduce falls, Injury prevention, Safety first, Early mobility)
2021 Hendrich Roll Out Plan

Topic	Date	Responsible Party
Complete Hendrich Epic Build		
Focus Groups/End User Testing—Playground Epic Environment		
Legal—Sign Working Agreement with A. Hendrich		
Develop Staff Education Plan • Learning Modules with Guided Tour • Assign Modules • Virtual Sessions • Branded Tips Sheets		
Test Automated Build—Side-by-Side Comparison (2 weeks)		
Learner Training—In-Person/Virtual Sessions • Network Safety Council • Network Quality and Safety • Network Nursing Quality and Safety • CNEs • Nurse Educators • Nurse Managers		
Research Proposal—IRB Application		
Create Reports with Business Intelligence and Epic Analyst		
Data Collection and Analysis		
Publish/Present		

The Need for Culture Change and Tips for Achieving It

The culture of "zero falls" is entrenched in many, if not most, healthcare organizations, and it will take effort and commitment to shift to a "safe mobility" culture. Incentives and accountabilities reinforce practices that keep patients from moving in order to keep them from falling: Risk managers look to reduce risk; leaders look for efficiency in delivering care; frontline nurses have been trained to rely on fall prevention measures, such as yellow fall risk armbands, call lights, nonskid slippers, and bed alarms, and may fear being blamed for a patient fall if they try to mobilize a patient. Do not underestimate the challenges organizations may face as they look to shift the culture.

Culture change starts with the creation of a sense of urgency (Schlesinger et al., 2014). To unite people in working together to achieve the desired future state, create and communicate a sense of urgency around the change effort. The urgency must be grounded in an understanding of the reason for the change and speak to the head and heart of those impacted by the change efforts. Ultimately, the organization needs to understand why change is no longer optional, and the need for change must exceed the resistance to it.

This chapter has already laid out the compelling reasons why a change to create a culture of safe mobility is urgent: Patients are harmed by immobility, with immediate deconditioning and negative downstream effects on their functional status and independence; the time and expertise of nurses can be put to better use by refocusing their efforts on the reduction of modifiable fall risk factors in collaboration with the interprofessional team rather than relying on a more mechanical fall prevention checklist approach that has limited effectiveness in actually preventing falls, let alone in helping patients sustain their mobility baseline. Resistance to change should be met with excitement about what can be achieved if the team pulls together to transform the way they do things.

As with any change effort, the shift to a culture of safe mobility will require leadership buy-in and champions committed to the change. One way to increase buy-in by leaders at all levels is to connect the effort with other strategic goals of the organization. For example, leaders will be committed to the effort if they see that safe mobility is intrinsically connected to patient safety and the quality and cost of care. The business case for safe mobility includes the avoidance of financial penalties and regulatory visits, improved patient satisfaction with growth in volume or covered lives, and the reduction of avoidable or needless readmissions in 30 days or less. As part of the change process, it is also important to get the right people at the table to serve as a "guiding coalition" (Schlesinger et al., 2014). This coalition can comprise both formal and informal leaders, front-line nurses and unlicensed assistive personnel, and other members of care teams involved in fall prevention.

Safe-mobility programs will require new learning for nurses and other members of the care team to have the skills and confidence to let go of familiar, non-value-added tasks. Adopting new practices may seem daunting at first but should ultimately result in better care. Leaders at all levels of the organization, including unit and department leaders, need to commit to replacing a punitive culture around patient falls with a "just culture," in which the organization recognizes that many safety events result from predictable interactions between human caregivers and the complex systems in which they work (Marx, 2001). A just culture values transparency in the reporting and examination of safety events so that processes can be improved.

If the organization creates a just culture, nurses and other members of the care team will feel empowered to report patient falls, work as a team to drill down to root causes, and unearth opportunities for improvement. The unit manager can use daily huddles to discuss any fall that occurred on the previous shift and guide the team to look at the patient's individual risk factors and the individualized interventions that have been / could be put in place to address that patient's risk factors. The discussion should extend beyond armbands and environmental precautions to consider the patient's evidence-based risk factors and the connection of these risk factors to the 4Ms. In alignment with the high-reliability principle of "preoccupation with failure," the discussion can also consider who might be the next patient to fall and what should be done to keep that patient safe. The unit manager is key to helping the team stay focused on the work, coaching and providing feedback, and being open to team input.

A shift in perspective that supports the creation of a culture of safe mobility is to recognize that an assisted fall is less likely to result in an injury and demonstrates that the team member was anticipating the needs of the patient (Venema et al., 2019). Falls are an expected risk of mobility, and an assisted fall may be more of a "good catch" than an error; it shows that the patient is being mobilized to prevent functional decline.

Engaging the patient in this work is key. An illuminating exercise for members of the care team is for them to ask patients if they know why they are wearing an armband, what the nonslip socks are for, or why they have a bed alarm. They may discover that patients do not really understand their fall risk and how they can work with the care team to mitigate that risk. The fall risk assessment that the nurse performs on admission provides an opportunity to engage the patient and family in understanding the identified fall risk factors and to plan together on how to prevent falls and practice safe mobility. Bedside handoff is also a good moment to engage the patient and family. The nurse handing off the patient reviews the fall risk factors and individualized interventions at the bedside with the receiving nurse and the patient. Patients, when possible, are encouraged to think through what they will do to keep safe and stay mobile at the hospital.

The shift from a "zero falls" culture to a "safe mobility" culture will require every tool in the change management toolbox, but the potential rewards—improved patient care, more engaged patients, more effective and efficient care teams—create a compelling case for change.

Additional Case Studies and Resources for Successful Mobility Programs

Providence St. Joseph Health, Oregon Region

Providence St. Joseph Health initiated a 4-week condensed curriculum known as the Geriatric Mini-Fellowship, which focuses on one of the 4Ms per week to equip community-based primary care providers (PCPs) with the competencies and skills to act on the 4Ms and deliver age-friendly geriatric care. Six PCPs across rural and urban settings are chosen to participate in the mini-fellowship each year. During the week for mobility training, they were first taught the epidemiology of falls, risk factors for falling, and fall risk assessments. They then applied their learnings in a simulated fall-risk clinic and analyzed fall risk efforts at their clinics to identify opportunities for improving workflows and screening rates. This experience has improved fall risk assessment and intervention among PCPs who had not been formally trained in geriatrics, thereby improving fall risk management practices for older patients. Trained fellows were 1.7 times more likely to screen for fall risk, 3.6 times more likely to discuss fall risk, and 5.8 times more likely to assess orthostatic blood pressure in older patients. Results were more significant among high-risk patients, such that PCPs were 4.1 times more likely to discuss fall risk and 6.3 times more likely to assess orthostatic blood pressure (Casey et al., 2020).

Anne Arundel Medical Center, Annapolis, Maryland

Anne Arundel Medical Center (AAMC) in Annapolis, Maryland, implemented an Acute Care for the Elderly (ACE) unit as part of the hospital's age-friendly initiative. Patients are encouraged to get out of bed and move at least three times per day, even if only a short distance. The ACE unit also launched "ACErcise," a group exercise program that encourages patients to do chair exercises and walk to and from their hospital rooms in groups, promoting socialization. During the COVID-19 pandemic, AAMC took the existing mobility initiatives a step further and formed the Prone and Mobility Team, which consists of a team of 36 physical therapists, physical therapy assistants, occupational therapists, and rehabilitation aides. This team mobilized patients while social distancing and also decreased social isolation by connecting patients virtually with family members, as that is what mattered to them. Clinicians continued to incorporate the other 4Ms into the care plan by paying increased attention to medications that negatively affected these older patients. Patient satisfaction throughout the COVID-19 pandemic was in the 92nd percentile, while HCAHPS was in the 82nd percentile (American Hospital Association, 2020).

St. Mary Mercy Livonia, Livonia, Michigan

St. Mary Mercy Livonia implemented Mobility Optimizes Virtually Everything (MOVE), in which each patient receives personalized mobility goals that they review with nurses and aides daily. The goal of MOVE is to have patients walk twice per day. Since staying mobile helps maintain muscle function and overall healing, it also reduces the risk of falls. After implementing MOVE at St. Mary Mercy, the patient fall rate in the two care units decreased from 2.7% to 0% from the last quarter of 2017 to the first quarter of 2018 (Grossfield, 2019).

Figure 6.7. Decision Tree to Mobilize a Patient

Decision Tree to Mobilize a Patient

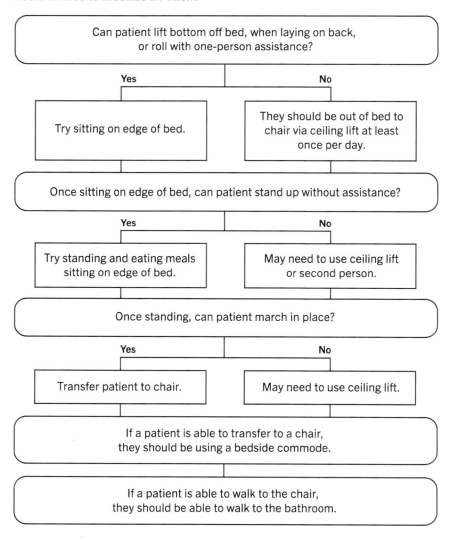

Figure 6.8. *Johns Hopkins Highest Level of Mobility Daily Goal (Johns Hopkins Medicine, 2017)*

View of goal setting row and pick choices:

Mobility Daily Goal (JH-HLM)

Select Single Option: (F5)

1 → Lie in bed
2 → Bed activity
3 → Sit at edge of bed
4 → Transfer to chair/commode
5 → Static standing (1 or more minutes)
6 → Walk 10 steps or more (ie. walked to restroom)
7 → Walk 25 feet or more (ie. walked outside of room)
8 → Walk 250 feet or more (ie. several laps on unit)

Comment (F6)

PCS flowsheet view:

Mobility

Johns Hopkins-Highest Level of Mobility

Mobility Daily Goal (JH-HLM) ← Set daily goal here!

Ambulation Distance (Feet)

Activity Level of Assistance

Assistive Device Utilized

Activity Intolerance Observed

Reason Patient Not Mobilized

Table 6.2. Mobility Measures (IHI, n.d.)

Percentage of care episodes in which patients who can ambulate had a multifactorial fall risk assessment at start/ resumption of care	*Numerator:* Count of care episodes in the denominator with a multifactorial fall risk assessment at start/resumption of care *Denominator:* Count of care episodes ending during the measurement period involving patients who can ambulate
Percentage of patients who were screened for future fall risk during the measurement period	*Numerator:* Count of patients in the denominator who were screened for future fall risk within the locally prescribed interval *Denominator:* Count of inpatient discharges or facility resident census in the measurement period
Percentage of patients with a history of falls who had a plan of care for falls documented within the past 12 months.	*Numerator:* Count of patients in the denominator with a documented plan of care for falls within the locally prescribed interval *Denominator:* Count of inpatient discharges or facility resident census in measurement period of patients with a history of falls (history of falls defined as two or more falls in the past year or any fall with injury in the past year)
Percentage of long-term episodes of care during which the patient improved inability to ambulate	*Numerator:* Number of care episodes in the denominator where the value recorded on the discharge assessment indicates less impairment in ambulation/locomotion at discharge than at start (or resumption) of care *Denominator:* Number of episodes of care in non-acute settings ending with a discharge during the reporting period

Recommendations and Summary

Though traditional fall prevention initiatives were well intentioned, the fear of increasing falls has resulted in a higher level of immobility in older adults. Immobility adversely affects mental and physical health outcomes, increasing length of stay, readmissions, institutionalization, and even death. Rather than focusing on fall prevention as an outcome, care settings should change their culture to emphasize safe mobility and interventions from the healthcare team to reduce modifiable risk factors when possible.

This culture change requires leader buy-in to adopt mobility as part of the larger operational and strategic plan (safety/risk, length of stay, reduced hospital-acquired complications, reimbursement penalties) and clinical champions from every unit. Nursing cannot be the sole owner of mobility and fall prevention. It will require education on modifiable risk factors and the complications caused by immobility for nursing staff, nonlicensed personnel, and other members of the interprofessional team if older adults are to be appropriately ambulated. Recognition programs that celebrate progress in the advancement of and compliance with mobility programs and "good fall catches" create a positive environment for the change we all wish to see.

Sensitivity to workflow and alarm fatigue is paramount while leveraging the EHR capabilities. Having frontline clinicians and teams determine how to adopt and integrate content into assessments and documentation is key. More work or new forms are often not needed; reducing redundancy and capturing preexisting record data into a new care model are. Improvement science tells us, "We improve what we measure." New progressive metrics should be readily available in the EHR for abstraction that will help to foster and measure culture and behavior changes. These measures might include

- comparing fall risk status on admission with the discharge day to detect worsening and/or improvements from the person's baseline;
- the number of referral follow-up appointments made before discharge for those with documented mentation changes or delirium occurrences;
- post-discharge deprescribing monitoring for those with medication changes as part of their transition in care; and
- planned ongoing and regular fall risk factor assessments by self or a primary care clinician to detect fall-risk status change related to risk factors as part of holistic clinic assessments.

The vision for a desired future state is one where every hospital uses an evidence-based fall risk tool that is integrated into the EHR, and the EHR, in turn, supports the creation of care plans by the inter-professional team to address modifiable fall risk factors identified by the tool. In this future state, every hospital has an early mobility pro-gram and team members are trained to implement safe-mobility pro-tocols. Ageism bias has been eliminated, with team members looking to a person's risk factors rather than their age or a history of fall-ing when developing a safe-mobility plan. Post-fall huddles balance safety and mobility as the team assesses a person's modifiable risk factors and how to support what matters most to the person. Upon admission, the person and their family are engaged as part of the care team, and transitions of care are planned with appropriate referrals that address the person's fall risk factors and improve mobility. On discharge, patients transition to primary care clinicians or other care facilities that have incorporated the 4Ms into their practice. This is what a transformation to a more person-centered, clinically relevant approach to fall prevention and safe mobility might look like and why it should be attractive to both frontline care teams and healthcare leaders.

References

Agency for Healthcare Research and Quality. (2019). *AHRQ national scorecard on hospital-acquired conditions: Updated baseline rates and preliminary results, 2014–2017.* https://www.ahrq.gov/sites/default/files/wysiwyg/professionals/quality-patient-safety/pfp/hacreport-2019.pdf

American Hospital Association. (2020). *The value initiative issue brief: Creating value with age-friendly health systems.* https://www.aha.org/system/files/media/file/2020/08/value-initiative-issue-brief-10-creating-value-with-age-friendly-health-systems.pdf

Barnes, D. E., Mehta, K. M., Boscardin, W. J., Fortinsky, R. H., Palmer, R. M., Kirby, K. A., & Landefeld, C. S. (2013). Prediction of recovery, dependence or death in elders who become disabled during hospitalization. *Journal of General Internal Medicine*, 28(2), 261–268. https://doi.org/10.1007/s11606-012-2226-y

Boyd, C. M., Landefeld, C. S., Counsell, S. R., Palmer, R. M., Fortinsky, R. H., Kresevic, D., Burant, C., & Covinsky, K. E. (2008). Recovery of activities of daily living in older adults after hospitalization for acute medical illness. *Journal of the American Geriatrics Society*, 56(12), 2171–2179. https://doi.org/10.1111/j.1532-5415.2008.02023.x

Boynton, T., Kumpar, D., & VanGilder, C. (2020). The Bedside Mobility Assessment Tool 2.0: Advancing patient mobility. *American Nurse Journal*, 15(7), 18–28. https://www.myamericannurse.com/wp-content/uploads/2020/07/an7-Mobility-618.pdf

Brown, C. J., Foley, K. T., Lowman, J. D., Jr., MacLennan, P. A., Razjouyan, J., Najafi, B., Locher, J., & Allman, R. M. (2016). Comparison of posthospitalization function and community mobility in hospital mobility program and usual care patients: A randomized clinical trial. *JAMA Internal Medicine*, 176(7), 921–927. https://doi.org/10.1001/jamainternmed.2016.1870

Brown, C. J., Friedkin, R. J., & Inouye, S. K. (2004). Prevalence and outcomes of low mobility in hospitalized older patients. *Journal of the American Geriatrics Society, 52*(8), 1263–1270. https://doi. org/10.1111/j.1532-5415.2004.52354.x

Casey, C. M., Caulley, J. M., Fox, A. F., & Hodges, M. O. (2020). Improving primary care fall risk management: Adoption of practice changes after a geriatric mini-fellowship. *Journal of Clinical Outcomes Management, 27*(6), 270–280. https://cdn.mdedge.com/files/s3fs-public/issues/ articles/jcom02706270.pdf

Chin-Yee, B., & Upshur, R. (2020). *The impact of artificial intelligence on clinical judgment: A briefing document.* https://www.ams-inc.on.ca/ wp-content/uploads/2020/02/The-Impact-of-AI-on-clinical-judgement. pdf

De La Cámara, M. Á., Jiménez-Fuente, A., & Pardos, A. I. (2020). Falls in older adults: The new pandemic in the post COVID-19 era? *Medical Hypotheses, 145*, 110321. https://doi.org/10.1016/j.mehy.2020.110321

Eckstrom, E., Parker, E. M., Lambert, G. H., Winkler, G., Dowler, D., & Casey, C. M. (2017). Implementing STEADI in academic primary care to address older adult fall risk. *Innovation in Aging, 1*(2), 1–9. https://doi.org/10.1093/ geroni/igx028

Escalon, M. X., Lichtenstein, A. H., Posner, E., Spielman, L., Delgado, A., & Kolakowsky-Hayner, S. A. (2020). The effects of early mobilization on patients requiring extended mechanical ventilation across multiple ICUs. *Critical Care Explorations, 2*(6), e0119. https://doi.org/10.1097/ CCE.0000000000000119

Fazio, S., Stocking, J., Kuhn, B., Doroy, A., Blackmon, E., Young, H. M., & Adams, J. Y. (2020). How much do hospitalized adults move? A systematic review and meta-analysis. *Applied Nursing Research, 51*, 151189. https://doi.org/10.1016/j.apnr.2019.151189

Florence, C. S., Bergen, G., Atherly, A., Burns, E., Stevens, J., & Drake, C. (2018). Medical costs of fatal and nonfatal falls in older adults. *Journal of the American Geriatrics Society, 66*(4), 693–698. https://doi.org/10.1111/ jgs.15304

Gill, T. M., Gahbauer, E. A., Murphy, T. E., Han, L., & Allore, H. G. (2012). Risk factors and precipitants of long-term disability in community mobility: A cohort study of older persons. *Annals of Internal Medicine, 156*(2), 131–140. https://doi.org/10.7326/0003-4819-156-2-201201170-00009

Greysen, S. R., Stijacic Cenzer, I., Auerbach, A. D., & Covinsky, K. E. (2015). Functional impairment and hospital readmission in Medicare seniors.

JAMA Internal Medicine, 175(4), 559–565. https://doi.org/10.1001/jamainternmed.2014.7756

Grossfield, E. (2019). *Staying mobile in the hospital helps to get better and get out.* Next Avenue. https://www.nextavenue.org/staying-mobile-in-hospital

Hendrich, A. L., Bender, P. S., & Nyhuis, A. (2003). Validation of the Hendrich II Fall Risk Model: A large concurrent case/control study of hospitalized patients. *Applied Nursing Research, 16*(1), 9–21. https://doi.org/10.1053/apnr.2003.016009

Hendrich, A. L., Bufalino, A., & Groves, C. (2020). Validation of the Hendrich II Fall Risk Model: The imperative to reduce modifiable risk factors. *Applied Nursing Research, 53,* 151243. https://doi.org/10.1016/j.apnr.2020.151243

Institute for Healthcare Improvement. (n.d.). *Mobility Measures* [Unpublished internal document].

Institute for Healthcare Improvement. (2020). *Age-friendly health systems: Guide to using the 4Ms in the care of older adults.* http://www.ihi.org/Engage/Initiatives/Age-Friendly-Health-Systems/Documents/IHIAgeFriendlyHealthSystems_GuidetoUsing4MsCare.pdf.

Jazayeri, D., Heng, H., & Slade, S. C., Seymour, B., Lui, R., Volpe, D., Jones, C., & Morris, M. E. (2021). Benefits and risks of non-slip socks in hospitals: A rapid review. *International Journal for Quality in Health Care, 33*(2), mzab057. https://doi.org/10.1093/intqhc/mzab057

Johns Hopkins Medicine. (2017). *Functional activity and mobility: Documentation for hospitalized adult.* https://www.johnshopkinssolutions.com/wp-content/uploads/2017/02/Functional-Activity-and-Mobility-Documentation-for-Hosp-Adult.pdf

Kortebein, P., Symons, T. B., Ferrando, A., Paddon-Jones, D., Ronsen, O., Protas, E., Conger, S., Lombeida, J., Wolfe, R., & Evans, W. J. (2008). Functional impact of 10 days of bed rest in healthy older adults. *The Journals of Gerontology. Series A: Biological Sciences and Medical Sciences, 63*(10), 1076–1081. https://doi.org/10.1093/gerona/63.10.1076

Marx, D. (2001). *Patient safety and the "just culture": A primer for health care executives.* Trustees of Columbia University in the City of New York. http://www.chpso.org/sites/main/files/file-attachments/marx_primer.pdf

Moreland, B., Kakara, R., & Henry, A. (2020). Trends in nonfatal falls and fall-related injuries among adults aged ≥65 years—United States,

2012–2018. *Morbidity and Mortality Weekly Report*, 69(27), 875–881. http://dx.doi.org/10.15585/mmwr.mm6927a5

Moskowitz, G., Egorova, N. N., Hazan, A., Freeman, R., Reich, D. L., & Leipzig, R. M. (2020). Using electronic health records to enhance predictions of fall risk in inpatient settings. *Joint Commission Journal on Quality and Patient Safety*, 46(4), 199–206. https://doi.org/10.1016/j.jcjq.2020.01.009

Phelan, E. A., Aerts, S., Dowler, D., Eckstrom, E., & Casey, C. M. (2016). Adoption of evidence-based fall prevention practices in primary care for older adults with a history of falls. *Frontiers in Public Health*, 4, 190. https://doi.org/10.3389/fpubh.2016.00190

Poe, S. S., Cvach, M. M., Gartrell, D. G., Radzik, B. R., & Joy, T. L. (2005). An evidence-based approach to fall risk assessment, prevention, and management: Lessons learned. *Journal of Nursing Care Quality*, 20(2), 107–116. https://doi.org/10.1097/00001786-200504000-00004

Poe, S. S., Dawson, P. B., Cvach, M., Burnett, M., Kumble, S., Lewis, M., Thompson, C. B., & Hill, E. E. (2018). The Johns Hopkins Fall Risk Assessment Tool: A study of reliability and validity. *Journal of Nursing Care Quality*, 33(1), 10–19. https://doi.org/10.1097/ncq.0000000000000301

Porter, R. B., Cullen, L., Farrington, M., Matthews, G., & Tucker, S. (2018). CE: Original research: Exploring clinicians' perceptions about sustaining an evidence-based fall prevention program. *American Journal of Nursing*, 118(5), 24–33. https://doi.org/10.1097/01.NAJ.0000532806.35972.29

Schlesinger, P., Sathe, V., Schlesinger, L., & Kotter, J. (2014). *Accelerate: Building strategic agility for a faster-moving world*. Harvard Business Review Press.

Shorr, R. I., Chandler, A. M., Mion, L. C., Waters, T. M., Liu, M., Daniels, M. J., Kessler, L. A., & Miller, S. T. (2012). Effects of an intervention to increase bed alarm use to prevent falls in hospitalized patients: A cluster randomized trial. *Annals of Internal Medicine*, 157(10), 692–699. https://doi.org/10.7326/0003-4819-157-10-201211200-00005

Shorr, R. I., Staggs, V. S., Waters, T. M., Daniels, M. J., Liu, M., Dunton, N., & Mion, L. C. (2019). Impact of the hospital-acquired conditions initiative on falls and physical restraints: A longitudinal study. *Journal of Hospital Medicine*, 14, E31–E36. https://doi.org/10.12788/jhm.3295

Smart, D. A., Dermody, G., Coronado, M. E., & Wilson, M. (2018). Mobility programs for the hospitalized older adult: A scoping review. *Gerontology & Geriatric Medicine*, 4, 1–18. https://doi.org/10.1177/2333721418808146

Venema, D. M., Skinner, A. M., Nailon, R., Conley, D., High, R., & Jones, K. J. (2019). Patient and system factors associated with unassisted and injurious falls in hospitals: An observational study. *BMC Geriatrics*, 19(1), 348. https://doi.org/10.1186/s12877-019-1368-8

Wald, H. L., Ramaswamy, R., Perskin, M. H., Roberts, L., Bogaisky, M., Suen, W., & Mikhailovich, A. (2019). The case for mobility assessment in hospitalized older adults: American geriatrics society white paper executive summary. *Journal of the American Geriatrics Society*, 67(1), 11–16. https://doi.org/10.1111/jgs.15595

Weick, K. E., & Sutcliffe, K. M. (2015). *Managing the unexpected: Sustained performance in a complex world.* John Wiley & Son.

CHAPTER 7

4Ms Care

Adapted from IHI's Age-Friendly Health Systems: Guide
to Using the 4Ms in the Care of Older Adults

The 4Ms are a powerful set that reinforce and interact together to ensure the best evidence is being used to provide age-friendly care. This chapter will describe an approach to getting underway with generating a strong workflow that will reduce the cognitive burden of trying to recall each element of geriatric care management while producing the same improved outcomes.

Getting Started: Putting the 4Ms Into Practice

A "recipe" for integrating the 4Ms into your standard care has steps and ingredients, just like a recipe to make a salad, main dish, or dessert. These steps include:

1. Understand your current state.
2. Design care consistent with the 4Ms.
3. Describe or adapt your workflow.

4. Provide care.
5. Study your performance.
6. Improve and sustain care.

Step 1: Understand Your Current State

The aim of an Age-Friendly Health System is to reliably apply the two key drivers of age-friendly care: assess and act on the 4Ms with all older adults. Almost all systems integrate some of the 4Ms into care, some of the time, with some older adults, in some place in their system. With an understanding of your current experience and capacity to engage in 4Ms care, you can build on that good work until the 4Ms are reliably practiced with all older adults.

The following steps help you prepare for your journey to becoming an Age-Friendly Health System by understanding your current state—knowing the older adults and the 4Ms in your health system currently—and then selecting a care setting and establishing a team to begin testing.

Know the Older Adults in Your Health System

In order to understand the care required in your health system, you have to know your denominator. What proportion of your patients are over 65? 75? 85? Estimate the number of adult patients you served in each age group in the last month (see Table 7.1).

Table 7.1. Adult Patients Served in the Last Month (by Age Group)

AGE GROUP	NUMBER	% OF TOTAL PATIENTS
18–64 years		
65–74 years		
75–84 years		
85+ years		
Total # of adult patients		100

4Ms CARE • 147

It is also essential that the care you are providing is culturally sensitive and ensures health equity. For adult patients aged 65 and older in your care, outlining their language, race/ethnicity, and religious and cultural preferences (see Table 7.2) and health literacy levels (see Table 7.3) is an important step to determine what matters and how to respect patient goals and preferences.

Table 7.2. *Language, Race/Ethnicity, and Religious and Cultural Preferences of Patients 65 Years and Older*

LANGUAGE	% OF TOTAL PATIENTS AGED 65+

RACE/ETHNICITY	% OF TOTAL PATIENTS AGED 65+

RELIGIOUS AND CULTURAL PREFERENCES	% OF TOTAL PATIENTS AGED 65+

Table 7.3. *Health Literacy Levels of Patients 65 Years and Older*

HEALTH LITERACY LEVEL	% OF TOTAL PATIENTS AGED 65+
Low	
Moderate	
High	

Know the 4Ms in Your Health System/Setting

To identify where the 4Ms are in practice in your health system, walk through activities as if you were an older adult or family caregiver. In an ambulatory setting, that may include making an appointment for an Annual Wellness Visit, preparing to come to an Annual Wellness Visit, observing an appointment, and understanding who on the care team takes responsibility for each of the 4Ms. In an inpatient setting, go through registration, spend time on a unit, and sit quietly in the hall of a unit. Look for the 4Ms in action. You will find aspects that make you proud and others that leave you disappointed. Try not to be judgmental. Find bright spots, opportunities, and champions of each of the 4Ms in your system. Use the form provided in Appendix E to note what you learn.

Select a Care Setting to Begin Testing

Once you know about your older adults and identify where the 4Ms currently exist in your health system, select a care setting in which to begin testing age-friendly interventions. Some questions to consider when selecting a site:

- Is there a setting that regularly cares for a larger number of older adults?
- Is there a desire to become age-friendly and improve care for older adults? Is there a champion?
- Is this setting relatively stable (i.e., not undergoing major changes already)?
- Does this setting have access to data? (See the Study Your Performance section below for more on measurement. Data is useful, though not required.)
- Can this setting be a model for the rest of the organization? (Modeling is not necessary but useful to scale-up efforts.)
- Is there a setting where your team members have experience with the 4Ms, either individually or in combination? Do

they already have some processes, tools, and/or resources to support the 4Ms?

- Is there a setting where the health literacy levels, language skills, and cultural preferences of your patients match the assets of the staff and the resources provided by your health system?

Set Up a Team

Based on experience, teams that include the roles and/or functions outlined in Table 7.4 are most likely to succeed.

Table 7.4. Team Member Roles

TEAM MEMBER	DESCRIPTION
An older adult and caregiver	Patients and families bring critical expertise to any improvement team. They have a different experience with the system than providers and can identify key issues. It is highly recommended that each team has at least one older adult patient or family member or other caregiver (ideally more than one) or a way to elicit feedback directly from patients (e.g., through a Patient and Family Advisory Council).
	Additional information about appropriately engaging patients and families in improvement efforts can be found on the Institute for Patient- and Family-Centered Care website.
Leader/sponsor	This person champions, authorizes, and supports team activities, as well as engaging senior leaders and other groups within the organization to remove barriers and support implementation and scale-up efforts. Although they may not do the "on-the-ground" work, the leader/sponsor is responsible for
	• building a case for change that is based on strategic priorities and the calculated return on investment;
	• encouraging the improvement team to set goals at an appropriate level;
	• providing the team with needed resources, including staff time and operating funds;
	• ensuring that improvement capability and other technical resources, especially those related to information technology (IT) and electronic health records (EHR), are available to the team; and
	• developing a plan to scale up successful changes from the improvement team to the rest of the organization.

Administrative partner	This person represents the disciplines involved in the 4Ms and works effectively with the clinicians, other technical experts, and leaders within the organization. It is recommended to place the manager of the unit where changes are being tested in this role so that individual can move nimbly to take necessary action and make the recommended changes in that unit and so that individual is invested in sustaining changes that result in improvement.
Clinicians who represent the disciplines involved in the 4Ms	These individuals may include a physician, nurse, physical therapist, social worker, pharmacist, chaplain, and/or others who represent the 4Ms in your context. Interprofessional representation on your team is critical; enlist more than one clinical champion. These champions have good working relationships with colleagues and are interested in driving change to achieve an Age-Friendly Health System. Consider professionals who are opinion leaders in the organization, who are sought by others for advice, and who are not afraid to test and implement change.
Others	• Improvement coach • Data analyst / EHR analyst • Finance representative

Step 2: Describe Care Consistent With the 4Ms

Using the worksheet provided in Appendix F, describe what it means to provide care consistent with the 4Ms. This worksheet allows you to integrate geriatric best practice interventions to assess, document, and act on the 4Ms together, while customizing your approach for your context. To be considered an Age-Friendly Health System, your system must explicitly describe how it will engage or assess people aged 65 and older for all 4Ms, document 4Ms information, and act on the 4Ms accordingly.

Questions to Consider

- How does your current state compare to the actions outlined in the 4Ms Care Description Worksheet?
- Which of the 4Ms do you already incorporate? How reliably are they practiced?

- For example: Do you already ask and document What Matters, review for high-risk medication use, screen for delirium, dementia, and depression, and screen for mobility for each older adult?
- Where are there gaps in 4Ms? What ideas do you have to fill the gaps?

In this step, describe the initial version of 4Ms care for the older adults you serve.

Set an Aim

Given your current state, set an aim for this initial effort. An aim articulates what you are trying to accomplish—what, how much, by when, and for whom. It serves as the focus for your team's work and enables you to measure your progress. Below is an aim statement template that requires you to think about the reach of 4Ms in the next 6 months.

AIM STATEMENT TEMPLATE

By [Date], [Name of Organization] will articulate how it operationalizes 4Ms care and will have provided that 4Ms care to [Number] patients 65 years or older.

Step 3: Design or Adapt Your Workflow

There are many ways to improve care for older adults. However, there is a finite set of key actions, summarized below, that touch on all 4Ms and dramatically improve care when implemented together (see Table 7.5). This list of actions is considered the gateway to your journey to becoming an Age-Friendly Health System. In Appendix G, you will find a list of these key actions and ways to get started with each one in your setting, as well as additional tips and resources. Be sure to plan how you will document and make visible the 4Ms across the care team and settings.

You may have many ideas in place already. You can continue, improve, and expand them where necessary. You may still need to test and implement other ideas. The key is to ensure these practices are reliable, happening every time in every setting for every older adult and their caregivers you serve.

Table 7.5. *Age-Friendly Health Systems Summary of Key Actions*

	ASSESS	ACT ON
	Know about the 4Ms for each older adult in your care	Incorporate the 4Ms into the plan of care
Hospital		
Key actions (to occur at least daily)	• Ask the older adult What Matters • Document What Matters • Review for high-risk medication use • Screen for delirium at least every 12 hours • Screen for mobility limitations	• Align the care plan with What Matters • Deprescribe or do not prescribe high-risk medications • Ensure sufficient oral hydration • Orient older adults to time, place, and situation • Ensure older adults have their personal adaptive equipment • Prevent sleep interruptions; use nonpharmacological interventions to support sleep • Ensure early, frequent, and safe mobility
Ambulatory		
Key actions (to occur at least annually or on change in condition)	• Ask the older adult What Matters • Document What Matters • Review for high-risk medication use • Screen for dementia • Screen for depression • Screen for mobility limitations	• Align the care plan with What Matters • Deprescribe or do not prescribe high-risk medications • Manage behaviors related to dementia; consider further evaluation and/or referrals • Identify and manage factors contributing to depression • Ensure safe mobility

Nursing Home		
Key actions (to occur regularly or on change in condition)	• Ask the older adult What Matters • Document What Matters • Review for high-risk medication use, polypharmacy, adverse drug events • Screen for delirium at least every 12 hours in a skilled nursing facility (SNF); every 24 hours and as needed in long-term care • Screen for dementia • Screen for depression • Screen for mobility	• Align the care plan with What Matters • Deprescribe or do not prescribe high-risk medications, and optimize all other medications • Ensure sufficient oral hydration • Orient older adults to time, place, and situation if/when appropriate • Ensure that older adults have their personal adaptive equipment • Prevent sleep interruptions; use nonpharmacological interventions to support sleep • Manage behaviors related to dementia; consider further evaluation and/or referrals • Identify and manage factors contributing to depression; consider further evaluation and/or referrals • Promote early, frequent, and safe mobility

Supporting Actions

- Use the 4Ms to organize care and focus on the older adult, wellness, and their strengths rather than solely on disease or on lack of functionality.
- Integrate the 4Ms into care or existing workflows.
- Identify what activities you can stop doing to reallocate resources for the 4Ms and when the 4Ms are reliably in practice.
- Document all 4Ms and consider grouping the 4Ms together in the medical record.
- Make the 4Ms visible across the care team and settings.

- Have an interdisciplinary care team that reviews the 4Ms in daily huddles and/or rounds.
- Educate older adults, caregivers, and the community about the 4Ms.
- Link the 4Ms to community resources and supports to achieve improved health outcomes.

Overall, look for opportunities to combine or redesign activities, processes, and workflows around the 4Ms. In this effort, you may find you can stop certain activities and reallocate resources to support age-friendly care.

If you have process-flow diagrams or value-stream maps of your daily care, edit these views of your workflow to include the key actions above and your description of age-friendly care.

You may start with a high-level workflow like the examples shown below (see Figures 7.1 and 7.2).

Then work through the details in the space below each high-level block to show how you will incorporate the 4Ms. Be specific about who will do what, where, when, and how, and how it will be documented. Examples are included in Appendix H. Outline what you still need to learn, and identify what you will test (e.g., using the Timed Up & Go [TUG] Test to evaluate mobility and fall risk).

Step 4: Provide Care

Learn as you move toward reliable 4Ms care. Begin to test the key actions with one older adult and their family caregivers as soon as you have notes for Step 2: Describe Care Consistent With the 4Ms, and Step 3: Design or Adapt Your Workflow. Do not wait to have your forms or EHR screens finalized before you test with one older adult. Use the Plan-Do-Study-Act (PDSA) tool to learn more from your tests. Then scale up your tests. For example:

Figure 7.1. *Age-Friendly Care Workflow Example for Hospitals: Core Functions*

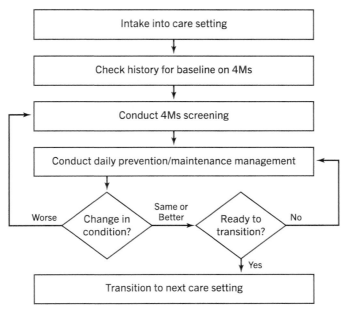

Figure 7.2. *Age-Friendly Care Workflow Example for Primary Care:*
Core Functions for New Patient, Annual Visit, or Change in Health Status

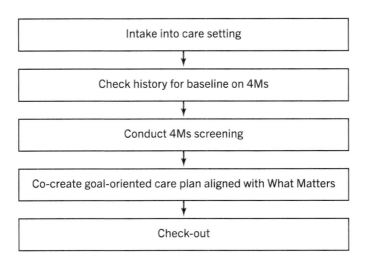

1.   Apply your draft standard procedure and workflow first with one patient. Can your team follow the procedure in your work environment?

2.   If necessary, modify your procedure. Then apply it with five patients. What lessons do you learn from applying 4Ms care with these patients? What impact does learning about all 4Ms have on care plans?

3.   If necessary, modify your procedure. Then apply with 25 patients and keep going. Are you getting close to being able to use your procedure for every patient? Are you getting good results?

Examples of PDSA cycles can be found in Appendix K.

Step 5: Study Your Performance

How reliable is your 4Ms care? What impact does your 4Ms care have? Here are the basic ingredients to study your performance.

Observe and Seek to Understand

Start your study with direct observation of your draft 4Ms care description in action.

- Can your team follow the description and successfully assess and act on the 4Ms with the older adults in your care?
- Do care plans reflect 4Ms care?

In the first month, do this for at least one patient each week. Then, for the next 6 months, observe 4Ms care for at least five patients each month.

Ask Your Team

At least once per month for the 7 months of your efforts, ask your team two open-ended questions and reflect on the answers:

- What are we doing well to assess and act on the 4Ms?
- What do we need to change to translate the 4Ms into more effective care?

Plan with your team how and when you will continue to reflect together using open-ended questions on an ongoing basis.

Ask Your Older Adults and Caregivers

At least once in the first month of your effort, ask an older adult and family caregiver two open-ended questions and reflect on the answers:

- What went well in your care today?
- What could we do better to understand what age-friendly care means to you?

Then try the questions with five additional older adults in the second month. Plan with your team how and when you will continue to talk with older adults, using open-ended questions on an ongoing basis.

Measure How Many Patients Receive 4Ms Care

There are three options to start measuring the number of patients receiving 4Ms care. Option 1 is recommended because it forces close attention to the 4Ms work and takes less effort than conducting retrospective chart audits or building a specific EHR report.

OPTION 1: REAL-TIME OBSERVATION

Use real-time observation and staff reporting of the work to tally your 4Ms counts on a whiteboard or paper. An example for patients seen in a primary care clinic might look like the chart below (see Figure 7.3).

Figure 7.3. *Example of Real-Time Observation in a Primary Care Clinic*

DATE	4MS CARE ACCORDING TO OUR SITE DESCRIPTION					
	All 4Ms	What Matters	Medications	Depression	Dementia	Mobility
Pt ID	*If N, check details*					
101	Y N	Y N	Y N	Y N	Y N	Y N
102	Y N	Y N	Y N	Y N	Y N	Y N
103	Y N	Y N	Y N	Y N	Y N	Y N
104	Y N	Y N	Y N	Y N	Y N	Y N
105	Y N	Y N	Y N	Y N	Y N	Y N
106	Y N	Y N	Y N	Y N	Y N	Y N
107	Y N	Y N	Y N	Y N	Y N	Y N
108	Y N	Y N	Y N	Y N	Y N	Y N
109	Y N	Y N	Y N	Y N	Y N	Y N
110	Y N	Y N	Y N	Y N	Y N	Y N
111	Y N	Y N	Y N	Y N	Y N	Y N
112	Y N	Y N	Y N	Y N	Y N	Y N
113	Y N	Y N	Y N	Y N	Y N	Y N
114	Y N	Y N	Y N	Y N	Y N	Y N
115	Y N	Y N	Y N	Y N	Y N	Y N

OPTION 2: CHART REVIEW

Use a tally sheet like the example discussed in Option 1 and review charts for evidence of 4Ms care. At the start of your work using the 4Ms, review charts of patients with whom you have tested 4Ms care (M) to confirm proper documentation. To estimate the number of patients receiving 4Ms care in a particular time period (e.g., monthly), randomly sample 20 charts from patients who received care during that time (out of M). Observe out of the 20 how many received your described care (C). Calculate the approximate number of patients receiving 4Ms care in the time period as follows in Figure 7.4.

Figure 7.4. *Volume Formula*

$$\text{Estimated \# of patients receiving 4Ms care} = \frac{M \times C}{20}$$

If a total count is not possible, you can sample (e.g., audit 20 patient charts) and estimate the total as the number of patients receiving 4Ms care / 20 × total number of patients cared for in the measurement period.

So, the formula would be:

[(# of patients receiving 4Ms care, C) / (# of patient charts
   audited, S)] × total number of patients cared for in
   measurement period, M or

(C/S) × M where

C = the number of patients receiving 4Ms care during sampled period

S = number of charts sampled

M = total number of patients cared for during the measurement
   period

OPTION 3: EHR REPORT

You may be able to run EHR reports, especially on assessment of the 4Ms, to estimate the number of patients receiving 4Ms care in a particular time period. It may take a lot of effort to create a suitable report, so we do not recommend this option as your first choice. However, for ongoing process control, some organizations may wish to develop reports that show 4Ms performance; you can request report development by your IT service while starting with Option 1 or 2.

Routine Counting of Patients

Once your site provides 4Ms care with high reliability (see Appendix I), the estimated number of patients receiving 4Ms care is simple: report the volume of patients receiving care from your site during the measurement period. See Appendix J for additional guidance in counting the number of patients receiving age-friendly care.

Step 6: Improve and Sustain Care

While we present the six steps as a sequence, in practice you can approach steps 2 through 6 as a loop aligned with Plan-Do-Study-Act cycles (see Figure 7.5).

For more information about how to sustain your 4Ms care, please see the IHI White Paper *Sustaining Improvement* (Scoville et al., 2016).

4Ms Cycle Integration

While we present the steps as a sequence, in practice steps 2 through 6 are a cycle aligned with the Plan-Do-Study-Act method. As you establish your age-friendly care, you may cycle through steps 2 through 6 many times over the course of several months in order to achieve a level of reliability and then turn your efforts to sustainability and monitoring (quality control) over time.

Figure 7.5. Integrating the 4Ms Into Care Using the PDSA Cycle

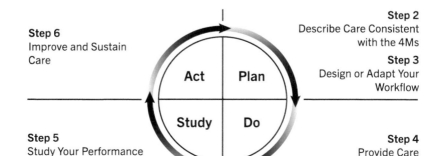

Figure 7.6. *Two Key Drivers of Age-Friendly Health Systems*

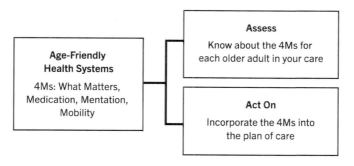

Hospital Approach

Table 7.6. *Assess: Know About the 4Ms for Each Older Adult in Your Care*

KEY CHANGES	GETTING STARTED
Ask the older adult What Matters most	This change focuses on clinical encounters, decision-making, and care planning for persons with complex care needs on What Matters most to them.
	If you do not have existing questions to start this conversation, try the following, and adapt as needed: "What do you most want to focus on while you are in the hospital/emergency department for [fill in health problem] so that you can do [fill in desired activity] more often or more easily?" (Naik et al., 2018; Patient Priorities Care, 2018; Tinetti et al., 2016).
	For older adults with advanced or serious illness, consider, "What are your most important goals if your health situation worsens?" (Ariadne Labs, 2017).
Document What Matters	Documentation can be on paper, on a whiteboard, or in the electronic health record (EHR) where it is accessible to the whole care team across settings (Sokol-Hessner et al., 2015).
Review high-risk medication use	Specifically, look for • benzodiazepines • opioids • highly anticholinergic medications, especially diphenhydramine • all prescription and over-the-counter sedatives and sleep medications • muscle relaxants • tricyclic antidepressants • antipsychotics (American Geriatrics Society, 2019; Hill-Taylor et al., 2013; Maher et al., 2014)

Screen for delirium at least every 12 hours	If you do not have an existing tool, try using the Ultra-Brief 2-Item Screener (UB-2; Fick et al., 2015; Fick et al., 2018).
Screen for mobility	If you do not have an existing tool, try using the Timed Up & Go (TUG) Test (Centers for Disease Control and Prevention & National Center for Injury Prevention and Control, 2017; Shah, 2017).

Table 7.7. Act On: Incorporate the 4Ms Into the Plan of Care

KEY CHANGES	GETTING STARTED
Align the care plan with What Matters most	Capture What Matters and the healthcare agent/proxy in the goal-oriented plan of care and align the care plan with the older adult's goals and preferences* (i.e., What Matters; Blaum et al., 2018; Patient Priorities Care, 2018; Tinetti et al., 2019).
Deprescribe or do not prescribe high-risk medications	Specifically avoid or deprescribe the medications listed below, which may interfere with What Matters and the Mentation and safe Mobility of older adults. These medications, individually and in combination, increase risk of confusion, delirium, unsteadiness, and falls (O'Mahony et al., 2015). • benzodiazepines • opioids • highly-anticholinergic medications, especially diphenhydramine • all prescription and over-the-counter sedatives and sleep medications • muscle relaxants • tricyclic antidepressants • antipsychotics (American Geriatrics Society, 2019; Lumish et al., 2018; Mattinson et al., 2010; Reuben et al., 2017) If the older adult is on one or more of these medications, discuss any concerns the patient may have, assess for adverse effects, and discuss deprescribing with the older adult (Deprescribing.org, 2021).
Ensure sufficient oral hydration	Identify a target amount of oral hydration appropriate for the older adult and monitor that it is met. Ensure water and other patient-preferred non-caffeinated fluids are available at the bedside and accessible to the older adult.
Orient older adults to time, place, and situation	For older adults with dementia, consider gentle reorientation or use of orienting cues; avoid repeated testing about the orientation if the older adult appears agitated (Marcantonio, 2017).

Ensure older adults have their personal sensory adaptive equipment	This includes equipment such as glasses, hearing aids, and dentures.
Prevent sleep interruptions; use nonpharmacological interventions to support sleep	• Avoid nighttime blood draws and vital signs when possible. • Use sleep kits (Hshieh, 2015; McDowell et al., 1998).
Ensure early and safe mobility**	Assess and manage impairments that reduce mobility (e.g., pain; impairments in strength, balance, or gait; avoid high-risk medications; catheters, IV lines, telemetry, and other tethers as soon as possible), including referral to physical therapy. Set and meet a daily mobility goal with each older adult.
Additional resources	• *"What Matters" to Older Adults? A Toolkit for Health Systems to Design Better Care With Older Adults* • Patient Priorities Care • *Serious Illness Conversation Guide* • Deprescribing.org • Hospital Elder Life Program (HELP)

*Health outcome goals are the activities that matter most to an individual, such as babysitting a grandchild, walking with friends in the morning, or continuing to work as a teacher. Healthcare preferences include the medications, healthcare visits, testing, and self-management tasks that an individual is able and willing to do.

**These activities are also key to preventing delirium and falls (Hospital Elder Life Program [HELP] for Prevention of Delirium, n.d.).

Ambulatory/Primary Care

Table 7.8. *Assess: Know About the 4Ms for Each Older Adult in Your Care*

KEY CHANGES	GETTING STARTED
Ask the older adult What Matters most	This change focuses clinical encounters, decision-making, and care planning for persons with complex care needs on What Matters most to them. If you do not have existing questions to start this conversation, try the following, and adapt as needed. "What is the one thing about your health or healthcare that you most want to focus on [fill in health problem OR the healthcare task] so that you can do [fill in desired activity] more often or more easily?" (Naik et al., 2018; Patient Priorities Care, 2018; Tinetti et al., 2016). For older adults with advanced or serious illness, consider, "What are your most important goals if your health situation worsens?" (Ariadne Labs, 2017).

Document What Matters	Documentation can be on paper, on a whiteboard, or in the electronic health record (EHR) where it is accessible to the whole care team across settings (Sokol-Hessner et al., 2015).
Review high-risk medication use	Specifically, look for these: • benzodiazepines • opioids • highly anticholinergic medications, especially diphenhydramine • all prescription and over-the-counter sedatives and sleep medications • muscle relaxants • tricyclic antidepressants • antipsychotics (American Geriatrics Society, 2019; Hill-Taylor et al., 2013; Maher et al., 2014)
Screen for delirium	If you do not have an existing tool, try using the Mini-Cog (Borson, 2021).
Screen for depression	If you do not have an existing tool, try using the Patient Health Questionnaire-2 (PHQ-2; Pfizer, 2021).
Screen for mobility	If you do not have an existing tool, try using the Timed Up & Go (TUG) Test (Centers for Disease Control and Prevention & National Center for Injury Prevention and Control, 2017; Shah, 2017).

Table 7.9. *Act On: Incorporate the 4Ms Into the Plan of Care*

KEY CHANGES	GETTING STARTED
Align the care plan with What Matters most	Capture What Matters and the healthcare agent/proxy in the goal-oriented plan of care and align the care plan with the older adult's goals and preferences* (i.e., What Matters; Blaum et al., 2018; Patient Priorities Care, 2018; Tinetti et al., 2019).
Deprescribe or do not prescribe high-risk medications	Specifically avoid or deprescribe the medications listed below, which may interfere with What Matters and the Mentation and safe Mobility of older adults. These medications, individually and in combination, increase risk of confusion, delirium, unsteadiness, and falls (O'Mahony et al., 2015). • benzodiazepines • opioids • highly anticholinergic medications, especially diphenhydramine • all prescription and over-the-counter sedatives and sleep medications • muscle relaxants • tricyclic antidepressants • antipsychotics (American Geriatrics Society, 2019; Lumish et al., 2018; Mattinson et al., 2010; Reuben et al., 2017) If the older adult is on one or more of these medications, discuss any concerns the patient may have, assess for adverse effects, and discuss deprescribing with the older adult (Deprescribing.org, 2021).

Consider further evaluation and manage manifestations of dementia, or refer to geriatrics, psychiatry, or neurology	Assess for modifiable contributors to cognitive impairment.

Consider further diagnostic evaluation if appropriate.

Follow current guidelines for treatment of dementia and resulting behavioral manifestations OR refer to geriatrics, psychiatry, or neurology for management of dementia-related issues.

Refer the older adult, family, and other caregivers to supportive resources, such as the Alzheimer's Association (Alzheimer's Association, 2021). |
| Identify and manage factors contributing to depression | Identify and manage factors that contribute to depressive symptoms:
<ul><li>sensory limitations (vision, hearing)</li><li>social isolation</li><li>bereavement</li><li>medications</li></ul>
Consider the need for counseling or pharmacological treatment of depression, or refer to a mental health provider if appropriate. |
| Ensure safe mobility | Assess and manage impairments that reduce mobility (e.g., pain; impairments in strength, balance, or gait; avoid high-risk medications; remove catheters, IV lines, telemetry, and other tethers as soon as possible), including referral to physical therapy.

Support older adults and other caregivers to create a home environment that is safe for mobility (Centers for Disease Control and Prevention & National Center for Injury Prevention and Control, 2017).

Support older adults to identify a daily mobility goal that supports What Matters.

Review and support progress toward the mobility goal. |
| Additional resources | • *"What Matters" to Older Adults? A Toolkit for Health Systems to Design Better Care With Older Adults*
• Patient Priorities Care
• *Serious Illness Conversation Guide*
• Deprescribing.org |

*Health outcome goals are the activities that matter most to an individual, such as babysitting a grandchild, walking with friends in the morning, or continuing to work as a teacher. Healthcare preferences include the medications, healthcare visits, testing, and self-management tasks that an individual is able and willing to do.

Recommendations and Summary

The initiation of any new approach to care is daunting, especially when it requires culture change related to the care of older adults. Incorporating their goals and preferences, as well as the advice of their family members, has been found to result in more efficient and effective care. The Age-Friendly Health Systems initiative is demonstrating the value of the 4Ms approach and the receptivity noted by older adults and their families when they feel they are truly being heard and can partner with care providers around the 4Ms.

References

Alzheimer's Association. (2021). https://alz.org/

American Geriatrics Society. (2019). *2019 AGS Beers Criteria pocketcard.* https://geriatricscareonline.org/ProductAbstract/2019-ags-beers-criteria-pocketcard/PC007

Ariadne Labs. (2017). *Serious illness conversation guide.* https://www.ariadnelabs.org/resources/downloads/serious-illness-conversation-guide/

Blaum, C. S., Rosen, J., Naik, A. D., Smith, C. D., Dindo, L., Vo, L., Hernandez-Bigos, K., Esterson, J., Geda, M., Ferris, R., Costello, D., Acampora, D., Meehan, T., & Tinetti, M. E. (2018). Feasibility of implementing patient priorities care for older adults with multiple chronic conditions. *Journal of the American Geriatrics Society, 66*(10), 2009–2016. https://doi.org/10.1111/jgs.15465

Borson, S. (2021). *Standardized Mini-Cog instrument.* https://mini-cog.com/mini-cog-instrument/standardized-mini-cog-instrument/

Centers for Disease Control and Prevention & National Center for Injury Prevention and Control. (2017). *Assessment: Timed Up & Go (TUG).* https://www.cdc.gov/steadi/pdf/TUG_Test-print.pdf

Deprescribing.org. (2021). *Deprescribing guidelines and algorithms.* https://deprescribing.org/resources/deprescribing-guidelines-algorithms

Fick, D. M., Inouye, S. K., Guess J., Ngo, L. H., Jones, R. N., Saczynski, J. S., & Marcantonio, E. R. (2015). Preliminary development of an ultrabrief two-item bedside test for delirium. *Journal of Hospital Medicine*, 10(10), 645–650. https://doi.org/10.1002/jhm.2418

Fick, D. M., Inouye, S. K., McDermott, C., Zhou, W., Ngo, L., Gallagher, J., McDowell, J., Penrod, J., Siuta, J., Covaleski, T., & Marcantonio, E. R. (2018). Pilot study of a two-step delirium detection protocol administered by certified nursing assistants, physicians, and registered nurses. *Journal of Gerontological Nursing*, 44(5), 18–24. https://doi.org/10.3928/00989134-20180302-01

Hill-Taylor, B., Sketris, I., Hayden, J., Byrne, S., O'Sullivan, D., & Christie, R. (2013). Application of the STOPP/START criteria: A systematic review of the prevalence of potentially inappropriate prescribing in older adults, and evidence of clinical, humanistic and economic impact. *Journal of Clinical Pharmacy and Therapeutics*, 38(5), 360–372. https://doi.org/10.1111/jcpt.12059

Hospital Elder Life Program (HELP) for Prevention of Delirium. (n.d.). https://www.hospitalelderlifeprogram.org

Hshieh, T. T., Yue, J., Oh, E., Puelle, M., Dowal, S., Travison, T., & Inouye, S. K. (2015). Effectiveness of multicomponent nonpharmacological delirium interventions: A meta-analysis. *JAMA Internal Medicine*, 175(4), 512–520. https://doi.org/10.1001/jamainternmed.2014.7779

Lumish, R., Goga, J. K., & Brandt, N. J. (2018). Optimizing pain management through opioid deprescribing. *Journal of Gerontological Nursing*, 44(1), 9–14. https://doi.org/10.3928/00989134-20171213-04

Maher, R. L., Hanlon, J., & Hajjar, E. R. (2014). Clinical consequences of polypharmacy in elderly. *Expert Opinion Drug Safety*, 13(1), 57–65. https://doi.org/10.1517/14740338.2013.827660

Marcantonio, E. R. (2017). Delirium in hospitalized older adults. *New England Journal of Medicine*, 377(15), 1456–1466. https://doi.org/10.1056/NEJMcp1605501

Mattison, M. L., Afonso, K. A., Ngo, L. H., & Mukamal, K. J. (2010). Preventing potentially inappropriate medication use in hospitalized older patients with a computerized provider order entry warning system. *Archives of Internal Medicine*, 170(15), 1331–1336. https://doi.org/10.1001/archinternmed.2010.244

McDowell, J. A., Mion, L. C., Lydon, T. J., & Inouye, S. K. (1998). A nonpharmacologic sleep protocol for hospitalized older patients.

Journal of the American Geriatrics Society, 46(6), 700–705. https://doi. org/10.1111/j.1532-5415.1998.tb03803.x

Naik, A. D., Dindo, L. N., Van Liew, J. R., Hundt, N. E., Vo, L., Hernandez-Bigos, K., Esterson, J., Geda, M., Rosen, J., Blaum, C. S., & Tinetti, M. E. (2018). Development of a clinically feasible process for identifying individual health priorities. *Journal of the American Geriatrics Society, 66*(10), 1872–1879. https://doi.org/10.1111/jgs.15437

O'Mahony, D., O'Sullivan, D., Byrne, S., O'Connor, M. N., Ryan, C., & Gallagher, P. (2015). STOPP/START criteria for potentially inappropriate prescribing in older people: Version 2. *Age and Ageing, 44*(2), 213–218. https://doi.org/10.1093/ageing/afu145

Patient Priorities Care. (2018). *Condensed conversation guide for identifying patient priorities (specific ask).* https://patientprioritiescare.org/wp-content/uploads/2018/11/Condensed-Conversation-Guide-for-Identifying-Patient-Priorities-28Specific-Ask29-in-the-Ambulatory-Setting.pdf

Pfizer. (2021). *Welcome to the Patient Health Questionnaire (PHQ) screeners.* http://www.phqscreeners.com/

Reuben, D. B., Gazarian, P., Alexander, N., Araujo, K., Baker, D., Bean, J. F., Boult, C., Charpentier, P., Duncan, P., Latham, N., Leipzig, R. M., Quintiliani, L. M., Storer, T., & McMahon, S. (2017). The strategies to reduce injuries and develop confidence in elders intervention: Falls risk factor assessment and management, patient engagement, and nurse co-management. *Journal of the American Geriatrics Society, 65*(12), 2733–2739. https://doi.org/10.1111/jgs.15121

Scoville, R., Little, K., Rakover, J., Luther, K., & Mate, K. (2016). *Sustaining Improvement* [White paper]. Institute for Healthcare Improvement. http://www.ihi.org/resources/Pages/IHIWhitePapers/Sustaining-Improvement.aspx

Shah, N. (2017). *The case against hospital beds.* Politico. https://www.politico.com/agenda/story/2017/11/08/the-case-against-hospital-beds-000575/

Sokol-Hessner, L., Zambeaux, A., Little, K., Macy, L., Lally, K. M., & McCutcheon Adams, K. (2015). *"Conversation ready": A framework for improving end-of-life care* [White paper]. Institute for Healthcare Improvement.

Sokol-Hessner, L., Zambeaux, A., Little, K., Macy, L., Lally, K. M., & McCutcheon Adams, K. (2019). *"Conversation ready": A framework for improving end-of-life care* [White paper, 2nd ed.]. Institute for Healthcare Improvement. http://www.ihi.org/resources/Pages/IHIWhitePapers/ConversationReadyEndofLifeCare.aspx

Tinetti, M., Dindo, L., Smith, C. D., Blaum, C., Costello, D., Ouellet, G., Rosen, J., Hernandez-Bigos, K., Geda, M., & Naik, A. (2019). Challenges and strategies in patients' health priorities-aligned decision-making for older adults with multiple chronic conditions. *PloS One*, 14(6), e0218249. https://doi.org/10.1371/journal.pone.0218249

Tinetti, M. E., Esterson, J., Ferris, R., Posner, P., & Blaum, C. S. (2016). Patient priority-directed decision making and care for older adults with multiple chronic conditions. *Clinics in Geriatric Medicine*, 32(2), 261–275. https://doi.org/10.1016/j.cger.2016.01.012

CHAPTER 8

4Ms Measures

A ge-Friendly Health Systems: Guide to Using the 4Ms in the Care of Older Adults describes a reliable approach for integrating the 4Ms (What **M**atters, **M**edication, **M**entation, **M**obility) into your standard care. Health systems that make the commitment to adopt this approach engage in a series of steps to ensure success. These steps include:

1. Understand your current state.
2. Describe care consistent with the 4Ms.
3. Design or adapt your workflow.
4. Provide care.
5. Study your performance.
6. Improve and sustain care.

The measures outlined in this measurement approach will help you with Step 5: Study Your Performance.

Data for Improvement

Below you will find a set of outcome and process measures with operational definitions. You can use these measures to understand whether the changes you are making result in improvement.

Test and study results from a small number of conversations with older adults, or family or other caregivers for adults unable to speak for themselves. Gathering this qualitative data will complement the core set of numerical measures.

Overview of Measures

Measures for skilled nursing facilities are in formation as of April 2021.

Table 8.1. Measures Overview

	HOSPITAL SITE OF CARE	AMBULATORY/PRIMARY CARE SITE OF CARE
4Ms measure		
Older adults receiving age-friendly (4Ms) care	X	X
Basic outcome measures		
30-day all-cause readmission rate	X	
Rate of emergency department (ED) visits		X
Consumer Assessment of Healthcare Providers and Systems (CAHPS)—select survey questions	HCAHPS	CG-CAHPS
Average length of stay	X	
Advanced outcome measures		
Older adults with diagnosis of delirium	X	
Survey of care concordance with What Matters (collaboRATE or similar tool adopted by your system to measure goal-concordant care)	X	X

Stratifying Data by Race and Ethnicity to Understand and Address Inequities

The persistence of important differences in treatment and health outcomes associated with race, ethnicity, and other social factors is significant. Health equity requires that health systems stratify key performance measures by these factors to reveal inequities and spur action to eliminate them. For Age-Friendly Health Systems, it is strongly encouraged that you stratify outcome measures for older adults, using the Office of Management and Budget core race and ethnicity factors to identify inequities in patient care and experience.

These definitions are helpful for teams when beginning the work of looking at data through an equity lens.

- **Health equity**: Everyone has a fair and just opportunity to be healthier, which requires removing obstacles to health such as poverty and discrimination, and their consequences, including powerlessness and the lack of access to good jobs with fair pay, as well as the lack of quality education and housing, safe environments, and healthcare (Braverman et al., 2017).

- **Health inequity**: Differences in health outcomes between groups within a population that are systemic, avoidable, and unjust (Wyatt et al., 2016).

Measures for Process Improvement

Teams working to provide 4Ms care to every older adult in their care typically track aspects of 4Ms care as they test changes to workflow in order to monitor if the changes are resulting in improvement. Appendix L specifies a set of process measures that teams have found useful to monitor the impact of tests and to guide management action.

4Ms Measures

HOSPITAL SITE OF CARE

Table 8.2. *Hospital Site of Care*

Measure name	Older adults receiving age-friendly (4Ms) care
Measure description	Number of patient interactions for individuals 65 years and older who receive age-friendly (4Ms) care as described by the hospital
Site	Hospital unit, hospital, or set of hospitals
Population measured	Patients 65 years and older
Measurement period	Monthly
Count	*Inclusion*: All patients 65 years and older with length of stay (LOS) greater than or equal to 1 day who are present on the unit between 12:01 a.m. on the first day of the measurement period and 11:59 p.m. on the last day of the measurement period who receive the unit's description of 4Ms care
Measure notes	The measure may be applied to units within a system as well as the entire system.
	See *Age-Friendly Health Systems: Guide to Using the 4Ms in the Care of Older Adults*, specifically the 4Ms Care Description Worksheet in Appendix F, to describe 4Ms care for your unit. To be considered age-friendly (4Ms) care, you must engage or screen all patients 65 years and older for all 4Ms, document the results, and act on them as appropriate.
	If a total count is not possible, you can sample (e.g., audit 20 patient charts) and estimate the total as the number of patients receiving 4Ms care / 20 × total number of patients cared for in the measurement period. If you are sampling, please note that when sharing data.
	Once you have established 4Ms care as the standard of care on your unit, validated by regular observation and process review, you can estimate the number of patients receiving 4Ms care as the number of patients cared for by the unit.
	You do not need to filter the number of patients by unique medical record number (MRN).

AMBULATORY/PRIMARY CARE SITE OF CARE

Table 8.3. *Ambulatory/Primary Care Site of Care*

Measure name	Older adults receiving age-friendly (4Ms) care
Measure description	Number of patient interactions for individuals 65 years and older who receive age-friendly (4Ms) care as described by the measuring unit
Site	Ambulatory/primary care
Population measured	Patients 65 years and older
Measurement period	Monthly
Count	*Inclusion*: All patients 65 years and older in the population considered to be patients of the ambulatory or primary care practice (e.g., patient assigned to a care team panel and seen by the practice within the past three years) who have an office visit, home visit, or telemedicine visit with the practice during the measurement period and who receive 4Ms care as defined by the site
Measure notes	The measure may be applied to units within a system as well as the entire system.
	See *Age-Friendly Health Systems: Guide to Using the 4Ms in the Care of Older Adults*, specifically the 4Ms Age-Friendly Care Description Worksheet, to describe 4Ms care for your unit. To be considered age-friendly (4Ms) care, you must engage or screen all patients 65 years and older for all 4Ms, document the results, and act on them as appropriate.
	Note that 4Ms care screening in primary care may be defined as screening within the previous 12 months.
	If a total count is not possible, you can sample (e.g., audit 20 patient charts) and estimate the total as the number of patients receiving 4Ms care / 20 × total number of patients cared for in the measurement period. If you are sampling, please note that when sharing data.
	Once you have established 4Ms care as the standard of care on your unit, validated by regular observation and process review, you can estimate the number of patients receiving 4Ms care as the number of patients cared for by the unit.
	You do not need to filter the number of patients by unique medical record number (MRN).

Hospital Outcome Measures

BASIC OUTCOME MEASURES

Table 8.4. Basic Hospital Outcome Measures

Measure name	30-day all-cause readmission rate
Measure description	Percentage of patients 65 years and older who are readmitted to hospital within 30 days following discharge
Site	Hospital unit, hospital, or set of hospitals
Population measured	Patients 65 years and older
Measurement period	Choose monthly or quarterly (monthly measurement can reveal signals of change faster than quarterly measurement; however, monthly measurement may yield low numbers of readmitted patients and make it difficult to interpret the measurement time series)
Denominator	*Inclusion*: Patient discharged from a specific set of care units in the measurement period *Exclusions*: None
Numerator	*Inclusion*: Number of patients in the denominator who are readmitted to a *specific set of hospitals* within 30 days of discharge for any reason *Exclusions*: None
Data source	Administrative and health records

Method details	Lower is better.
	
	The "specific set of hospitals" is key to calculation of the rate.
	
	• Here is an example definition from a hospital system with two large hospitals (A and B) and three small satellite hospitals:
	  • *Count the number of patients who had an inpatient stay in either hospital A or B and were readmitted to any of the five hospitals in our system within 30 days for any reason.*
	  • For this system, the specific set of hospitals consists of the two large hospitals and the three small hospitals.
	  • If a system has a data-sharing arrangement with hospitals not in its system, then the defined set of hospitals can be larger than the number of hospitals in the system.
	
	The readmission measure need not be identical across units of care. The intention is that each hospital or system will be able to monitor the impact of changes over time, not to create rankings or league tables across systems.

4Ms MEASURES • 177

Method details *(continued)*	Recent literature raises the issue that focus on 30-day readmissions, especially for conditions covered by the Centers for Medicare & Medicaid Services (CMS) Hospital Readmissions Reduction Program (HRRP), may cause an increase in mortality (Braverman et al., 2017).
	• "Among Medicare beneficiaries, the HRRP was significantly associated with an increase in 30-day post-discharge mortality after hospitalization for heart failure (HF) and pneumonia, but not for acute myocardial infarction (AMI). Given the study design and the lack of significant association of the HRRP with mortality within 45 days of admission, further research is needed to understand whether the increase in 30-day post-discharge mortality is a result of the policy" (Wadhera et al., 2018).

Table 8.5. HCAHPS Overall Experience Measures at Hospital Site

Measure name	Hospital Consumer Assessment of Healthcare Providers and Systems (HCAHPS) overall experience
Measure description	Top-box percentages for two HCAHPS questions for patients 65 years and older: (a) rating of hospital (0-10) and (b) recommendation to friends and family
Site	Hospital unit, hospital, or set of hospitals
Population measured	Patients 65 years and older
Measurement period	Quarterly
Denominator	Patients responding to HCAHPS survey
Numerator	Patients responding "top-box" to specified questions
Data source	HCAHPS data
Method details	"Top-box" is explained here: https://www.hcahpsonline.org/en/summary-analyses/-analyses/
	Stratification of responses by age is the only difference between the standard HCAHPS measures and the proposed measures.
	• Rather than using the entire set of responses to calculate patient experience, responses will need to be put into age strata and then calculated.
	• Stratification may lead to smaller numbers than recommended for detailed analysis.

| Method details *(contined)* | • Obtain 12 months of survey responses stratified by age group to determine median number of responses. If the median monthly number of responses is 10 or more per month in each stratum, run charts of the HCAHPS scores are likely to be informative. If median monthly numbers are less than 10 per month per stratum, pool the monthly numbers into quarterly values. |
| | While any of the individual questions or composite scores (e.g., physician communication) may be tracked, we propose focus on the two questions related to overall experience and willingness to recommend. |

Table 8.6. Average Length of Stay Measures at Hospital Site

Measure name	Average length of stay
Measure description	Average length of stay for patients 65 years and older
Site	Hospital unit, hospital, or set of hospitals
Population measured	Patients 65 years and older discharged from the hospital site during the measurement period, where age is determined at date of admission
Measurement period	Monthly
Denominator	*Inclusion*: Patients who are discharged from the hospital site during the measurement period or who die in hospital site during the measurement period
	Exclusions: None
Numerator	*Inclusion*: Sum of length of stay for each patient in the denominator, calculated as (a) date of discharge – date of admission + 1 for patients who are discharged, or (b) date of death – date of admission + 1 for patients who die during the measurement period
	Exclusions: None
Measure notes	The measure outlined here is a raw measure. There are no proposed exclusions or adjustments for risk.
	If the hospital uses a length-of-stay measure as part of its regular reporting, calculated by a different formula, the hospital should continue to use that definition applied to patients 65 years and older.
	We encourage hospitals to review the distribution of length of stay records to understand impact of care and changes to care on the patients with relatively long stays.

Advanced Outcome Measures

Table 8.7. *Advanced Hospital Outcome Measures*

Measure name	Older adults with diagnosis of delirium
Measure description	Percentage of patients 65 years and older with positive result on delirium assessment
Site	Hospital unit, hospital, or set of hospitals
Population measured	Patients 65 years and older
Measurement period	Monthly
Denominator	Inclusion: Patients with length of stay greater than or equal to 1 day who are present on each unit used in calculation of the measure between 12:01 a.m. on the first day of the measurement period and 11:59 p.m. on the last day of the measurement period Exclusions: None
Numerator	Inclusion: Patients with positive result on delirium assessment Exclusions: None
Data source	Health records
Method details	Lower is better. Useful delirium rate data presupposes agreement on protocols for delirium screening, diagnosis, and documentation, linked to design and application of appropriate workflows in all nursing units. • This measurement "pre-work" should be matched with protocols for delirium prevention and response, with appropriate workflows. • For a case example, see the work of Allen et al. on the "Implementation of a System-Wide Quality Improvement Project to Prevent Delirium in Hospitalized Patients" (as cited in Wyatt et al., 2016). An alternative to the use of health records to identify patients with delirium is to use claims data, querying ICD-10 codes in series F05, F13 (.121, .221, .231, .921, .931), and F19 (.121, .221, .231, .921, .931). Claims data typically will lag clinical treatment and actions; hence, claims-based measurement may be less useful for improvement work. Please note that initial experience with claims data indicates that it will underestimate delirium incidence relative to health records in sites that use screening tools reliably, with positive screens followed by clinical determination.

Method details (continued)	For units with small numbers of patients, consider these alternatives to the rate measure, which require counting of patient days: number of patient days with delirium per 1,000 patient days or number of patient days between cases of delirium.
	As your system improves consistency of documentation of delirium, delirium rate is likely to increase at least in the short term. Communicate this likelihood to your team and managers.

Table 8.8. Survey of Care Concordance Measures at Hospital Site

Measure name	Survey of care concordance with What Matters
Measure description	Percentage collaboRATE top-box score for patients 65 years and older
Site	Hospital unit, hospital, or set of hospitals
Population measured	Patients 65 years and older
Measurement period	Choose weekly or monthly (weekly measurement will support faster testing/learning cycles but has consequently higher measurement burden and may not be feasible)
Denominator	Number of completed surveys returned from patients
	Inclusion: Patients with length of stay greater than or equal to 1 day present on the unit between 12:01 a.m. on the first day of the measurement period and 11:59 p.m. on the last day of the measurement period
	Exclusions: None
Numerator	*Inclusion*: Count of surveys with top-box answers to all three questions ("all or nothing" score)
	Exclusions: None
Method details	For patients cognitively unable to respond to the questions, use the proxy version of collaboRATE.
	PDF versions of the collaboRATE scale are available at http://www.glynelwyn.com/collaborate-measure.html. We recommend the 10-point-scale version, available in multiple languages and in proxy form.
	Measure development notes suggest (a) a minimum of 25 completed surveys to compute a top-box percentage and (b) the importance of respondent confidentiality: http://www.glynelwyn.com/scoring-collaboRATE.html.
	To support informed analysis and interpretation, units should track the total number of patients approached to obtain the number of completed surveys.

Method details *(continued)*	To address survey burden for staff and patients, there are two options for sampling: Ask every kth patient such that $N / (m \times k) \geq 25$ for the measurement period OR gather responses from $25 \times m$ consecutive patients during the measurement period (a "pulse" approach). Here N is the expected number of patients in the population in the measurement period, and m is a factor that accounts for refusal to respond to the survey. Typical ranges of m are 2.5 to 4 (G. Elwyn, personal communication, May 30, 2018).
	Paper/manual data tools will work for initial testing but are not likely to scale. Organizations will need to develop information technology to allow patients to respond to the questions and to summarize the measurement with low effort.

Ambulatory/Primary Care Outcome Measures
Basic Outcome Measures

Table 8.9: Basic Ambulatory/Primary Care Outcome Measures

Measure name	Rate of emergency department (ED) visits
Measure description	Emergency department visits per 1,000 for patients 65 years and older
Site	Primary care
Population measured	Patients 65 years and older
Measurement period	Monthly
Denominator	*Inclusion*: All patients in the population considered to be patients of the primary care practice (e.g., patient assigned to a care team panel and seen by the practice within the past three years)
	Exclusions: None
Numerator	*Inclusion*: Number of ED visits by patients in the denominator in the measurement month
	Exclusions: None
Data source	Health records
Method details	Lower is better.
	The calculation of the denominator depends on the definition of association of patients to the practice (e.g., patient assigned to a care team panel and seen by the practice within the past three years).

Method details *(continued)*	The calculation of the numerator depends on the sharing of medical record information between the primary care practice and a specific set of EDs. Integrated health systems typically will have fewer obstacles in calculating the numerator for patients seen in EDs within their system. Independent primary care practices often will have information on their patients from "nearby" EDs, defined by custom.

	• As this measure is proposed to be calculated from health records rather than claims data, we expect that a small number of ED visits may be missed in a month (e.g., visits by patients who are traveling far from home and have a visit to an ED that does not share information with the primary care practice). However, we expect the small number of missed visits to be relatively constant month-to-month, with consequently modest impact on usefulness of the measure as an indicator of ED utilization by older patients.
	• Example calculation: The proposed measurement period is monthly. Calculate the denominator, calculate the numerator, and normalize the rate.
	   • In August 2018, 2,000 patients considered to be patients of the primary care clinic were aged 65 years and older. For those 2,000 patients, there were 110 ED visits. So calculate:
	   • $(110/2{,}000) \times 1{,}000 = 55$ ED visits per 1,000 patients aged 65 years and older

Table 8.10. CG-CAHPS Measures at Ambulatory/Primary Care Site

Measure name	Consumer Assessment of Healthcare Providers and Systems—Clinical and Group Survey (CG-CAHPS) rating of communication (composite)
Measure description	Top-box percentage for CG-CAHPS communication questions composite for patients 65 years and older
Site	Primary care
Population measured	*Patients in two age strata*: 65–74, 75 years and older (corresponding to structure of the standard age stratification question included in CG-CAHPS core questions)
Measurement period	Monthly
Denominator	4
Numerator	Top-box percentage for each of the component questions in the communications composite

Data source	CG-CAHPS data
Method details	The questions in the communication composite are numbered 11, 12, 14, and 15 in the basic CG-CAHPS version 3.0: https://www.ahrq.gov/sites/default/files/wysiwyg/cahps/surveys-guidance/cg/survey3.0/adult-eng-cg30-2351a.pdf. • In the last 6 months, how often did this provider explain things in a way that was easy to understand? • In the last 6 months, how often did this provider listen carefully to you? • In the last 6 months, how often did this provider show respect for what you had to say? • In the last 6 months, how often did this provider spend enough time with you? Calculation of "top-box" for composite scores is explained here as a simple average of individual question top-box scores: https://cahpsdatabase.ahrq.gov/cahpsidb/Public/Files/Doc6_CG_How_Results_are_Calculated_2012.pdf Stratification of responses by age is the only difference between the standard CG-CAHPS measures and the proposed measures. • Rather than using the entire set of responses to calculate patient experience, responses will need to be put into age strata and then calculated. • Stratification may lead to smaller numbers than recommended for detailed analysis. • Obtain 12 months of survey responses stratified by age group to determine median number of responses. If the median monthly number of responses is 10 or more per month in each stratum, run charts of the CG-CAHPS scores are likely to be informative. If median monthly numbers are less than 10 per month per stratum, pool the monthly numbers into quarterly values. Measure is to be aggregated over all providers in the ambulatory or primary care practice. Paper/manual data tools will work for initial testing but are not likely to scale. Organizations will need to develop information technology to allow patients to respond to the questions and to summarize the measurement with low effort.

Advanced Outcome Measure

Table 8.11. Advanced Ambulatory/Primary Care Outcome Measures

Measure name	Survey of care concordance with What Matters
Measure description	Percentage collaboRATE top-box score for patients 65 years and older
Site	Primary care
Population measured	Patients 65 years and older
Measurement period	Choose weekly or monthly (weekly measurement will support faster testing/learning cycles but has consequently higher measurement burden and may not be feasible)
Denominator	Number of completed surveys returned from patients
	Inclusion: Patients in the population seen for any reason by the primary care unit during the measurement period
	Exclusions: None
Numerator	*Inclusion*: Count of surveys with top-box answers to all three questions ("all or nothing" score)
	Exclusions: None
Method details	For patients cognitively unable to respond to the questions, use the proxy version of collaboRATE.
	PDF versions of the collaboRATE scale are available at http://www.glynelwyn.com/collaborate-measure.html. We recommend the 10-point-scale version, available in multiple languages and in proxy form.
	Measure development notes suggest (a) a minimum of 25 completed surveys to compute a top-box percentage and (b) the importance of respondent confidentiality: http://www.glynelwyn.com/scoring-collaboRATE.html.
	To support informed analysis and interpretation, units should track the total number of patients approached to obtain the number of completed surveys.
	To address survey burden for staff and patients, there are two options for sampling: Ask every kth patient such that $N / (m \times k) \geq 25$ for the measurement period OR gather responses from $25 \times m$ consecutive patients during the measurement period (a "pulse" approach). Here N is the expected number of patients in the population in the measurement period, and m is a factor that accounts for refusal to respond to the survey. Typical ranges of m are 2.5 to 4 (G. Elwyn, personal communication, May 30, 2018).

4Ms MEASURES • 185

Method details *(continued)*	Paper/manual data tools will work for initial testing but are not likely to scale. Organizations will need to develop information technology to allow patients to respond to the questions and to summarize the measurement with low effort.

Overview of Process Measures

Table 8.12. Process Measures Overview

PROCESS MEASURE	HOSPITAL SITE OF CARE	AMBULATORY/PRIMARY CARE SITE OF CARE
What Matters documentation	X	X
Older adults on targeted medications	X	X
Delirium screening	X	
Dementia screening		X
Depression screening		X
Mobility screening	X	X

Hospital Process Measures

Table 8.13. Hospital Process Measures

Measure name	What Matters documentation
Measure description	Percentage of patients 65 years and older with documentation of What Matters
Site	Hospital unit, hospital, or set of hospitals
Population measured	Patients 65 years and older
Measurement period	Choose weekly or monthly (weekly measurement will support faster testing/learning cycles but has consequently higher measurement burden and may not be feasible)
Denominator	*Inclusion*: Patients with length of stay greater than or equal to 1 day who are present on the unit between 12:01 a.m. on the first day of the measurement period and 11:59 p.m. on the last day of the measurement period *Exclusions*: None
Numerator	*Inclusion*: Patients in the denominator with documentation of What Matters per the unit's definition of What Matters *Exclusions*: None
Data source	Health records

Method details	For patients unable to speak for themselves, your What Matters engagement should include interaction with an appropriate healthcare agent to understand What Matters.
	
	• Note about patients who decline to engage in discussion of What Matters in a specific encounter.
	  • Our recommendation: Your procedure should allow for patients to decline to discuss What Matters. A patient who declines to answer "counts" in the numerator.
	  • You will have to judge whether the percentage of patients who decline to answer is acceptable. If too high, then you have a target for study and improvement.
	
	Asking What Matters is defined by the unit for the patients it serves. At minimum, asking What Matters involves (a) querying the medical record for existing documentation of What Matters and care wishes, and (b) engaging the patient or healthcare agent in discussion of What Matters as defined by the unit.

Method details (continued)	Documentation standard is defined by the unit for the patients it serves; the standard describes documentation content and method of recording content.
	If an automated report is possible, calculate the denominator and numerator.
	If a complete manual tally is possible, calculate the denominator and numerator.
	If neither an automated report nor a complete tally is possible, sample records at the end of the measurement period and calculate the denominator and numerator. You can apply a stopping rule to further reduce measurement burden.
	What Matters documentation focuses on What Matters to the older adult; it is not intended to be a specific measure of advance care planning (such as NQF 0326).

Table 8.14. *Targeted Medications Measures at Hospital Site*

Measure name	**Older adults on targeted medications (Allen et al., 2011)**
Measure description	Percentage of patients 65 years and older with active use of one or more medications on target list
Site	Hospital unit, hospital, or set of hospitals
Population measured	Patients 65 years and older
Measurement period	Monthly
Denominator	*Inclusion*: Patients with length of stay greater than or equal to 1 day who are present on the unit between 12:01 a.m. on the first day of the measurement period and 11:59 p.m. on the last day of the measurement period
	Exclusions: None
Numerator	*Inclusion*: Patients in the denominator with active use of one or more medications on target list
	Exclusions: None
Data source	Health records / pharmacy administration records

Method details	This measure is still under development. We anticipate further testing to refine the measure.
	The target list of medications combines the medications named in measures developed by Pharmacy Quality Alliance (PQA, www.pqaalliance.org), specifically Polypharmacy: Use of Multiple Anticholinergic Medications in Older Adults (POLY-ACH) and Concurrent Use of Opioids and Benzodiazepines (COB). Tables are used with permission of PQA with the understanding that this initiative measure does not represent a current measure endorsed by PQA.
	• Over-the-counter (OTC) drugs, sleep aids, and sedatives can also be problematic. If any OTC medications have ingredients on the target list, then use of these OTC medications will trigger inclusion of a patient in the numerator.
	• There are clinically appropriate uses for medications on the target list, individually and in combination. The medication measure is intended to help you characterize the extent of medication use.
	• To more closely align with PQA measures, we considered splitting this single medication measure into two measures, one focused on anticholinergic medications and the other on concurrent use of opioids and benzodiazepines. Based on current expert discussion and recommendations, we opted for a single measure.
	Active use is defined by medications administered to the patient between admission and discharge (as defined by the pharmacy administration records).

Table 8.15. *Delirium Screening Measures at Hospital Site*

Measure name	Delirium screening
Measure description	Percentage of patients 65 years and older screened for delirium
Site	Hospital unit, hospital, or set of hospitals
Population measured	Patients 65 years and older
Measurement period	Choose weekly or monthly (weekly measurement will support faster testing/learning cycles but has consequently higher measurement burden and may not be feasible)

Denominator	*Inclusion*: Patients with length of stay greater than or equal to 1 day who are present on the unit between 12:01 a.m. on the first day of the measurement period and 11:59 p.m. on the last day of the measurement period
	Exclusions: None
Numerator	*Inclusion*: Patients in the denominator screened for delirium according to the standard procedure established on the unit
	Exclusions: None
Data source	Health records
Method details	Standard procedure should include a screen for delirium at least every 12 hours using an instrument such as the Ultra-Brief 2-Item Screener (UB-2) and documentation in the medical record.
	Note that the screening protocol complements delirium prevention and management protocols that include, for example, medications, mobility, oral hydration, orientation, and nonpharmacological sleep support.

Table 8.16. Mobility Screening at Hospital Site

Measure name	Mobility screening
Measure description	Percentage of patients 65 years and older screened for mobility
Site	Hospital unit, hospital, or set of hospitals
Population measured	Patients 65 years and older
Measurement period	Choose weekly or monthly (weekly measurement will support faster testing/learning cycles but has consequently higher measurement burden and may not be feasible)
Denominator	*Inclusion*: Patients with length of stay greater than or equal to 1 day who are present on the unit between 12:01 a.m. on the first day of the measurement period and 11:59 p.m. on the last day of the measurement period
	Exclusions: None
Numerator	*Inclusion*: Patients in the denominator screened for mobility according to the standard procedure established on the unit
	Exclusions: None
Data source	Health records

Method details	The standard procedure should include, at a minimum:
	1. Assess mobility status of the patient in one of three categories: (a) bedbound at admission, (b) chairbound at admission, or (c) neither (a) nor (b).
	2. If status (c), further assess the patient with a validated tool (e.g., Timed Up & Go [TUG] Test, physical therapy evaluation).
	3. Document assessment in the medical record.

Ambulatory/Primary Care Process Measures

Table 8.17. *What Matters Documentation Measures at Ambulatory/Primary Care Site*

Measure name	What Matters documentation
Measure description	Percentage of patients 65 and older with documentation of What Matters
Site	Primary care
Population measured	Patients 65 years and older
Measurement period	Choose weekly or monthly (weekly measurement will support faster testing/learning cycles but has consequently higher measurement burden and may not be feasible)
Denominator	*Inclusion*: All patients in the population considered to be patients of the primary care practice (e.g., patient assigned to a care team panel and seen by the practice within the past three years) who have an office visit, home visit, or telemedicine visit with the practice during the measurement period
	Exclusions: None
Numerator	*Inclusion*: Patients in the denominator with documentation of What Matters within 12 months of the most recent office visit, home visit, or telemedicine visit in the measurement month, per the primary care unit's definition of What Matters
	Exclusions: None
Data source	Health records

Method details	For patients unable to speak for themselves, your What Matters engagement should include interaction with an appropriate healthcare agent to understand What Matters.

- Note about patients who decline to engage in discussion of What Matters in a specific encounter.
  - Recommendation: Your procedure should allow for patients to decline to discuss What Matters. A patient who declines to answer in the course of your standard engagement "counts" in the numerator.
  - You will have to judge whether the percentage of patients who decline to answer is acceptable. If too high, then you have a target for study and improvement.

The process of asking What Matters is defined by the primary care practice for the patients it serves. At minimum, asking What Matters involves (a) querying the medical record for existing documentation of What Matters and care wishes, and (b) engaging the patient or healthcare agent in discussion of What Matters as defined by the unit.

Documentation standard is defined by the primary care practice for the patients it serves; the standard describes documentation content and method of recording content.

If an automated report is possible, calculate the denominator and numerator.

If a complete manual tally is possible, calculate the denominator and numerator.

If neither an automated report nor a complete tally is possible, sample records at the end of the measurement period and calculate the denominator and numerator. You can apply a stopping rule to further reduce measurement burden.

What Matters documentation focuses on What Matters to the older adult; it is not intended to be a specific measure of advance care planning (such as NQF 0326).

Table 8.18. Targeted Medications Measures at Ambulatory/Primary Care Site

Measure name	Older adults on targeted medications (Teri & Wagner, 1991)
Measure description	Percentage of patients 65 years and older with active use of one or more medications on target list
Site	Primary care
Population measured	Patients 65 years and older

Measurement period	Monthly
Denominator	*Inclusion*: All patients in the population considered to be patients of the primary care practice (e.g., patient assigned to a care team panel and seen by the practice within the past three years) who have an office visit, home visit, or telemedicine visit with the practice during the measurement period *Exclusions*: None
Numerator	*Inclusion*: Patients in the denominator with active use of one or more medications on target list *Exclusions*: None
Data source	Health records
Method details	This measure is still under development. We anticipate further testing to refine the measure. The target list of medications combines the medications named in measures developed by Pharmacy Quality Alliance (PQA, www.pqaalliance.org), specifically Polypharmacy: Use of Multiple Anticholinergic Medications in Older Adults (POLY-ACH) and Concurrent Use of Opioids and Benzodiazepines (COB). Tables are used with permission of PQA with the understanding that this initiative measure does not represent a current measure endorsed by PQA. • Over-the-counter (OTC) drugs, sleep aids, and sedatives can also be problematic. If any OTC medications have ingredients on the target list, then use of these OTC medications will trigger inclusion of a patient in the numerator. • There are clinically appropriate uses for medications on the target list, individually and in combination. The medication measure is intended to help you characterize the extent of medication use. • To more closely align with PQA measures, we considered splitting this single medication measure into two measures, one focused on anticholinergic medications and the other on concurrent use of opioids and benzodiazepines. Based on current expert discussion and recommendations, we opted for a single measure. Active use is defined by active medications in the medical record (e.g., "Current Medications" items in a discharge note or items viewed by patient in patient portal. In Epic MyChart, Health > Medications. In Cerner, clinicians can access medications through use of the Dynamic Work List function and filter on current medications).

Table 8.19. Dementia Screening at Ambulatory/Primary Care Site

Measure name	Dementia screening
Measure description	Percentage of patients 65 years and older screened for dementia
Site	Primary care
Population measured	Patients 65 years and older
Measurement period	Choose weekly or monthly (weekly measurement will support faster testing/learning cycles but has consequently higher measurement burden and may not be feasible)
Denominator	*Inclusion*: All patients in the population considered to be patients of the primary care practice (e.g., patient assigned to a care team panel and seen by the practice within the past three years) who have an office visit, home visit, or telemedicine visit with the practice during the measurement period
	Exclusions: Patients with diagnosis of dementia (major neurocognitive disorder); patients who refuse the screen, with documentation of refusal, and do not have documentation of a screen within the past 12 months
Numerator	*Inclusion*: Patients in the denominator with documentation of dementia screening within 12 months of the most recent office visit, home visit, or telemedicine visit during the measurement period
	Exclusions: None
Data source	Health records
Method details	Exclusion of patients who refuse the screen, with documentation of refusal, and do not have a screen in the past 12 months is technically a denominator exception. However, since the effect is to remove such patients from the denominator count, we use the single term "exclusion."
	Based on clinical judgment, patients may be screened more frequently than once every 12 months.
	A recommended screening instrument is the Mini-Cog.
	While the US Preventive Services Task Force in March 2014 concluded that then-current evidence was "insufficient to assess the balance of benefits and harms of screening for cognitive impairment," screening for dementia is a core part of the 4Ms and is currently promoted by CMS as part of Annual Wellness exams (Brown et al., 2009).

Table 8.20. Depression Screening at Ambulatory/Primary Care Site

Measure name	Depression screening
Measure description	Percentage of patients 65 years and older screened for depression
Site	Primary care
Population measured	Patients 65 years and older
Measurement period	Choose weekly or monthly (weekly measurement will support faster testing/learning cycles but has consequently higher measurement burden and may not be feasible)
Denominator	*Inclusion*: All patients in the population considered to be patients of the primary care practice (e.g., patient assigned to a care team panel and seen by the practice within the past three years) who have an office visit, home visit, or telemedicine visit with the practice during the measurement period
	Exclusions: Patients with active diagnosis of depression or bipolar disorder; patients currently in hospice; patients who refuse the screen, with documentation of refusal, and do not have documentation of a screen within the past 12 months
Numerator	*Inclusion*: Patients in the denominator with documentation of depression screening within 12 months of the most recent office visit, home visit, or telemedicine visit with the practice during the measurement period
	Exclusions: None
Data source	Health records
Method details	HEDIS 2018 measure "Depression Screening and Follow-Up for Adolescents and Adults (DSF)" provides relevant background for screening tools and exclusions in the context of annual measurement using electronic clinical data records. NQF 0418, "Preventive Care and Screening: Screening for Depression and Follow-Up Plan," based on claims data, targets the same population and process actions.
	Persons with dementia require special screening. "Depression screening in persons with dementia is hindered at times by the patient's inability to self-report symptoms and tendency to underestimate degree of depression, and discrepant caregiver reports (Wadhera et al., 2018). The assessment of depression in dementia is complicated by the considerable overlap in its clinical presentation with that of dementia" (Allen et al., 2011).

Method details (continued)	Organizations should seek to develop and apply a "pragmatic approach" to depression screening. "There is little evidence regarding the optimal timing for screening. The optimum interval for screening for depression is also unknown; more evidence for all populations is needed to identify ideal screening intervals. A pragmatic approach in the absence of data might include screening all adults who have not been screened previously and using clinical judgment in consideration of risk factors, comorbid conditions, and life events to determine if additional screening of high-risk patients is warranted" (Teri & Wagner, 1991).

Table 8.21. Mobility Screening at Ambulatory/Primary Care Site

Measure name	Mobility screening
Measure description	Percentage of patients 65 years and older screened for mobility
Site	Primary care
Population measured	Patients 65 years and older
Measurement period	Choose weekly or monthly (weekly measurement will support faster testing/learning cycles but has consequently higher measurement burden and may not be feasible)
Denominator	*Inclusion*: All patients in the population considered to be patients of the primary care practice (e.g., patient assigned to a care team panel and seen by the practice within the past three years) who have an office visit, home visit, or telemedicine visit with the practice during the measurement period *Exclusions*: None
Numerator	*Inclusion*: Patients in the denominator with documentation of a mobility screening within 12 months of the most recent office visit, home visit, or telemedicine visit *Exclusions*: None
Data source	Health records
Method details	The mobility screening standard should include, at a minimum: Assess mobility status of patient in one of two categories: (a) non-ambulatory or (b) ambulatory. If ambulatory, further assess the patient with a validated tool (e.g., Timed Up & Go [TUG], Performance-Oriented Mobility Assessment [POMA], physical therapy evaluation).

Method details (continued)	Document assessment in the medical record. If (a) non-ambulatory, document degree of assistance needed. If (b) ambulatory, document results from assessment tool.
	Based on clinical judgment, patients may be screened more frequently than once every 12 months.

TABLES OF MEDICATIONS

The tables POLY-ACH-A, COB-A, and COB-B together represent the target list of medications in the measure Patients on Targeted Medications.[2]

Table 8.22. *Anticholinergic Medications (From PQA Measure Polypharmacy: Use of Multiple Anticholinergic Medications in Older Adults [POLY-ACH])*[3]

Antihistamines		
• brompheniramine	• dexbrompheniramine	• hydroxyzine
• carbinoxamine	• dexchlorpheniramine	• meclizine
• chlorpheniramine	• dimenhydrinate	• pyrilamine
• clemastine	• doxylamine	• triprolidine
• diphenhydramine (oral)		
• cyproheptadine		

---

2   The Patients on Targeted Medications measure is adapted with permission based on selected elements of PQA measures, POLY-ACH, and COB. In this adapted form, these monitoring measures no longer represent the PQA measures. PQA retains all rights to ownership of PQA measures and can rescind or alter the measures at any time. All uses of PQA measures are subject to such conditions as PQA specifies, and certain uses of the measures may be subject to a licensing agreement specifying the terms of use and the licensing fee. Users of the measure shall not have the right to alter, enhance, or otherwise modify the measures.

3   Note (in general—unless otherwise specified): Includes combination products that contain a target medication listed and the following routes of administration: oral, transdermal, rectal, sublingual, and buccal. Injectable and inhalation routes of administration are not included (not able to accurately estimate days' supply needed for measure logic). For combination products that contain more than one target medication, each target medication (active ingredient) should be considered independently.

Antiparkinsonian Agents

- benztropine
- trihexyphenidyl

Skeletal Muscle Relaxants

- cyclobenzaprine
- orphenadrine

Antidepressants

- amitriptyline
- amoxapine
- clomipramine
- desipramine
- doxepin (> 6 mg/day)[4]
- imipramine
- nortriptyline
- paroxetine
- protriptyline
- trimipramine

Antipsychotics

- chlorpromazine
- clozapine
- loxapine
- olanzapine
- perphenazine
- thioridazine
- trifluoperazine

Antiarrythmic

- disopyramide

Antimuscarinics (urinary incontinence)

- darifenacin
- fesoterodine
- flavoxate
- oxybutynin
- solifenacin
- tolterodine
- trospium

Antispasmodics

- atropine (excludes ophthalmic)
- belladonna alkaloids
- clidinium-chlordiazepoxide[5]
- dicyclomine
- homatropine (excludes ophthalmic)
- hyoscyamine
- methscopolamine
- propantheline
- scopolamine (excludes ophthalmic)

Antiemetic

- prochlorperazine
- promethazine

4 Includes combination products and prescription opioid cough medications.
5 Note: Chlordiazepoxide is not a target medication as a single drug.

Table 8.23. Opioids[6] (From PQA Measure Concurrent
Use of Opioids and Benzodiazepines [COB])

Opiods		
• benzhydrocodone	• hydrocodone	• opium
• buprenorphine[7]	• hydromorphone	• oxycodone
• butorphanol	• levorphanol	• oxymorphone
• codeine	• meperidine	• pentazocine
• dihydrocodeine	• methadone	• tapentadol
• fentanyl	• morphine	• tramadol

Table 8.24. Benzodiazepines[8] (From PQA Measure Concurrent
Use of Opioids and Benzodiazepines [COB])

Benzodiazepines		
• alprazolam	• diazepam	• oxazepam
• chlordiazepoxide	• estazolam	• quazepam
• clobazam	• flurazepam	• temazepam
• clonazepam	• lorazepam	• triazolam
• clorazepate	• midazolam	

This measure is not intended for clinical decision-making. This measure is intended for retrospective evaluation of populations of patients and should not be used to guide clinical decisions for individual patients. For clinical guidance on opioid prescribing, see the Centers for Disease Control and Prevention (CDC) "Guideline for Prescribing Opioids for Chronic Pain" and Guideline Resources.

---

6   Includes combination products and prescription opioid cough medications. Excludes the following: injectable formulations; sufentanil (used in a supervised setting); and single-agent and combination buprenorphine products used to treat opioid use disorder (i.e., buprenorphine sublingual tablets, Probuphine® Implant kit subcutaneous implant, and all buprenorphine/naloxone combination products).

7   Note: Excludes single-agent and combination buprenorphine products used to treat opioid use disorder (i.e., buprenorphine sublingual tablets, Probuphine® Implant kit subcutaneous implant, and all buprenorphine/naloxone combination products).

8   Includes combination products. Excludes injectable formulations.

Impact on the Care Team: An Informal Qualitative Measure

Balancing measures detect unintended consequences of new inter-ventions. This balancing measure assesses the impact of 4Ms care on the care team. The care team needs to know whether or not their approach to assessing and acting on the 4Ms is feasible in the short term and sustainable over the long term.

For example:

- Does engaging older adults in What Matters conversations cause stress to certain team members?
- Does the task of documentation create a burden?
- Does acting on what is learned from the "assess" stage fall short too often?

Too much stress or burden leads to inconsistent engagement in providing care consistent with the 4Ms and can contribute to staff burnout. You don't need a formal survey or questionnaire to learn about work burden and barriers to reliable 4Ms care. Leaders should instead commit to regularly asking care team members (e.g., once a month) two questions:

1. What are we doing well in providing care consistent with the 4Ms?
2. What could we do better to provide care consistent with the 4Ms?

Tips for Using the Two Questions

- To encourage care team members to continue to respond to the two questions, it is critical to show that leaders are listening to their responses and acting on them. One approach is to engage the team in testing one or more ideas and discuss together what was learned, with the aim to make the 4Ms work easier.

- If the question responses are collected during a team huddle or meeting and recorded on a flipchart or whiteboard, take a digital photo so there is a time-stamped record.

References

Allen, K., Fosnight, S., Wilford, R., Benedict, L., Sabo, A., Holder, C., Jackovitz, D. S., Germano, S., Gleespen, L., Baum, E. E., Wilber, S., & Hazelett, S. (2011). Implementation of a system-wide quality improvement project to prevent delirium in hospitalized patients. *Journal of Clinical Outcomes Management*, 18(6), 253–258.

Braverman, P., Arkin, E., Orleans, T., Proctor, D., & Plough, A. (2017). *What is health equity?* Robert Wood Johnson Foundation.

Brown, E. L., Raue, P. J., Halpert, K., Adams, S., & Titler, M. G. (2009). Evidence-based guideline detection of depression in older adults with dementia. Journal of Gerontological Nursing, 35(2), 11–15. https://doi.org/10.3928/00989134-20151015-03

Teri, L., & Wagner, A. W. (1991). Assessment of depression in patients with Alzheimer's disease: Concordance among informants. *Psychology and Aging*, 6(2), 280–285. https://doi.org/10.1037/0882-7974.6.2.280

US Preventive Services Task Force. (2020). Screening for cognitive impairment in older adults: US Preventive Services Task Force recommendation statement. *JAMA*, 323(8), 757–763. https://doi.org/10.1001/jama.2020.0435

Wadhera, R. K., Joynt Maddox, K. E., Wasfy, J. H., Haneuse, S., Shen, C., & Yeh, R. W. (2018). Association of the Hospital Readmissions Reduction Program with mortality among Medicare beneficiaries hospitalized for heart failure, acute myocardial infarction, and pneumonia. *JAMA*, 320(24), 2542–2552. https://doi.org/10.1001/jama.2018.19232

Wyatt, R., Laderman, M., Botwinick, L., Mate, K., & Whittington, J. (2016). *Achieving health equity: A guide for health care organizations* [White paper]. Institute for Healthcare Improvement. http://www.ihi.org/resources/Pages/IHIWhitePapers/Achieving-Health-Equity.aspx

CHAPTER 9

The Business Case for Becoming an Age-Friendly Health System

by Victor Tabbush, UCLA

The first part of this book explores how patients and clinicians would benefit from shifting to an Age-Friendly Health System (Fulmer et al., 2018). That's the medical case. This section will discuss the business case by looking at the return on investment achieved by systems that have made the change. This chapter will offer best practices for making the case for adopting an age-friendly approach in your own system.

The benefits of becoming an Age-Friendly Health System tend to fall into different categories depending on the care setting. In the inpatient setting, the major driver is reduced costs, resulting from fewer iatrogenic complications, fewer undesired medical interventions, and improved patient safety. These cost savings are reflected in the form of fewer and shorter hospital stays and lower costs per day. In the outpatient setting, by contrast, the gains come chiefly from added revenues resulting from expanding appropriate outpatient services.

In both settings, the increased use of cost-effective services can contribute to the business case for age-friendly care. Redesigning services can optimize the site of care by organizing care based on the What Matters element: the particular priorities and care preferences of older adults and their family caregivers. This approach often supports the transition of older adults from hospitals to lower-cost ambulatory care and home settings, ultimately reducing overutilization and increasing practices such as palliative care and home-based care.

The 4Ms are the focus of the Age-Friendly Health Systems model because there is extremely strong evidence for their effectiveness. Performed together, they undergird and reinforce one another.

How to Make the Business Case for Becoming an Age-Friendly Health System

Making the business case means providing evidence regarding financial returns—the instrumental value—from investing in becoming an Age-Friendly Health System. The business case does not include improved outcomes or satisfaction—the intrinsic value—that result for patients and their families. If the Age-Friendly Health System can show instrumental value, however, its intrinsic value is more likely to be sustained.

Making the business case consists of six steps that are identical across care settings—inpatient, outpatient, or in the home (see Figure 9.1).

Figure 9.1. Steps in Making the Business Case for
Becoming an Age-Friendly Health System

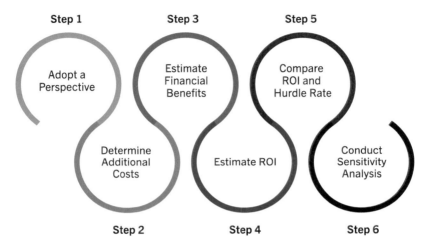

Step 1: Adopt a Perspective

The first step is to determine whose costs and whose financial benefits to consider. While the 4Ms may generate financial gains for a variety of stakeholders, only the financial consequences for the investing party (i.e., the healthcare organization making the investment) count in this analysis.

Step 2: Determine the Additional Costs of Becoming an Age-Friendly Health System

The next step is to assess any additional costs of providing age-friendly care relative to the status quo. The costs will generally be dominated by staffing expenses, although training, consulting costs, information technology (IT), supplies, and additional space and equipment are other possible expense categories. In many cases, health systems may redeploy existing staff resources to perform age-friendly care activities, and implementing the 4Ms could be cost-neutral.

Step 3: Estimate Financial Benefits

The financial benefits of becoming an Age-Friendly Health System fall into three broad categories. These categories, along with their respective drivers, are depicted in Figure 9.2 and explained below.

Figure 9.2. Financial Benefits of Becoming an Age-Friendly Health System

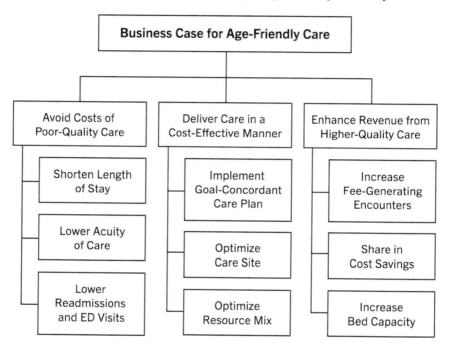

Avoid Costs of Poor-Quality Care

An Age-Friendly Health System reduces costs in part by reducing poor-quality medical care. Cost avoidance stems principally from reductions in the incidence, duration, and acuity of hospital and post-acute care as well as readmissions and emergency department visits. (Whether the party that causes the savings also benefits from them is another matter, as mentioned above in Step 1.)

Deliver Care in a Cost-Effective Manner

An Age-Friendly Health System can prosper financially by providing the right goal-concordant care, in the right place, and in the right way. For example:

- intensive ambulatory care in the home for high-need older adults can substitute for more costly emergency department care;
- inquiring into What Matters may result in fewer days in the intensive care unit (ICU), less specialty care, and more palliation; and
- simple and inexpensive hydration, mobilization, and reorientation activities can replace less effective and more expensive antipsychotics in managing delirium.

Enhance Revenue From Higher-Quality Care

An Age-Friendly Health System can augment revenue by increasing the number of appropriate encounters and interventions. One source of potential revenue is the Medicare Annual Wellness Visit (AWV) and resulting encounters, such as advance care planning and health screenings.

Revenues can be augmented, too, through the quality improvement that characterizes age-friendly care. First, such care improves the patient experience, which positively influences survey results for the Consumer Assessment of Healthcare Providers and Systems (CAHPS) and Hospital CAHPS. Improved survey scores may assist in meeting quality improvement standards imposed by the Centers for Medicare & Medicaid Services (CMS) or health plans (*Salary.com*, 2021). Second, value-enhancing care may lead to an improved reputation and increased market share. Shared savings and other arrangements designed to reward improvements in the quality of care are increasingly common and create further opportunities for bolstering revenues. Finally, age-friendly care can lead to fewer hospital admissions and readmissions and reduced length of stay (LOS). Capacity can then be released and the beds back-filled by other revenue-generating patients if such demand is available.

Step 4: Estimate the Return on Investment

Once gross benefits (i.e., the dollar sum of cost avoidance, new revenues, and financial gains from more cost-effective delivery models) are estimated, an Age-Friendly Health System will need to subtract the additional costs of implementing the 4Ms in order to determine the net income.

Return on investment (ROI), often expressed as a percentage, is defined as net income divided by the program outlay (Leslie et al., 2008). See Appendix M for further details on ROI.

Step 5: Compare the ROI to a Hurdle Rate

Some health systems may be content with a cost-neutral program, while other systems may require a positive return that recognizes what the required resources could have earned in alternative uses. An organization will typically set a higher hurdle rate (i.e., the minimum required rate of return on a project or investment) when a high degree of uncertainty surrounds the accuracy of the ROI assessment. In that circumstance, the investment is riskier, and that risk may need to be balanced by the prospect of a larger return.

Step 6: Conduct Sensitivity Analysis

The values of the key variables in the ROI assessment will inevitably be subject to uncertainty and debate. So, instead of reporting a single ROI, it is wise for an Age-Friendly Health System advocate to suggest a probable range. A simple approach is to report the projected ROIs for at least two scenarios. In the first scenario, all independent variables that shape the ROI are assigned "pessimistic" values; in the second, these variables are either conservative or at their most likely levels. If the 4Ms are predicted to generate an ROI in excess of the hurdle rate, even under the more pessimistic set of assumptions, the business case might be considered more convincing.

Factors That Strengthen the Business Case for Becoming an Age-Friendly Health System

The strength of any business case is crucially dependent on the context and local information. However, six factors tend to strengthen the business case for any healthcare initiative, including becoming an Age-Friendly Health System (see Figure 9.3).

1. High Baseline Medical Utilization

The greater the predicted utilization under usual care, the greater the potential for an Age-Friendly Health system to deliver benefits in terms of averted medical events. Targeting individuals most at risk for future medical utilization will likely yield a higher ROI than targeting individuals who are lighter utilizers.

2. Expensive Medical Events

The total expense of medical utilization prior to implementation of the 4Ms represents the baseline from which cost savings will be calculated. Crucially, hospital admissions and readmissions constitute about 80% of the annual per capita medical costs for high-risk Medicare beneficiaries. Curtailing relatively cheap primary care visits does little to enhance the ROI; by the same token, should becoming an Age-Friendly Health System result in a larger number of primary care visits, any direct adverse impact on the ROI is likely to be minimal.

Figure 9.3. Factors Shaping a Favorable ROI

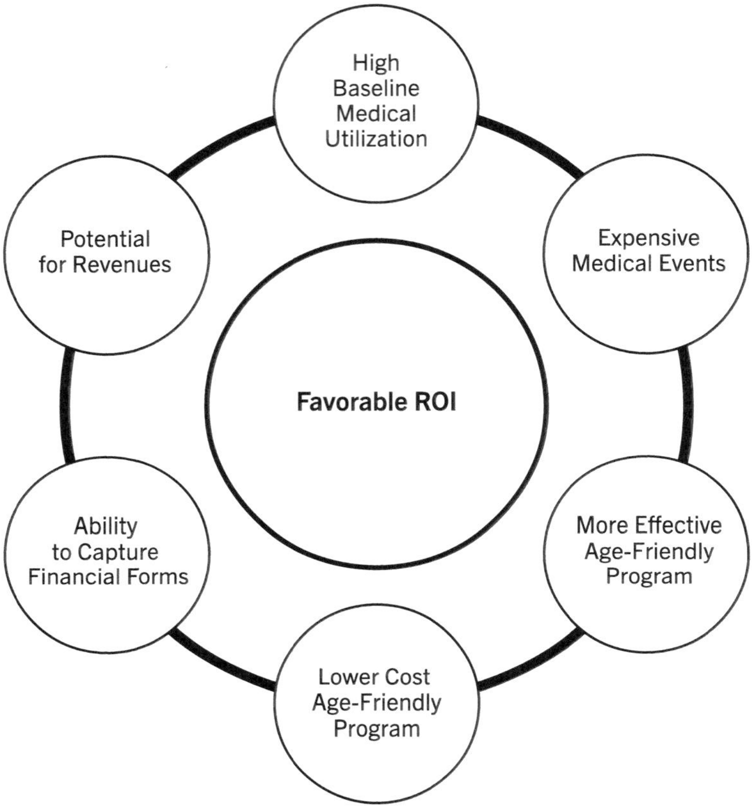

3. More Effective Age-Friendly Health System Program

Effectiveness in this context means the extent to which the 4Ms reduce unnecessary, unwanted medical utilization. The effectiveness of the Age-Friendly Health System program will depend on a number of factors, including the caliber of the leadership of the age-friendly care team; the motivation, skill, and experience of those who deliver the care; the comprehensiveness with which all 4Ms are reliably integrated into care delivery; and the number of resources dedicated to the program.

4. Lower Implementation Costs of an Age-Friendly Health System Program

Costs are lower when

- the Age-Friendly Health System program is not forced to absorb a large portion of organizational overhead;
- the program is expected to run for several years, allowing for any up-front expenses to be spread out over time;
- the scale of the program is larger, allowing fixed costs of operation to be spread over more patients, thereby achieving economies of scale; and
- the health system can reallocate existing resources to 4M-related tasks and activities.

5. Ability of the Investing Party to Capture the Financial Returns

The cost savings may not accrue entirely to the organization that invests in age-friendly care. How a health system derives its revenues and the degree to which it is at risk for costs of medical utilization are profound influences on the strength of the business case. With an increased emphasis by CMS on at-risk contracting (e.g., value-based purchasing, accountable care organizations, Shared Savings Programs, and bundled payments), the business case for becoming an Age-Friendly Health System will be increasingly attractive.

6. Potential for the Age-Friendly Health System to Generate Additional Revenues

Additional revenues have financial consequences similar to reduced costs; both increase the ROI and make the business case stronger. Some financial analysts place a higher weight on a dollar gained than on a dollar saved, because it is so difficult to measure savings from averted medical events. The comparative certainty contributes to the financial appeal of an age-friendly AWV to a medical group. As noted earlier, there are several other circumstances under which an Age-Friendly Health System can contribute to the health system's top-line revenues.

Case Studies

The following report presents two case studies of organizations working toward becoming Age-Friendly Health Systems. The first case study, in the outpatient context at St. Vincent Medical Group, focuses on Medicare's Annual Wellness Visit. The case demonstrates the income-generating power of an age-friendly AWV, which leads to advance care planning, appropriate screenings, and other encounters, all of which generate additional revenue. At St. Vincent, these services collectively have the potential to generate an estimated annual net income of about $3.6 million.

The second case study, in the inpatient setting at Hartford Hospital, examines the business case for an age-friendly delirium prevention and treatment program. The case study focuses on the program's efforts to reduce the high costs of hospital stays complicated by delirium. The condition can add more than $20,000 to the cost of a stay by lengthening it and increasing the daily intensity of care. Hartford Hospital's Age-Friendly program reduces costs and also generates revenue by freeing up hospital beds that can then be filled by other revenue-generating patients.

These case studies provide important lessons for health systems contemplating adopting the 4Ms framework. The most important is that in order to make a convincing demonstration of ROI from the 4Ms, reliable and relevant clinical and financial data must be collected. The business case methodology described in this report will help an organization seeking to become an Age-Friendly Health System identify the relevant data, analyze it, and describe its financial implications.

Outpatient Case Study: St. Vincent Medical Group, Indianapolis, Indiana

St. Vincent Medical Group in Indiana is part of Ascension, a pioneer health system in the Age-Friendly Health Systems initiative. Ascension, one of the largest nonprofit health systems in the US, has more than 2,600 sites of care, including 139 hospitals and more than 40 senior living facilities, across 19 states and the District of Columbia.

During an interview with IHI, Ascension leaders stated that a priority in its Advanced Strategic Direction is to improve the profitability of Medicare reimbursement across the system, and they believe that becoming an Age-Friendly Health System can contribute to narrowing the gap between Medicare revenues and costs. Specifically, Ascension is looking to expand the Medicare AWV to as many as 90% of eligible beneficiaries as a vehicle to address operating margins that are otherwise expected to decline over the coming years.

Ascension Medical Group (AMG), a physician-led provider organization within the Ascension system, reached a stretch target set in 2018 that 75% of eligible patients would complete an AWV in the previous 12 months by the end of FY2019. The financial impact of expanding the AWV was substantial, as this case study of St. Vincent Medical Group illustrates. St. Vincent Medical Group offers primary care in more than 100 sites throughout Indiana. The payment context for St. Vincent includes all Medicare payment plans.

AWVs were introduced by CMS in 2011 as part of the Affordable Care Act. Coverage is provided for a yearly visit to conduct a health risk assessment and to develop or update a beneficiary's personalized prevention plan (Pantilat et al., 2007). In March 2018, in collaboration with AMG, St. Vincent Center for Healthy Aging created a 4Ms-focused encounter template for the AWV. Within St. Vincent Medical Group, initial and subsequent AWVs are conducted by physicians or Medicare Wellness Nurses (MWNs), who are exclusively dedicated to providing these AWV encounters; approximately one-half of AWVs are conducted by each (Inouye et al., 1999).

St. Vincent ensures that What Matters is an explicit conversation with the patient. In part to reduce costs, St. Vincent is increasing the proportion of AWVs conducted by MWNs. In addition, St. Vincent aligned with AMG and expanded the percentage of eligible beneficiaries who participated in such visits from 40.5% in 2018 to 75% by the end of FY2019. Both aims appear realistic given that the daily capacity of the MWN is six visits, but current MWN productivity averages about four visits per day.

The St. Vincent case study illustrates the potential financial returns from approaching the AWV using a local adaptation of the 4Ms framework.

Financial Returns From the Annual Wellness Visit

Under a fee-for-service system, the direct financial returns from providing the AWV can be attractive. These returns accrue from

- the net income from the AWV itself;
- the subsequent income-generating encounters that the AWV drives; and
- potentially improved quality scores in value-based reimbursement programs.

Another financial benefit, albeit indirect, is the decrease in unnecessary use of physician time.

The fee received by St. Vincent for each AWV is currently about $140, a blended average that considers the mix of initial and subsequent visits. The cost of an MWN-provided AWV is estimated to be about $92. Thus, the net income margin for MWN-provided visits is $48.

Additional financial benefits may derive from an increased number of advance care plans and preventive screenings resulting from the AWVs that would not have otherwise occurred. The next two sections discuss the financial gains from these two sources. (Note: It is also possible that AWVs generate additional income from added evaluation and management encounters, but that is not included as part of the analysis below.)

Net Income From the Advance Care Plan

The advance care plan (ACP) is a voluntary, face-to-face conversation between a physician (or other qualified healthcare professional, such as a physician assistant, nurse practitioner, or certified clinical nurse specialist) and a patient concerning advance directives pertaining to future medical treatment, if the patient is not able to make decisions independently at that time.

Effective January 1, 2016, CMS began paying for the ACP under the Medicare Physician Fee Schedule (PFS). Since the AWV often touches on the patient's end-of-life goals, especially when What Matters is explicitly raised, that visit can prompt a subsequent ACP. Data from St. Vincent show that when an age-friendly AWV is provided (i.e., the AWV explicitly focuses on the 4Ms as the orientation for the visit), the probability of a subsequent ACP increases from 19.8% to 38.1%, thereby adding to the financial gains from the AWV.

There are two codes for the ACP:

- code 99497 is designed as compensation for a 30-minute encounter and pays a clinician approximately $80; and
- code 99498 allows for an extension of the initial period and pays an additional $71.

At St. Vincent, both ACP codes are almost always used for what are typically lengthier consultations. The combined payments total about $150.

When conducted by a physician assistant, nurse practitioner, or certified clinical nurse specialist—all of whom are qualified to conduct ACPs—the cost of the ACP is estimated to be about $83. This figure is based on an annual wage of $100,000 for these providers and an assumed capacity of conducting five encounters per day. Allowing for an additional $17 (20%) for possible indirect costs associated with each ACP results in a net income margin for each ACP of about $50. In some cases the physician may conduct the ACP, which could minimally impact the net margin.

Net Income From Preventive Screenings

There are 25 billable preventive screenings that can be prescribed under Medicare Part B. The AWV provides an opportunity to determine the appropriateness of services such as colorectal cancer screening, breast cancer screening, bone mass measurements, depression screening, and others. Thus, the AWV drives preventive screenings, which, for many medical groups, contribute to quality measures in addition to driving revenues directly.

As shown in Table 9.1 below, based on 2018 data from St. Vincent, the impact of the age-friendly AWV on the uptake of the four most common screenings can be quite large. For example, for falls screening, the provision of the AWV adds 31.5 percentage points to the probability that this screening will occur. For the purpose of illustration, if we assume that the net income from this screening is $10, then the expected additional value of the AWV from the falls screening would be $3.15 (31.5% of $10). (Similar calculations for the three other screenings are reflected in the overall results in Table 9.2.)

Table 9.1. *St. Vincent Medical Group Screening Rates: With Annual Wellness Visit (AWV) Versus Without AWV*

SCREENING TYPE	TOTAL ANNUAL NUMBER OF SCREENINGS	SCREENING RATE WITH AWV	SCREENING RATE WITHOUT AWV	TOTAL NUMBER OF ADDITIONAL SCREENINGS DUE TO THE AWV
Falls	30,129	76.6%	45.1%	6,890
Depression	21,747	77.5%	38.7%	6,551
Colorectal cancer	23,508	86.6%	61.0%	3,748
Breast cancer	12,406	93.3%	67.5%	1,864

Overall Potential ROI From the AWV

By the end of 2019, St. Vincent Medical Group aims to expand the proportion of its eligible population that receives age-friendly AWVs to 75% of all eligible seniors, deploy their MWNs to conduct these visits, and increase the productivity of MWNs from four to six visits per day. If all of these efforts succeed, St. Vincent's annual net income potential from age-friendly AWVs is projected to be about $3.0 million. When the net income from screenings and from the ACPs attributable to the AWVs is included, that number rises to about $3.6 million (see Table 9.2).

Table 9.2. *St. Vincent Medical Group Annual Net Income Potential From Age-Friendly AWVs*

SOURCE OF NET INCOME	AMOUNT
Age-friendly annual wellness visits	$3,003,000
Screenings	$250,000
Advance care plans	$385,000
Total	$3,638,000

Summary
Under its Age-Friendly program, the expansion of ambulatory visits—
and, in particular, age-friendly AWVs—is creating significant income-
generating opportunities for St. Vincent and for the other medical
groups in the Ascension system. If the net income from advance care
plans and health screenings is added to the net income from the age-
friendly AWVs, these changes have the potential to generate annual
net income for St. Vincent of about $3.6 million.

Note that other medical groups can replicate these calculations
using their own data by accessing the IHI Age-Friendly Health
Systems Outpatient ROI Calculator, an Excel-based tool developed
for assessing the business case for an age-friendly AWV.

Inpatient Case Study:
Hartford Hospital, Hartford, Connecticut

The business case for implementing the 4Ms in a hospital setting is
predicated mainly on the healthcare costs avoided through the elimination of poor-quality care. Figure 9.4 shows the most common and
costly adverse events that the 4Ms may potentially avert. In the figure, although each event is linked to one specific "M," in practice all
4Ms work synergistically against each negative outcome.

Consequently, the business case for the 4Ms should account for all
the negative events they potentially avert, events predicted to occur
under typical hospital care. To illustrate how health systems can construct the business case, the following case study focuses on a single
adverse event: the incidence of delirium. However, the approach to
making the business case for averting other adverse events with the
4Ms is identical.

The business case for preventing delirium is based on lowering
the hospital LOS and the daily cost. (The case would be even stronger were a hospital to bear some financial responsibility for its post-
discharge or downstream sequelae: hospital-acquired delirium has

been shown to increase nursing home placement and overall health-care costs subsequent to hospital discharge [Leslie et al., 2008].)

This case study focuses on Hartford Hospital's ADAPT (Actions for Delirium Assessment Prevention and Treatment) program. Hartford Hospital is a participant in the IHI Age-Friendly Health Systems Action Community. ADAPT has generated sufficient data to make a plausible business case for its age-friendly approach to care. Hartford Hospital, an 867-bed teaching facility, is part of Hartford HealthCare, a comprehensive healthcare network in Connecticut. ADAPT was introduced there in 2012 and is currently led by Christine M. Waszynski, DNP, APRN, GNP-BC, and Robert S. Dicks, MD, FACP. ADAPT is now being implemented in multiple hospital units where more than 4,000 patients were seen in 2018.

Figure 9.4. Adverse Events Potentially Averted by Implementing the 4Ms

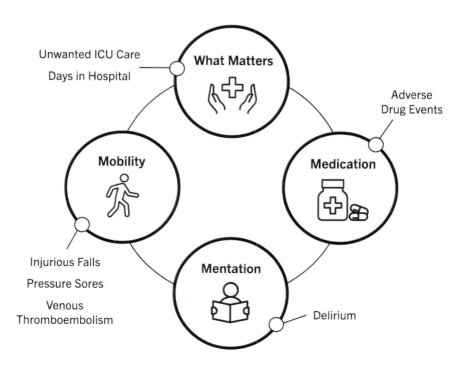

ADAPT Strategies

ADAPT's delirium care pathway is straightforward: screen all patients for delirium, prevent cases from developing, treat those that do, and manage cases that cannot be resolved. ADAPT is similar in most respects to the Hospital Elder Life Program (HELP), the widely studied and accepted standard of delirium care. ADAPT's evidence-based strategies are firmly grounded in the 4Ms framework of an Age-Friendly Health System. In addition to Mentation, the main category into which delirium falls, the pathway explicitly includes the individualized plan of care (What Matters), mobilization and falls prevention (Mobility), and avoiding or stopping potentially inappropriate medications (Medication).

Prevalence of Delirium at Hartford Hospital

ADAPT screens almost all patients for delirium because the hospital's data show that no age group or service line is immune to the condition. In 2018, diagnosed delirium varied between 5% and 50% in all hospitalized patients in the participating units. Delirium-positive rates vary by service, with coronary artery bypass grafting (CABG) being the highest, followed by trauma, at slightly under 40%. Joint replacement had the lowest rate, at about 5%. Current rates reflect implementation of ADAPT strategies, in the absence of which delirium rates presumably would have been higher.

Cost Avoidance With ADAPT Implementation

While the absence of data from a randomized control group makes it challenging to rigorously establish the ROI from ADAPT, the heavy financial burden that delirium imposes on this hospital, together with the low costs of ADAPT, sets up a plausibly strong business case for the efforts to prevent it.

Delirium cases are enormously expensive at Hartford Hospital. From July 2015 to June 2016, 35,700 hospital days were attributed to delirium, with hospital-incurred costs of about $96 million. These delirium-related costs stem from an increased LOS combined with a higher cost per day, as shown in Table 9.3. Considering these two factors, delirium is responsible for adding more than $22,000 to a hospital stay. Hartford Hospital data and published studies support the position that delirium alone, rather than other factors, is responsible for the dramatic increase in hospital LOS (Ely et al., 2001).

The payer mix and payment systems under which Hartford Hospital operates ensure that the financial savings from ADAPT's prevention efforts accrue to the larger Hartford HealthCare system. Older patients are primarily traditional Medicare beneficiaries, although a small number fall under per diem or per case rates paid by health plans with which the system contracts. Under fee-for-service, lowering length of stay creates a financial benefit.

Table 9.3. Hartford Hospital Per-Patient Costs Associated With Delirium

	WITH DELIRIUM	WITHOUT DELIRIUM	DIFFERENCE
Hospital length of stay	12 days	4 days	8 days
Daily cost	$2,798	$2,225	$573
Total cost of stay[9]	$31,284	$8,900	$22,384

It can be misleading, however, to use the cost figure of roughly $22,000 (above, in Table 9.3) as the financial return from preventing a case of delirium. The cost savings includes only the variable costs of that day, not the full costs, which include fixed elements that are unaffected by shorter stays.

9   Note: The cost of a stay with delirium is based on the extra cost per day applying just to the 8 added days.

Thus, a conservative estimate, based on the assumption that fixed costs constitute 50% of the total, is that the financial benefit of an avoided delirium case is about $11,000 (Pantilat et al., 2007). Demonstrating a positive ROI requires evidence that the cost of preventing a case is less than that amount. The cost of preventing a delirium case is a calculation that requires knowledge of (a) the costs of implementing ADAPT and (b) its effectiveness in reducing the incidence of delirium.

ADAPT requires minimal outlays: about $5 per patient for items (such as reader glasses, stuffed animals, personalized music, and sleep eye masks) to improve function or provide comfort. There are, of course, indirect time-based costs for personnel. Additional time is required for ADAPT leadership tasks, for training (about two hours per nurse), for configuring the electronic health record, and for gathering and reporting data.

To date, Hartford Hospital has not attempted to convert these time requirements into a dollar equivalent. However, ADAPT's leaders estimate that the total amount, including out-of-pocket and indirect costs, comes to no more than $50 per patient. (Note that this cost is considerably lower than the costs for HELP. In 1999, HELP was reported to cost $327 per patient, the equivalent of $630 in 2019 dollars [Inouye et al., 1999]. The cost disparity is due to two factors: first, ADAPT relies more heavily on volunteers; and second, unlike HELP, ADAPT does not have specific personnel whose only function is to oversee the program.)

While no concrete data have yet been reported on ADAPT's effectiveness, it is highly likely that it is cost-beneficial. A financial tool called breakeven analysis, used in the context of data gaps, suggests this likelihood. With this tool, we calculated the percentage of delirium cases that ADAPT must prevent in order to be cost-neutral. Then we compared this breakeven threshold to what might be reasonably expected.

If the breakeven threshold is a lower number of prevented cases than expected, it is plausible that the program will generate a positive financial return. When the analysis is performed even under the conservative assumptions, the breakeven threshold is minimal and likely to be far beneath what might be reasonably expected. The breakeven threshold is only 2% when the cost per patient is $100 and the value of a case prevented is $5,000. Research from HELP supports the view that up to 40% of delirium cases are preventable (Inouye et al., 1999).

From the Hartford Hospital data and analysis applied to it, one might reasonably conclude that even under the most conservative scenarios, ADAPT should at least break even and probably perform far better than that. ADAPT, HELP, and other similar age-friendly initiatives to address delirium while also averting other iatrogenic events, such as falls, infections, and pressure sores, make a plausibly strong business case for their adoption. While the financial dimension is generally not the decisive factor for adopting the 4Ms, an attractive ROI should serve to encourage the scale-up and spread of age-friendly hospital care.

Organizations can use the IHI Age-Friendly Health Systems Inpatient ROI Calculator, with their own data, to evaluate the business case for their inpatient 4Ms programs. This Excel-based calculator contains not only costs of delirium, but also some of the other potentially avoidable costs.

Lessons and Challenges

A review of the two case studies yields crucial lessons. These should serve to inform a business case for any organization that has become, or is considering becoming, an Age-Friendly Health System.

Lesson 1: There Is No Single Business Case for Becoming an Age-Friendly Health System

It would be misleading to claim that there is a single, consistently attractive business case for becoming an Age-Friendly Health System. There are simply too many variables that affect the ROI, including the setting (outpatient, inpatient, or in the home), how reliably the 4Ms are applied, the specifics of the population served, and the payment system under which the health system operates. The last two factors are so important that each warrants a separate lesson.

Lesson 2: The Crucial Factor Underlying a Strong Business Case Is the Healthcare Organization's Responsibility for a Large Portion of the Total Cost of Care

An Age-Friendly Health System is more likely to generate an attractive ROI if it is at risk for a substantial portion of the total cost of care and if it is rewarded for quality service delivery. But even under a fee-for-service system, hospitals are exposed to financial risk stemming from length of stay and cost per day.

Lesson 3: Risk Stratification of the Population Eligible for Age-Friendly Care May Be Advisable

To the extent that age-friendly care involves a marginal cost relative to usual care, it will generally make financial sense to focus such care on patients with the greatest need and who incur the highest cost. (This financial consideration may conflict with the clinical imperative to provide better care to all, irrespective of their degree of need.) Extending the services to those at lower risk for expensive medical events may reduce the overall ROI, potentially beneath a financially acceptable hurdle. In the inpatient setting, for example, the risk of delirium is far greater for patients in postoperative thoracic surgery than in elective orthopedic surgery.

Lesson 4: The 4Ms Work Collectively as a Set of Evidence-Based Elements—It Is Not Possible to Assess the Individual Contribution Each of the 4Ms Makes to the ROI

The 4Ms work collectively and synergistically. For example, delirium prevention and treatment (Mentation) deliver significant financial benefits to hospitals. But a focus on Mentation alone may not reliably produce this outcome; Medication and Mobility also play important roles. And in the ambulatory setting, the Annual Wellness Visit is profitable by virtue of focusing on all 4Ms, including What Matters.

Lesson 5: Every Site Needs to Collect Its Own Data

While published data on certain age-friendly activities may be available, it is strongly preferred that each site collect its own data since results will differ in each context. It is often challenging to collect the relevant data, but each health system needs to develop a plan for evaluating financial outcomes. That plan should begin by identifying the inputs for which data need to be collected.

The ROI calculators that IHI has made available will help health systems address this challenge by identifying the data requirements for making their own business case. These calculators will also generate estimates of ROI ranges when the data are difficult to collect and when there is uncertainty regarding their magnitudes.

Recommendations and Summary

While financial benefits are not the primary reason to become an Age-Friendly Health System, the business case can be compelling. Making the best possible business case requires certain general considerations, described in this chapter, as well as a deep understanding of your specific healthcare setting. We hope the resources provided will furnish you with the tools to get started on your journey to providing age-friendly care.

References

Ely, E. W., Gautam, S., Margolin, R., Francis, J., May, L., Speroff, T., Truman, B., Dittus, R., Bernard, R., & Inouye, S. K. (2001). The impact of delirium in the intensive care unit on hospital length of stay. *Intensive Care Medicine*, 27(12), 1892–1900. https://doi.org/10.1007/s00134-001-1132-2

Fulmer, T., Mate, K. S., & Berman, A. (2018). The age-friendly health system imperative. *Journal of the American Geriatrics Society*, 66(1), 22–24. https://doi.org/10.1111/jgs.15076

Inouye, S. K., Bogardus, S. T., Jr., Charpentier, P. A., Leo-Summers, L., Acampora, D., Holford, T. R., & Cooney, L. M., Jr. (1999). A multicomponent intervention to prevent delirium in hospitalized older patients. *New England Journal of Medicine*, 340(9), 669–676. https://doi.org/10.1056/NEJM199903043400901

Leslie, D. L., Marcantonio, E. R., Zhang, Y., Leo-Summers, L., & Inouye, S. K. (2008). One-year health care costs associated with delirium in the elderly population. *Archives of Internal Medicine*, 168(1), 27–32. https://doi.org/10.1001/archinternmed.2007.4

Pantilat, S. Z., Rabow, M. W., Kerr, K. M., & Markowitz, A. J. (2007). *Palliative care in California: The business case for hospital-based programs*. California Healthcare Foundation, University of California-San Francisco, Palliative Care Program. https://www.chcf.org/wp-content/uploads/2017/12/PDF-PalliativeCareBusinessCase.pdf

Salary.com. (2021). *Leading the charge*. https://www.salary.com/about-us/

Tabbush, V., Pelton, L., Mate, K., & Duong, T. (2019). *The business case for becoming an age-friendly health system. Institute for Healthcare Improvement*. http://www.ihi.org/Engage/Initiatives/Age-Friendly-Health-Systems/Documents/IHI_Business_Case_for_Becoming_Age_Friendly_Health_System.pdf

CHAPTER 10

Role of the Electronic Health Record in Aging

Integrating the 4Ms into the electronic health record (EHR) is a mechanism to ensure reliable practice of these essential elements across care settings.
                    —The Age-Friendly Health Systems initiative

This implementation guide was designed by IHI as a resource for health systems to build the 4Ms, and associated care practices, into the EHR. It addresses how to incorporate both the "assess" and "act on" drivers of the 4Ms into the EHR. The guidance in this guide is not specific to a particular EHR vendor; however, specific suggestions are provided for use with Epic. Please note that the EHR processes are continually updated and consult with your vendor as needed.

Figure 10.1. Two Key Drivers of Age-Friendly Health Systems

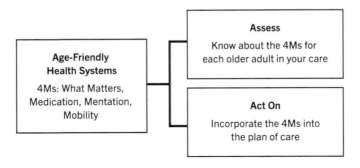

Inpatient Implementation

When using these guidelines to implement the 4Ms in your EHR, validate both content and workflow inside your organization. Provide 4Ms documentation for all specialties across the continuum of care.

Figure 10.2. Beginning Epic Build

In Epic: Begin your build by creating a CER (rule) record. Choose a criterion of patient age, excluding patients under 65 years of age (e.g., "Patient Age is not less than 65 years"). This rule will be used as your filter where CER rules are accepted throughout your build. Skip this step if all components of the 4Ms will be used for all patients regardless of age. The same rule may be shared between inpatient and outpatient contexts.

Create a 4Ms report for use within the Patient Summary activity. Ensure all 4Ms documentation can be found for review by clinicians in the 4Ms report.

What Matters

What Matters means *knowing and aligning care with each older adult's specific health outcome goals and care preferences including, but not limited to, end-of-life care and across settings of care. What Matters* and *www.ihi.org/AgeFriendly* website have more detailed guidance about how to put What Matters into practice as part of the 4Ms.

Assess

First, in admission-required documentation flowsheets, create a row titled "What Matters to the older adult/family caregiver" to capture What Matters. Next, provide prompts in row details (additional information) for clinicians to ask about What Matters to the older adult and their goals related to health and healthcare. If you do not have existing prompts, try the following, and adapt as needed:

- For all older adults: "Older adult / family caregiver focus for stay."
- For older adults with advanced or serious illness: "Most important goals if condition worsens."

Document the older adult's answer in the EHR or enable a space in your inpatient patient portal. A multi-response answer may be used to list the most common responses to What Matters. Examples of potential answer choices include family connections, comfort, understanding care plans, clinical care needs, or other (with space for comments). Validate a comprehensive list of options across the continuum of care.

A flowsheet row may be used for a specific response of What Matters to older adults in their own words, such as attending an upcoming family event or rejoining a group or class each week. Include the information documented here on the older adult's summary report in a conspicuous location. Ensure it appears to care team members across the continuum of care.

Figure 10.3. Using Epic for What Matters

In Epic: Build two multi-select flowsheet rows as detailed above for general What Matters options and a third for details of the older adult's response of What Matters. Build a flowsheet group for your What Matters questions and embed the flowsheet rows. Include the group containing the flowsheet rows in the admission navigator and within the flowsheets activity. Build a print group (LPG) to display the older adult or family caregiver answers to clinicians.

A print group (LPG) should show these items at the top of a rounding report, Kardex/SBAR/Snapshot, or similar report in addition to the 4Ms report.

If using MyChart Bedside, create a questionnaire available to older adults and enable the older adult or family caregiver to answer. Repsonses should be enabled to file to the above flowsheets with clinician validation.

Figure 10.4. Using Cerner for Patient Assessment

In Cerner: For those using an Admission History PowerForm for the initial patient assessment: Create a new section that walks clinicians through assessing the 4Ms of the older adult. Age flex the Discrete Task Assay (DTA) (65 and older) and make crucial fields required. (See Appendix A for a suggested build.)

For clients using iView for the initial patient assessment: Create an order (suggested name: 4Ms Assessment). This order will create a task for the nurse. The task will open an area in iView (Doc Set) that will contain a series of fields common to most Cerner builds. These fields allow the nurse to document the initial assessment of the 4Ms. (See Appendix B for a suggested build; however, you may choose to create net new fields in your Doc Set.)

Use separate DTAs for inpatient and ambulatory assessments, to allow for different prompts for the older adults in the assessments for each of the two settings.

The results of this documentation in either form will flow to a specialty results tab in Results Review, Interdisciplinary Summary Pages, Nursing, and Care Management Summary Pages.

Act On

Use the information documented in the assessment to align the care plan with What Matters. The answers to the What Matters flowsheet will drive an alert or advisory that will, in turn, prompt clinicians to add care plans appropriate to the older adult's priorities. For example, if an older adult identifies managing pain as a priority, a pain management care plan should be suggested or automatically added based on the earlier flowsheet documentation.

An option for "other" should be available both for initial documentation of the older adult's information as well as within care plan documentation. Clinicians should individualize the care plan for each older adult, considering the person's goals and preferences. Add appropriate patient education for enabling the older adult's goals and preferences. Some content may be generated from flowsheet and/or care plan documentation via alerts, prompts, or behind-the-scenes rules.

Figure 10.5. Using Epic Best Practice Advisory

In Epic: Create a Best Practice Advisory (BPA) to suggest care plans corresponding with the What Matters documentation. The BPA criteria should look to the FLO documentation (e.g., if fall risk is reported as What Matters to the older adult, fire a care plan relating to fall risk reduction). In the attached care plan, suggest corresponding patient education documentation via BPA as well. If validated in your organization, patient education may be auto-added from appropriate care plan documentation.

Figure 10.6. Using Cerner Interdisciplinary Plan of Care

In Cerner: Create a 4Ms Interdisciplinary Plan of Care (IPOC). See Appendix C for an example build.

Based on documentation in either the PowerForm or iView, suggest the IPOC. If using the PowerForm in an inpatient setting, a label can be placed on the PowerForm to remind nurses to initiate the 4Ms IPOC.

Continue to address IPOC once daily during the admission.

Add Patient Education during the Admissions that appropriately addresses the older adult's identified concerns and goals.

Consider incorporating What Matters to the older adult into the clinician admission note template, along with space for actions taken. For organizations with existing templates or significant customization amongst clinicians, consider publishing a link that can pull in the older adult's answers from flowsheets.

Figure 10.7. Using Epic SmartLink/SmartPhrase

In Epic: Create a SmartLink or SmartPhrase (for example .FLOW[FLO ID]) and incorporate it into standard clinician note templates, or train to the new SmartLink/SmartPhrase and assist clinicians in adding to their existing, personalized templates.

Figure 10.8. Using Cerner PowerNote/Dynamic Documentation

In Cerner: If organization clinicians are using PowerNote, consider creating shared macros that contain language that conveys the clinician has acknolwedged the older adult's wishes. Smart templates can also be coded to pull documented elements of the 4Ms into the clinician note, such as DTAs from the PowerForm assessments of What Matters, Mobility, and dementia screens. Home medications will pull into the note.

If using Dynamic Documentation (DynDoc), the same smart template recommendation can be employed, and the same home medication information will be pulled into the note.

All care team members should be able to view What Matters within the older adult's chart. Incorporate this information into the 4Ms report mentioned at the beginning of this document. In addition to incorporating What Matters, consider including code status, advance directives, and Medical Orders for Life-Sustaining Treatment (MOLST) / Physician Orders for Life-Sustaining Treatment (POLST) documentation to encourage its use in clinical decision-making. Alternatively, or additionally, create a navigator dedicated to 4Ms documentation and review. If a navigator is created, consider restricting to patients 65 and older.

Figure 10.9. Using Cerner for What Matters

In Cerner: Most organizations are collecting advance directive information at the time of admission as a regulatory requirement. Addressing What Matters for the older adult is a separate conversation. Document and assess it separately.

Medication

If medication is necessary, use age-friendly medication that does not interfere with What Matters to the older adult, Mentation, or Mobility across settings of care. *Age-Friendly Health Systems: Guide to Using the 4Ms in the Care of Older Adults* (pp. 31, 34–35) provides information about Assessing and Acting On Medication in the context of being an Age-Friendly Health System in an inpatient setting.

Assess

Review for high-risk medication use. Potentially inappropriate medications for older adults include the following:

- benzodiazepines
- opioids
- highly anticholinergic medications (e.g., diphenhydramine)
- all prescription and over-the-counter sedatives and sleep medications
- muscle relaxants
- tricyclic antidepressants
- antipsychotics

Act On

Figure 10.10. *Using Epic for Medication Reconciliation*

In Epic: Include medication reconciliation in the admission navigator and required admission documentation as validated by your organization. Ensure suggestions inside order sets reflect age-appropriate medication choices and doses. Reconciliation and new medication orders should fire alternative alerts to clinician and pharmacists.

From the Kardex/SBAR/Snapshot report, 4Ms report, and clinician review reports (such as a rounding report), an age-filtered print group should appear for medications presenting greater risk to patients 65 and older.

Analysts may use Age/Sex medication warnings if using Medi-Span or Multlex and use Geriatric medication warnings if using FDB. These can be build as Medication Rules (RXR) records by your medication warning builder and attached to the medication class as appropriate. Ensure your medication warning builder confirms the alerts are set appropriately so they are not filtered out. See the Alternative Alerts section of Galaxy for more information or discuss with your Willow IS or TS.

Figure 10.11. Using Cerner for Medication Reconciliation

In Cerner: Medication Reconciliation is a required step for physicians during the admission process.

Consider creating an age-appropriate Admission PowerPlan that offers a medication profile that is more suitable for the older population. Consider including orders for nonpharmacologic alternatives for sleep and relaxation.

Avoid or deprescribe the high-risk medications listed above. If the older adult takes one or more of the medications listed, discuss any concerns the patient may have, assess for adverse effects, and discuss deprescribing with the older adult.

Figure 10.12. Using Epic for Medication Alerts

In Epic: Highlight high-risk medications. Consider adding a BPA to deprescribe either when any medications on the list are highlighted or when prescribing any medications on the list.

Figure 10.13. Using Cerner for Medication Alerts

In Cerner: If your health system is open to creating medication alerts, consider including alerts to remind clinicians to avoid or deprescribe the high-risk medications during the ordering process. These will alert physicians about high-risk medications when added to the scratchpad.

Mentation

Prevent, identify, treat, and manage dementia, depression, and delirium across settings of care. *Age-Friendly Health Systems: Guide to Using the 4Ms in the Care of Older Adults* (pp. 32, 35–36) provides information about Assessing and Acting On Mentation in the context of being an Age-Friendly Health System in an inpatient setting.

Assess

Screen for delirium at least every 12 hours. Incorporate your delirium screening tool into required admission and shift documentation.

If you do not have an existing tool, try using the Ultra-Brief 2-Item Screener (UB-2; Fick et al., 2018).

Figure 10.14. Using Epic for Delirium Screening

In Epic: Build a delirium screen required documentation rule containing your delirium screening flowsheet rows or group. If you do not have a delirium screen tool currently in place, you may build the UB-2 and incorporate the associated rows into your required documentation rules. Add the delirium screen to Head to Toe/Adult PCS flowsheet template if not already present.

Example of the UB-2 used at other organizations using Epic may be found on the Community Library.

Add your delirium screen required documentation rule to both the admission and shift tabs within required documentation, preferably at the system level. Filter out patients under 65.

Figure 10.15. Using Cerner for Mentation Assessments

In Cerner: For nursing, mentation assessment is performed in either iView or PowerForm. Continued documentation against the 4Ms IPOC will serve as a reminder for nurses to address the most important aspects of care with this group of patients (See Appendix C for an example 4Ms IPOC). There are several mentation assessment tools that can be built into iView, depending on organization's alignment and preference. However, Confusion Assessment Method for the ICU (CAM-ICU) is the only screening tool found in model content.

For clinicians, mentation assessment is performed in Dynamic Documentation (DynDoc). Orders can be placed via PowerPlan to direct patient care to the specific mentation issues.

Act On

Note that interventions below may support other goals within the 4Ms framework in addition to Mentation.

ENSURE SUFFICIENT ORAL HYDRATION

Make fields available to clinicians for documentation when prompting or encouraging older adults to drink (in addition to fields for oral fluid intake) within the Intake and Output and Daily Cares flowsheet templates or another location specified by your organization. Ensure an option is available for documentation of fluid restriction and/or nothing by mouth (NPO) status.

ORIENT OLDER ADULTS TO TIME, PLACE, AND SITUATION
Document orientation status in flowsheets. If the older adult is disoriented, provide a row or use the orientation row with additional options for staff to document use of gentle reorientation and/or orienting cues.

ENSURE OLDER ADULTS HAVE THEIR
PERSONAL ADAPTIVE EQUIPMENT
Include a flowsheet row titled "Adaptive equipment accessible" for registered nurses (RNs) or aides to document that the older adult's items are within reach. As multi-select items, include glasses, hearing aids, dentures, walkers, and other. Consider other choices as defined by your organization. Make your documentation available from the Daily Cares flowsheet template.

PREVENT SLEEP INTERRUPTIONS AND USE
NONPHARMACOLOGICAL INTERVENTIONS TO SUPPORT SLEEP
Ensure that EHR documentation windows reflect policy and that clinicians can avoid sleep interruptions for older adults' assessments by clustering care.

Offer a flowsheet row with nonpharmacological interventions as options in Bedtime Readiness: sleep aids (e.g., earplugs, sleep masks, muscle relaxation), lights dimmed, noise minimized, music, sleep kit offered, and other for RN or aide documentation. This may be included in the Daily Cares flowsheet template or another place of your organization's choosing.

Figure 10.16. Using Epic for Mentation Documentation

In Epic: Build flowsheet rows for mentation documentation as needed. Include these both in the most relevant flowsheet template for documentation as well as required shift documentation (with exception of bedtime readiness). Ensure all documentation flows to the patient summary reports defined (e.g., 4Ms, SnapShot, etc.) for clinician review.

Figure 10.17. Using Cerner for Mentation Documentation

In Cerner: Include these care strategies in the 4Ms IPOC design and make them available documentation in iView.

Mobility

Ensure that older adults move safely every day to maintain function and do What Matters. *Age-Friendly Health Systems: Guide to Using the 4Ms in the Care of Older Adults* (pp. 32–33, 37) provides information about Assessing and Acting On Mobility in the context of being an Age-Friendly Health System in an inpatient setting.

Assess

Screen for mobility limitations. Incorporate your mobility screening tool into required admission documentation. If you do not have an existing tool, try using the Timed Up & Go (TUG) Test (Centers for Disease Control and Prevention & National Center for Injury Prevention and Control, 2017).

Act On

Ensure early, frequent, and safe mobility. Manage impairments that reduce mobility. Include pain scores, catheters, IV lines, telemetry orders, or other tethers such as continuous pulse oximetry, electroencephalogram (EEG), or restraints on the patient overview, rounding, and nursing handoff reports along with mobility documentation.

Within the care plan, provide a place for the RN to document the older adult's daily mobility goal and the steps needed to achieve the day's goal.

Patient activity should be documented with activities of daily living.

Figure 10.18. Using Epic for Mobility Assessments

In Epic: Use your mobility scoring/screening flowsheet documentation to fire a BPA to suggest care plan documentation. Consider adding patient education based on care planning as validated by your organization.

Examples of the Timed Up & Go assessment used at other organizations using Epic may be found in the Community Library.

Figure 10.19. Using Cerner for Discharge Plans

In Cerner: If making a specific Geriatric PowerPlan, add Case Management and Social Work referrals orders as pre-checked to make the plan standard.

Add specific patient education to discharge instructions, as validated by your organization (e.g., fall prevention, mobility, or medication education).

Transitions of Care

Utilizing Your EHR to Implement the 4Ms in Transitions of Care

At discharge, manage impairments that reduce mobility, and support creation of a safe home environment. Checklists may assist older adults and family caregivers in creating an aging-in-place-friendly home. Consider adding checklists, such as the "Check for Safety—A Home Fall Prevention Checklist for Older Adults" from the Centers for Disease Control and Prevention (CDC) & National Center for Injury Prevention and Control, and handouts, such as the "MyMobility Plan" from the CDC, in patient handouts printed directly from the EHR with the After Visit Summary (CDC & National Center for Injury Prevention and Control, 2017a, 2020).

Ensure older adults have timely outpatient follow-ups scheduled with primary care, specialists, and/or physical therapy and occupational therapy as necessary. Additionally, provide options for referrals to area agencies on aging (AAAs), community-based organizations, and/or centers for independent living (CILs).

Figure 10.20. Using Epic for Discharge Plans

In Epic: Ensure clinicians have appropriate consult orders available and suggested within discharge order sets.

Figure 10.21. Using Cerner for Follow-Up Scheduling

In Cerner: Follow-up can be scheduled during the Depart Process to ensure there is no gap in care and that the older adult or family caregiver understands how to complete this task.

Care management should ensure that adaptive/assistive devices and medications are available to older adults and that support systems are in place for assisting older adults in pursuing continued appropriate prevention, identification, treatment, and management of dementia, depression, and delirium. Further, ensure care managers have available documentation for medication availability and understanding following education.

Figure 10.22. Using Epic for Care Management

In Epic: Consider implementing a system list for care managers displaying patients 65 and older with discharge orders. Further, consider implementing the cognitive computing risk of fall (v. August 2018) and readmission models, available within Galaxy. Care managers should have discharge planning tools to encourage follow-up with outpatient resources. Scheduled appointments should be displayed on the After Visit Summary (AVS) along with suggested patient education handouts. Flowsheets should be available to document confirmation that adaptive/assistive equipment is present and older adult and/or family caregiver is educated on its use.

Figure 10.23. Using Cerner for Care Management

In Cerner: If your organization is using Cerner's Care Management Component, a custom worklist can be created for patients 65 and older. Care managers will be crucial in developing a discharge plan and assessment that best serves the patient's need, in alignment with What Matters to the patient.

Ambulatory Implementation

Utilizing Your EHR to Implement the 4Ms in the Outpatient Primary Care Setting With Older Adults

When using these guidelines for implementing the 4Ms in your EHR, validate both content and workflow inside your organization. Provide 4Ms documentation for all specialties across the continuum of care.

Figure 10.24. Beginning Epic Build

In Epic: Begin your build by creating a CER (rule) record. Choose a criterion of patient age, excluding patients under 65 years of age (e.g., "Patient Age is not less than 65 years"). This rule will be used as your filter where CER rules are accepted throughout your build. Skip this step if all components of the 4Ms will be used for all patients regardless of age. The same rule may be shared between inpatient and outpatient contexts.

The following components will be integrated into a SmartSet recommended for patients ages 65 and over.

Figure 10.25. Beginning Cerner for 4Ms Use

In Cerner: If the organization has the ability to create screening questionnaires in advance of the patient's scheduled visit, consider creating a 4Ms document for the patient to complete prior to the appointment. If your older adult population is less inclined to use patient portal technology, consider mailing the questionnaires in advance. The answers can be transcribed by the medical assistant or RN into the EHR to make the data discrete and actionable.

What Matters

Assess

Figure 10.26. Using Epic for What Matters

In Epic: Build two multi-select flowsheet rows as detailed above for general What Matters options and a third for details of the older adult's response of What Matters. Build a flowsheet group for your What Matters questions and embed the flowsheet rows. Include the group containing the flowsheet rows in the admission navigator and within the flowsheets activity. Build a print group (LPG) to display the older adult/family caregiver answers to clinicians.

A print group (LPG) should show these items at the top of a rounding report, Kardex/SBAR/Snapshot, or similar report in addition to the 4Ms report.

If using MyChart Bedside, create a questionnaire available to older adults and enable the older adult or family caregiver to answer. Responses should be enabled to file to the above flowsheets with clinician validation.

Use the Advance Care Planning activity or incorporate it into a single centralized tool to encourage comprehensive viewing and documentation of advance directives, proxies, MOLST/POLST, etc.

Figure 10.27. Using Cerner for Patient Assessment

In Cerner: For organizations using an Ambulatory Intake PowerForm or Annual Wellness Visit Form, create a new section that walks clinicians through assessing the 4Ms of the patient. (See Appendix D for a suggested build.)

If your organization uses both forms, remember to add the section to both.

Use separate DTAs to for inpatient and ambulatory assessments, to allow for different prompts for the older adults in the assessments for each of the two settings.

Using the screening tool of the organization's choice, insert another section in the Intake Form to assess Mobility and dementia.

A speciality flow sheet can be added to the Results tab for quick review by clinicians before developing the patient's plan.

Act On

Use the information documented in the assessment to align the care plan with What Matters. Within clinician notes, include documentation of what will be done to address What Matters to each older adult.

Figure 10.28. Using Epic for What Matters Documentation

In Epic: Incorporate the What Matters flowsheet into medical assistant (MA)/RN workflows. MyChart questionnaire answers should populate these rows if answered previously by the older adult or proxy. The older adult's answers to What Matters should be shown in the Summary reports shown to all clinicians.

Include older adult answers in the clinician note. Default a SmartText into the clinician note that includes information on the clinician actions addressing What Matters to the older adult. In the event that only one clinician will be seeing the older adult, use a SmartData Element (SDE) within a SmartList in the note template to capture the information that would otherwise be captured via flowsheet, above. Pull in MA/RN flowsheet documentation via SmartLink (use the metadata button to link to the provider SDE). Pursue MA/RN documentation wherever possible.

Additionally, consider building a What Matters "dotphrase" to document information as reported by the older adult.

Figure 10.29. Using Cerner PowerNote / Dynamic Documentation

In Cerner: If organization clinicians are using PowerNote, consider creating shared macros that contain language that conveys the clinician has acknowledged the older adult's wishes. Smart templates can also be coded to pull documented elements of the 4Ms into the clinician note, such as DTAs from the PowerForm assessments of What Matters, Mobility, and dementia screens. Home medications will pull into the note.

If using Dynamic Documentation (DynDoc), the same smart template recommendation can be employed, and the same home medication information will be pulled in the note.

Medication
Assess

Review for high-risk medication use. Potentially inappropriate medications for older adults include the following:

- benzodiazepines
- opioids

- highly anticholinergic medications (e.g., diphenhydramine)
- all prescription and over-the-counter sedatives and sleep medications
- muscle relaxants
- tricyclic antidepressants
- antipsychotics

Display medication alternative alerts to all specialties across the continuum of care for older adults 65 and older.

Figure 10.30. Using Epic for Medication Management

In Epic: Confirm home medications during rooming for every older adult. Ensure suggestions inside smart sets reflect age-appropriate medication choices and doses. Reconciliation and new medication orders should fire alternative alerts to clinicians and pharmacists.

From the patient reports, including the 4Ms report and clinician review reports, an age-filtered print group should appear for medications presenting greater risk to patients 65 and older.

Analysts may use Age/Sex medication warnings if using Medi-Span or Multilex and use Geriatic medication warnings if using FDB. These can be built as Medication Rules (RXR) records by your medication warning building and attached to the medication class as appropriate. Ensure your medication warning builder confirms that the alerts are set appropriately so that they are not filtered out. See the Alternative Alerts section of Galaxy for more information or discuss with your Willow IS or TS.

Act On

Figure 10.31. Using Epic for Medication Alerts

In Epic: Highlight high-risk medications. Consider adding a BPA to deprescribe either when any medications on the list are highlighted or when prescribing any medications of the list.

Figure 10.32. Using Cerner for Medication Alerts

In Cerner: If your health system is open to creating medication alerts, consider including alerts to remind clinicians to avoid or deprescribe the high-risk medications during the ordering process. These will alert physicians about high-risk medications when added to the scratchpad.

You can also consider open chart alerts based on age that remind the clinician to avoid high-risk medications.

Mentation

Assess

Screen for dementia or cognitive impairment and depression. Incorporate your dementia and depression screening tools into your intake and office-visit assessment tools. If you do not have an existing tool for dementia screening, try using the Mini-Cog screening tool (Mini-Cog, n.d.). If you do not have an existing tool for depression screening, consider implementing the Patient Health Questionnaire-2 (PHQ-2) within your organization (Pfizer, 2021).

Figure 10.33. Using Epic for Mentation Assessments

In Epic: Build dementia and depression screening tools and incorporate into your rooming activity and/or enable items to be pulled from a MyChart questionnaire populated by the older adult. These items should be filtered for older adults 65 and older.

Examples of Mini-Cog and PHQ-2 screens used at other organizations using Epic may be found on the Community Library.

Figure 10.34. Using Cerner for Mentation Assessments

In Cerner: PHQ-2 and PHQ-9 are common sections in most Intake Forms.

Other standardized assessments can be built into the Intake Form.

Act On

DEMENTIA

Consider the impact of dementia on other problems, such as difficulty remembering complicated medication regimens or other treatments, and assist older adults and family caregivers with education and support.

When clinicians add dementia or similar issues to the problem list, enable suggestions for After Visit Summary text and supportive resources on which clinicians can also counsel (e.g., the Alzheimer's Association) or consultation with specialty providers as necessary.

Figure 10.35. *Using Epic for Mentation Support*

In Epic: Use the addition of dementia and similar problems to suggest patient instructions for inclusion in the After Visit Summary via SmartSet. Use the problem list to further suggest referrals to geriatics, psychiatry, or neurology where appropriate.

Figure 10.36. *Using Cerner for Mentation Support*

In Cerner: Patient education is suggested based on diagnosis. Ensure the appropriate education is selected to meet the older adult's needs. If the organization lacks education specific to Mentation and Mobility, create custom discharge instructions and upload them into Cerner. Medication leaflets are generated with new prescriptions and can be pulled into patient education as needed.

DEPRESSION

Based on the results of the depression screen, clinicians should manage factors that contribute to depressive symptoms, including sensory limitations (vision, hearing), social isolation, losses of aging (job, income, societal roles), bereavement, and medications.

Consider the need for counseling and/or pharmacological treatment of depression, or refer to a mental health provider if appropriate.

Consider implementing tools suggesting items for the problem list based on the completed screen score, including order sets or order set components, note templates, or components of an After Visit Summary.

Mobility

Assess

Screen for mobility limitations. Incorporate your mobility screening tool into assessments or questionnaires. If you do not have an existing tool, try using the Timed Up & Go (TUG) Test.

Figure 10.37. Using Epic for Mobility Assessment

In Epic: Create a mobility score that can be documented via questionnaire in MyChart or by clinicians during assessment.

Example of the Timed Up & Go assessment used at other organizations using Epic may be found on the Community Library.

Figure 10.38. Using Cerner for Mobility Assessment

In Cerner: Consider adding mobility assessment sections to the Ambulatory Intake and Annual Wellness Visit PowerForms. Age flex the build to make these required fields for those 65 and older.

Act On

Ensure safe mobility. Manage impairments that reduce mobility, and support creation of a safe home environment. Include pain scores; strength, balance, or gait; and hazards in home, such as stairs, loose carpet or rugs, and loose or broken handrails on the patient overview reports along with mobility documentation.

When appropriate, consider adding orders for consult to physical and/or occupational therapy to order suggestions for impairments that often limit mobility.

Figure 10.39. Using Epic for Mobility Support

In Epic: Use the recommendations of your scoring system(s) to suggest SmartGroups for additional orders to address consults or therapies for mobility concerns. Suggest handouts and patient instructions based on the scoring system as well.

Implement mobility goal tracking and reporting from older adults with follow-up and support from clinical staff.

Figure 10.40. Using Epic for Mobility Goal Tracking and Documentation

In Epic: Consider implementing patient tracking of API or FHIR integration with MyChart.

Include a section within your follow-up visit workspaces for mobility goals and progress since the older adult's last visit. Flowsheets may be used for tracking over time and pulled into clinician visit notes where appropriate.

Reporting: Utilizing Your EHR to Report on 4Ms Utilization and Outcomes

Inpatient Settings

Within the inpatient context, build reports to review compliance with your definition of the 4Ms. Include patient list reports, short- and mid-term documentation compliance, and reporting of medication ordering alerts in addition to long-term outcome reporting. Filter these reports to include older adults aged 65 and older. Preferably, implement views allowing for filtering to see breakdowns of older adults aged 65–74, 75–84, and 85 and over. Compliance should be reviewed per policy and protocol at your organization by nursing and physician leadership, in addition to quality and reporting staff, to pursue opportunities for improvement.

For long-term reports, include 30-day readmission rates, Hospital Consumer Assessment of Healthcare Providers and Systems (HCAHPS), and length-of-stay metrics as well as options for filtering older adults aged 65–74, 75–84, and 85 and over in addition to an overall view of older adults 65 and older. In addition to EHR reporting, pull baseline harms reporting (not documented within an EHR) for comparison with levels following 4Ms implementation.

For any existing reports, run reports to save baseline data of patient outcomes before 4Ms implementation for later comparison.

Figure 10.41. Using Epic for Patient Reports

In Epic: Use patient list report columns to reflect completed admission and shift documentation. These should look to your organization's required documentation rules, which should be filtered for appropriate required documentation for older adults 65 and older (as detailed above).

Create Reporting Workbench reports for all admitted and recently discharged patients ages 65 and older. In these reports, show compliance of documentation, with a focus on flowsheet documentation. Further, Willow alternative alert reporting should be reviewed by physician and pharmacy leadership regularly.

Create clarity reports if not already implemented for readmissions, HCAHPS, and emergency department visit rates for patients ages 65 and over.

Consider breakdowns for reviewing data across patients 65–74, 75–84, and 85 and over.

Ambulatory Settings

Within the outpatient context, build reports to review compliance with your definition of the 4Ms. Include short- and mid-term documentation compliance in addition to reporting of medication ordering alerts. Filter these reports to older adults aged 65 and older. Preferably, implement views allowing for filtering to see breakdowns of older adults aged 65–74, 75–84, and 85 and over. Compliance should be reviewed per policy and protocol at your organization by nursing and physician leadership, in addition to quality and reporting staff, to pursue opportunities for improvement.

Figure 10.42. Using Cerner for Patient Reports

In Cerner: Create a custom DA2 report, or CCL report if a more detailed report is desired, that aggregates data from areas of the chart that include age-friendly documentation. Suggested reports that can be developed based on organizations' 4Ms implementation preference include:

- 4M PowerPlan usage (if this report has been developed)
- 4M IPOC utilization
- 4M DTA utilization
- Patient volume based on age to perform manual audits on Medication Reconciliation, Discharge Medication List, and patient follow-up

Figure 10.43. Using Cerner for Patient Reports

In Cerner: All of these data elements can be easily pulled into a custom DA2 report.

For long-term reports, include information regarding older adults with and without referral or treatment orders based on a corresponding scoring system. For example, when possible, report on older adults with and without a referral to physical or occupational therapy based on the corresponding TUG score. In additional long-term reports, include data on falls, Consumer Assessment of Healthcare Providers and Systems Clinician and Group Survey (CG-CAHPS), and emergency department visit rates for older adults aged 65 and over seen since implementation of the 4Ms and within a given reporting period (e.g., 1, 3, and 6 months).

Figure 10.44. Using Epic for Long-Term Reports

In Epic: Create Reporting Workbench reports for all admitted and recently discharged patients ages 65 and older. In these reports, show compliance of documentation, with a focus on scoring within flowsheet documentation. Consider implementing a reporting to review use of an implemented What Matters SmartText within clinician notes in comparison to the number of patients ages 65 and older seen.

Willow alternative alert reporting should be reviewed by physician and pharmacy leadership regularly. Before implementation of 4Ms criteria, save baseline data or patients on high-risk medications for later comparison post-live (e.g., 1, 3, and 6 months).

Create clarity reports looking to patients with documentation indicating a need for follow-up and appropriate completion. Examples may include referral to physical or occupational therapy based on documented TUG score, or organizationally-validated scales. Ensure an appropriate careplan is started based on the Mini-Cog screen score indicating need for treatment. Create clarity reports if not already implemented for falls, CG-CAHPS, and emergency department visit rates for patients 65 and over seen since implementation of the 4Ms and within a given reporting period (e.g., 1, 3, and 6 months).

Consider breakdowns for reviewing data across patients 65–74, 75–84, and 85 and over.

Recommendations and Summary

- Incorporate both the "assess" and "act on" drivers of the 4Ms into the EHR.

- Provide prompts for clinicians to ask about What Matters to the older adult and their goals related to health and healthcare, and document the answers in the EHR.

- Use the information documented in the assessment to align the care plan with What Matters.

- Review the EHR for high-risk medication use and avoid or deprescribe the high-risk medications listed. If the older adult takes one or more of the medications listed, discuss any concerns the patient may have, assess for adverse effects, and discuss deprescribing with the older adult.

- Screen for delirium at least every 12 hours. Incorporate your delirium screening tool into required admission and shift documentation.

- Make fields available to clinicians for documentation when prompting or encouraging older adults to drink. Use the Intake and Output and Daily Cares flowsheet templates or another location specified by your organization.

- Document orientation status in flowsheets. If the older adult is disoriented, provide a row or use the orientation row with additional options for staff to document use of gentle reorientation and/or orienting cues.

- Include a flowsheet row titled "Adaptive equipment accessible" for registered nurses (RNs) or aides to document that the older adult's items are within reach.

- Ensure that EHR documentation windows reflect policy and that clinicians can avoid sleep interruptions for older adults' assessments by clustering care.

- Offer a flowsheet row with nonpharmacological interventions as options in Bedtime Readiness: sleep aids (e.g., earplugs, sleep masks, muscle relaxation), lights dimmed, noise minimized, music, sleep kit offered, and other for RN or aide documentation.

- Screen for mobility limitations. Incorporate your mobility screening tool into required admission documentation.

- Ensure early, frequent, and safe mobility. Manage impairments that reduce mobility. Include pain scores, catheters, IV lines, telemetry orders, or other tethers such as continuous pulse oximetry, electroencephalogram (EEG), or restraints on the patient overview, rounding, and nursing handoff reports along with mobility documentation.

- At discharge, manage impairments that reduce mobility, and support creation of a safe home environment. Consider adding checklists, such as the "Check for Safety—A Home

Fall Prevention Checklist for Older Adults" from the Centers for Disease Control and Prevention (CDC) & National Center for Injury Prevention and Control, and handouts, such as the "MyMobility Plan" from the CDC, in patient handouts printed directly from the EHR with the After Visit Summary.

While there is still a larger need to ensure that all EHRs support the documentation and implementation of the 4Ms model, this guide was designed to help health systems get started. All content and workflow should be validated inside your health system, and all policies and procedures should be updated to reflect any adopted build. Further, building the 4Ms in the EHR is simply a starting point. Health systems and all organizations that use EHRs should consider the barriers to making electronic data usable and interoperable, understand how these tools might integrate into existing clinical workflows, and plan to train staff on how workflows will change. The goal is to ensure the 4Ms can be documented and used in a reliable and efficient way to ensure that care is consistent with the 4Ms across care settings.

References

Centers for Disease Control and Prevention. & National Center for Injury Prevention and Control (2017a). *Check for safety: A home fall prevention checklist for older adults.* https://www.cdc.gov/steadi/pdf/STEADI-Brochure-CheckForSafety-508.pdf

Centers for Disease Control and Prevention & National Center for Injury Prevention and Control. (2017b). *Timed Up & Go (TUG).* https://www.cdc.gov/steadi/pdf/TUG_Test-print.pdf

Centers for Disease Control and Prevention & National Center for Injury Prevention and Control. (2020). *MyMobility plan.* https://www.cdc.gov/motorvehiclesafety/pdf/older_adult_drivers/CDC-AdultMobilityTool-9.27.pdf

Fick, D. M., Inouye, S. K., McDermott, C., Zhou, W., Ngo, L., Gallagher, J., McDowell, J., Penrod, J., Siuta, J., Covaleski, T., & Marcantonio, E. R. (2018). Pilot study of a two-step delirium detection protocol administered by certified nursing assistants, physicians, and registered nurses. *Journal of Gerontological Nursing, 44*(5), 18–24. https://doi.org/10.3928/00989134-20180302-01

Institute for Healthcare Improvement. (2019). *Age-friendly health systems: Guide to electronic health record requirements for adoption of the 4Ms. An implementation guide for health system with cerner examples.* http://www.ihi.org/Engage/Initiatives/Age-Friendly-Health-Systems/Documents/IHI_Age_Friendly_Health_Systems_Cerner_Implementation_Guide.pdf

Mini-Cog. (n.d.). *Using the Mini-Cog.* https://mini-cog.com/about/using-the-mini-cog/

Pfizer. (2021). *Welcome to the Patient Health Questionnaire (PHQ) screeners.* https://www.phqscreeners.com/

CHAPTER 11

Transitions of Care

C urrent trends within the US healthcare system, such as the focus on specialization and single-disease management programs, also contribute to the likelihood of adverse outcomes for individuals with comorbidities undergoing transitions.

High rates of preventable hospitalizations and ED visits are among the most burdensome consequences. In a recent Medicare Payment Advisory Commission (MedPAC) Report to the Congress, all-cause 30-day rehospitalization rates for Medicare beneficiaries decreased from an average of 19% to below 18%, at least in part due to major changes in incentives (Hirschman et al., 2015). However, among Medicare beneficiaries with four or more chronic conditions, the 30-day rehospitalization rate was 36% (Lochner et al., 2013).

While some rehospitalizations are appropriate and unavoidable, between 13% and 20% of those experienced by chronically ill older adults are conservatively estimated to be preventable (Bentler et al., 2014; Nyweide et al., 2013). In addition to the tremendous human burden, societal costs associated with supporting older adults are significant. In 2011, an average of $2,097 was spent annually on healthcare for Medicare beneficiaries aged 65 and older with up to one chronic condition compared to $11,628 for those with four to five conditions and $31,543 for those with six or more conditions. In 2010, healthcare services for Medicare beneficiaries with four or more chronic conditions accounted for 74% of total Medicare spending (Centers for Medicare & Medicaid Services, 2012). The vast majority of these costs were due to high rates of often avoidable hospitalizations and rehospitalizations (MedPAC, 2014).

These are often the result of care transitions, characterized as changes in the level and location of care with a handoff from one healthcare team to another, which often lead to conflicting instructions, medication discrepancies, and lack of follow-up appointments with primary care providers after hospitalizations (Foust et al., 2012). This fractured and inappropriate care may be unaligned with individuals' goals and preferences, resulting in poor outcomes (National Quality Forum, 2012). Current trends within the US healthcare system, such as the focus on specialization and single-disease management programs, also contribute to the likelihood of adverse outcomes for individuals with comorbidities undergoing transitions.

Six overlapping categories of problems have been associated with negative outcomes among hospitalized older adults with multiple chronic conditions (MCCs) who transition to post-acute settings or their homes: lack of patient engagement; absent or inadequate communication; lack of collaboration among team members; limited follow-up and monitoring; poor continuity of care; and serious gaps in services as patients move between healthcare professionals (clinicians) and across care settings (Bowles et al., 2010; Naylor, 2012). Among this patient group, these system issues have been linked to poor ratings of the care experience and further declines in health status (Naylor et al., 2004).

In general, recipients of long-term services and supports (LTSS) frequently transition between LTSS settings (e.g., assisted living facilities, nursing homes) and hospitals for acute changes in health. In interviews with 57 recently hospitalized LTSS recipients and their family caregivers describing barriers and facilitators to high-quality care to support older adults through these care transitions, a study found that LTSS recipients and family caregivers do not receive needed information about the reasons for their transfers to hospitals, medical diagnoses, and planned treatments to address acute changes in health. Findings indicate an urgent need for nurses and other healthcare team members to talk with LTSS recipients (and family caregivers) and ensure they are engaged and informed participants in care. There is also a need for research to test evidence-based transitional care for high-risk LTSS recipients and their family caregivers.

Components of Comprehensive and Effective Transitional Care

A study funded by the Patient-Centered Outcomes Research Institute (PCORI), Achieving Patient-Centered Care and Optimized Health In Care Transitions by Evaluating the Value of Evidence (Project ACHIEVE), found eight core components essential to Transitional Care: patient engagement, caregiver engagement, complexity and medication management, patient education, caregiver education, patients' and caregivers' well-being, care continuity, and accountability (Naylor et al., 2017). Although the degree of attention given to each component will vary based on the specific needs of patients and caregivers, workgroup members agree that health systems need to address all components to ensure optimal transitional care for all Medicare beneficiaries.

Table 11.1. Categories of Patients' and Caregivers' Issues
Throughout Transitions and Specific Examples of the Issues

CATEGORY	EXAMPLES
Lack of patient or caregiver engagement	• Patients' or caregivers' levels of engagement are not assessed. • Transition planning does not include patients or caregivers. • Plans of care do not include patient (e.g., ability to work in garden) or caregiver (e.g., confidence in capacity to manage loved one's care) goals or preferences. • Patients and caregivers lack necessary information to participate in decision-making regarding their plans of care.
Poor continuity of care	• Patients and caregivers do not know whom to call with questions or concerns following transitions to home. • Information regarding the plan of care is not transmitted among organizations, healthcare team members, patients, and caregivers.
Inadequate preparation	• Health literacy or language barriers are not identified or addressed. • Patients and caregivers are not provided adequate time to absorb instructions or demonstrate knowledge and skills regarding follow-up care or symptom or medication management. • Caregivers are not adequately prepared and lack confidence, resources, and support to care for patients.
Gaps in services	• Healthcare team members lack organizational support needed to ensure seamless transitions. • Coordination of services between hospitals and community providers is often inadequate.
Absent or inadequate communication	• Absence of relationships between patients and caregivers and healthcare professionals has negative effect on patients' level of trust and adherence to care plans.
Limited collaboration	• Patients and caregivers are not considered part of the healthcare team. • Healthcare team members do not communicate with one another or fail to resolve differences regarding critical elements of care plans.
Multiple health and social challenges	• Patients often have multiple coexisting health conditions complicated by functional deficits, cognitive impairment, substance abuse, or depression—as well as social problems, such as poverty—that affect needs and outcomes. • Seriously ill patients often are not provided with the opportunity and support needed to explore palliative care and end-of-life decisions.
Complex treatment regimens	• Errors of omission and commission involving complex medication plans are common. • Patients and caregivers often feel overwhelmed and experience emotional distress because of responsibilities for managing complex care needs at home.

Table 11.2. Strategies to Implement Project ACHIEVE
Transitional Care Core Components

COMPONENT	STRATEGIES	CATEGORIES OF PATIENTS' AND CAREGIVERS' ISSUES
Patient engagement	• Conducting comprehensive assessment to identify patients' goals • Demonstrating respect for patients as partners in developing care plans reflective of their goals • Monitoring patients' progress at achieving their goals • Enabling timely bidirectional communication and care continuity • Continually evaluating patients' levels of engagement	• Lack of patient and/or caregiver engagement • Poor continuity of care • Absent or inadequate communication • Limited collaboration
Caregiver engagement	• Conducting comprehensive assessments to identify caregivers and determine their preferences and capabilities • Demonstrating respect for caregivers as partners in developing care plans reflective of their goals • Monitoring caregivers' progress at achieving their goals and helping patients to meet their needs • Enabling timely bidirectional communication and care continuity • Continually evaluating caregivers' levels of engagement	• Lack of patient and/or caregiver engagement • Poor continuity of care • Absent or inadequate communication • Limited collaboration
Complexity / medication management	• Identifying high-risk patients • Anticipating and planning for common transitional care problems • Managing common coexisting chronic conditions and other health and social risks • Preventing the occurrence of post-hospital syndrome • Aligning health and community services with patients' and caregivers' goals throughout transitions • Ensuring that medication management plan is based on evidence • Respecting patients' choices in adherence to plan • Providing appropriate information and training so that patient is knowledgeable and confident • Evaluating access to medications • Monitoring to avoid medication errors	• Lack of patient and/or caregiver engagement • Inadequate preparation • Gaps in services • Limited collaboration • Multiple health and social challenges • Complex treatment regimens

Patient education	• Identifying and addressing health literacy and language • Presenting health information in easily accessible, accurate, and usable formats • Confirming patients' understanding of instructions	• Lack of patient and/or caregiver engagement • Inadequate preparation • Multiple health and social challenges • Complex treatment regimens
Caregiver education	• Involving caregivers in planning care • Respecting and valuing caregivers' contributions to team • Providing appropriate information and training to help caregivers feel knowledgeable and confident • Referring caregivers to community-based resources for support	• Lack of patient and/or caregiver engagement • Inadequate preparation • Multiple health and social challenges • Complex treatment regimens • Gaps in services
Patients' and caregivers' well-being	• Fostering early identification and interventions to address emotional distress • Recognizing caregivers' common concerns regarding reactions to caregiving role, including fear of harming their loved ones • Identifying and implementing effective strategies to support patients' and caregivers' emotional well-being	• Lack of patient and/or caregiver engagement • Poor continuity of care • Inadequate preparation • Absent or inadequate communication • Multiple health and social challenges
Care continuity	• Ensuring follow-up with primary care clinicians and specialists, home care or community-based services, etc. • Communicating effectively among inpatient team and community-based healthcare team • Encouraging members of healthcare team to engage patients and caregivers in trusting, reciprocal, respectful relationships	• Lack of patient and/or caregiver engagement • Poor continuity of care • Absent or inadequate communication
Accountability (clinician, team, organizational)	• Fulfilling each clinician's responsibilities in comprehensive, timely manner • Collaborating as a team to ensure that patients' and caregivers' goals and preferences are met • Providing reliable performance-improvement support for transitional care programs	• Lack of patient and/or caregiver engagement • Poor continuity of care • Gaps in services • Absent or inadequate communication • Limited collaboration

Continuity of Care: The Transitional Care Model

One rigorously tested model that has consistently demonstrated effectiveness in addressing the needs of this complex population while reducing healthcare costs is the Transitional Care Model (TCM). The TCM is a nurse-led intervention targeting older adults at risk for poor outcomes as they move across healthcare settings and between clinicians.

The TCM intervention focuses on improving care; enhancing patient and family caregiver outcomes; and reducing costs among vulnerable, chronically ill older adults identified in health systems and community-based settings, such as patient-centered medical homes (PCMHs). Over the past two decades, this nurse-led, team-based model of care has been designed, tested, and refined by a multidisciplinary team of clinical scholars and health services researchers based at the University of Pennsylvania. The TCM emphasizes identification of patients' health goals, design and implementation of a streamlined plan of care, and continuity of care across settings and between providers throughout episodes of acute illness (e.g., hospital to home; Naylor et al., 2014).

Under this model, care is both delivered and coordinated by the same master's-prepared advanced practice registered nurse (APRN) in collaboration with patients, their family caregivers, physicians, and other health team members. The TCM supplements care provided to patients in the hospital and substitutes for care provided by professional nurses in patients' homes.

Table 11.3. Transitional Care Model Components and Definitions

COMPONENT	DEFINITION
Screening	Targets adults transitioning from hospital to home who are at high risk for poor outcomes.
Staffing	Uses APRNs who assume primary responsibility for care management throughout episodes of acute illness.
Maintaining relationships	Establishes and maintains a trusting relationship with the patient and family caregivers involved in the patient's care.
Engaging patients and caregivers	Engages older adults in design and implementation of the plan of care aligned with their preferences, values, and goals.
Assessing/managing risks and symptoms	Identifies and addresses the patient's priority risk factors and symptoms.
Educating/promoting self-management	Prepares older adults and family caregivers to identify and respond quickly to worsening symptoms.
Collaborating	Promotes consensus on plan of care between older adults and members of the care team.
Promoting continuity	Prevents breakdowns in care from hospital to home by having same clinician involved across these sites.
Fostering coordination	Promotes communication and connections between healthcare and community-based practitioners.

Table 11.4. *Domains and Examples of Standardized Tools Used for Clinical Assessment Over Time*

DOMAIN	TOOLS	COMPLETED WITH
Cognitive	Six-item screener	Patient
Delirium	Confusion Assessment Method Diagnostic Algorithm (CAM) or Family CAM (FAM-CAM; Steis et al., 2012)	Patient, family caregiver (CG)
Function	• Timed Up & Go (TUG) Test • Basic activities of daily living • Instrumental activities of daily living	Patient
Symptoms	• Symptom Bother Scale • Edmonton Symptom Assessment Scale-Pain and Anxiety (Selby et al., 2010) • Patient Health Questionnaire-9 (PHQ-9)	Patient
Patient engagement	Healthcare Empowerment Inventory (HCEI; Johnson et al., 2012)	Patient, family CG
Care preferences	Absence or presence of advance directive: • type of advance directive (e.g., Living Will, Physician Orders for Life Sustaining Treatment [POLST], Durable Power of Attorney for Health Care [DPOAHC]) • interest in discussing care • preferences if not documented	Patient, family CG, electronic medical record (EMR)
Health literacy	Brief Health Literacy Scale (BHLS; Wallston et al., 2014)	Patient, family CG
Substance abuse	Alcohol Use Disorders Identification Test (AUDIT-C)—cut-point of ≥ 5 risky alcohol use in geriatric population (Draper et al., 2015)	Patient
Polypharmacy and medication behavior	• Number of medications taken daily or schedule complexity • High-risk medications	Patient, EMR
Self-monitoring	Verify self-monitoring being completed by patient as part of self-management • watch patient do what they need to for self-care (e.g., checking blood glucose, weighing self, checking blood pressure) • this should consistently go in the Subjective, Objective, Assessment and Plan (SOAP) note	Patient, family CG
Nutrition	• Unexplained weight loss of ≥ 10 pounds or ≥ 5% of body weight or persistent weight loss • Mini Nutrition Assessment (MNA)	Patient, EMR, family CG

Skin integrity	Braden Scale for Predicting Pressure Sore Risk (Braden, 2012)	Patient, family CG
Social support	• Living situation • Availability of caregivers • Community resources used	Patient, EMR
Caregiver needs	Next Step in Care Assessment—guided conversation (United Hospital Fund, 2015) • availability, training needs, worries	Family CG

Recommendations and Summary

Successful transitions of care are based on excellent communication between and among care team members and across all sites of care that will be engaged, including the possibility of skilled nursing facilities, hospice, and home care organizations. It is vital to work closely with family members as well as those who will be providing long-term services and supports for optimal information exchange and quality outcomes for the older adult.

Many issues have plagued continuity of information and care, including lack of patient engagement, absent or inadequate communication, lack of collaboration among team members, limited follow-up and monitoring, poor continuity of care, and serious gaps in services as patients move between healthcare professionals (clinicians) and across care settings. Project ACHIEVE features eight core components that seek to address these issues: patient engagement, caregiver engagement, complexity and medication management, patient education, caregiver education, patients' and caregivers' well-being, care continuity, and accountability. The Transitional Care Model similarly comprises screening, staffing, maintaining relationships, engaging patients and caregivers, assessing and managing risk symptoms, educating and promoting self-management, collaborating, promoting continuity, and fostering coordination. We recommend using one of these models to develop and optimize care for high-risk older adults.

References

Bentler, S. E., Morgan, R. O., Virnig, B. A., & Wolinsky, F. D. (2014). The association of longitudinal and interpersonal continuity of care with emergency department use, hospitalization, and mortality among Medicare beneficiaries. *PloS One*, 9(12), e115088. https://doi.org/10.1371/journal.pone.0115088

Bowles, K. H., Pham, J., O'Connor, M., & Horowitz, D. A. (2010). Information deficits in home care: A barrier to evidence-based disease management. *Home Health Care Management & Practice*, 22(4), 278–285. https://doi.org/10.1177/1084822309353145

Braden, B. J. (2012). The Braden Scale for predicting pressure sore risk: Reflections after 25 years. *Advances in Skin & Wound Care*, 25(2), 61. https://doi.org/10.1097/01.asw.0000411403.11392.10

Centers for Medicare & Medicaid Services. (2012). *Chronic conditions among Medicare beneficiaries, chartbook* [2012 edition]. www.cms.gov/Research-Statistics-Data-and-Systems/Statistics-Trends-and-Reports/Chronic-Conditions/Downloads/2012Chartbook.pdf

Draper, B., Ridley, N., Johnco, C., Withall, A., Sim, W., Freeman, M., Contini, E., & Lintzeris, N. (2015). Screening for alcohol and substance use for older people in geriatric hospital and community health settings. *International Psychogeriatrics*, 27(1), 157–166. https://doi.org/10.1017/s1041610214002014

Foust, J. B., Naylor, M. D., Bixby, M. B., & Ratcliffe, S. J. (2012). Medication problems occurring at hospital discharge among older adults with heart failure. *Research in Gerontological Nursing*, 5(1), 25–33. https://doi.org/10.3928/19404921-20111206-04

Hirschman, K. B., Shaid, E., McCauley, K., Pauly, M. V., & Naylor, M. D. (2015). Continuity of care: The transitional care model. Online *Journal of Issues in Nursing*, 20(3), manuscript 1. https://www.doi.org/10.3912/OJIN.Vol20No03Man01

Johnson, M. O., Dawson-Rose, C., Dilworth, S. E., & Neilands, T. B. (2012). Advances in the conceptualization and measurement of health care empowerment: Development and validation of the Health Care Empowerment Inventory. *PloS One*, 7(9), e45692. https://doi.org/10.1371/journal.pone.0045692

Lochner, K. A., Goodman, R. A., Posner, S., & Parekh, A. (2013). Multiple chronic conditions among Medicare beneficiaries: State-level variations in prevalence, utilization, and cost, 2011. *Medicare & Medicaid Research Review*, 3(3), mmrr.003.03.b02. https://doi.org/10.5600/mmrr.003.03.b02

Medicare Payment Advisory Commission. (2014). *A data book: Health care spending and the Medicare program.* MedPAC.

National Quality Forum. (2012). *Multiple chronic conditions measurement framework.* https://www.qualityforum.org/WorkArea/linkit.aspx?LinkIdentifier=id&ItemID=71227

Naylor, M. D. (2012). Advancing high value transitional care: The central role of nursing and its leadership. *Nursing Administration Quarterly*, 36(2), 115–126. https://doi.org/10.1097/naq.0b013e31824a040b

Naylor, M. D., Brooten, D. A., Campbell, R. L., Maislin, G., McCauley, K. M., & Schwartz, J. S. (2004). Transitional care of older adults hospitalized with heart failure: A randomized, controlled trial. *Journal of the American Geriatrics Society*, 52(5), 675–684. https://doi.org/10.1111/j.1532-5415.2004.52202.x

Naylor, M. D., Hirschman, K. B., Hanlon, A. L., Bowles, K. H., Bradway, C., McCauley, K. M., & Pauly, M. V. (2014). Comparison of evidence-based interventions on outcomes of hospitalized, cognitively impaired older adults. *Journal of Comparative Effectiveness Research*, 3(3), 245–257. https://doi.org/10.2217/cer.14.14

Naylor, M. D., Shaid, E. C., Carpenter, D., Gass, B., Levine, C., Li, J., Malley, A., McCauley, K., Nguyen, H. Q., Watson, H., Brock, J., Mittman, B., Jack, B., Mitchell, S., Callicoatte, B., Schall, J., & Williams, M. V. (2017). Components of comprehensive and effective transitional care. *Journal of the American Geriatrics Society*, 65(6), 1119–1125. https://doi.org/10.1111/jgs.14782

Nyweide, D. J., Anthony, D. L., Bynum, J. P. W., Strawderman, R. L., Weeks, W. B., Casalino, L. P., & Fisher, E. S. (2013). Continuity of care and the risk of preventable hospitalization in older adults. *JAMA Internal Medicine*, 173(20), 1879–1885. https://doi.org/10.1001/jamainternmed.2013.10059

Selby, D., Cascella, A., Gardiner, K., Do, R., Moravan, V., Myers, J., & Chow, E. (2010). A single set of numerical cutpoints to define moderate and severe symptoms for the Edmonton Symptom Assessment System. *Journal of*

Pain and Symptom Management, 39(2), 241–249. https://doi.org/10.1016/j.jpainsymman.2009.06.010

Steis, M. R., Evans, L., Hirschman, K. B., Hanlon, A., Fick, D. M., Flanagan, N., & Inouye, S. K. (2012). Screening for delirium using family caregivers: Convergent validity of the Family Confusion Assessment Method and interviewer-rated Confusion Assessment Method. *Journal of the American Geriatrics Society, 60*(11), 2121–2126. https://doi.org/10.1111/j.1532-5415.2012.04200.x

United Hospital Fund. (2015). *What do family caregivers need?* https://www.nextstepincare.org/Provider_Home/What_Do_I_Need/

Wallston, K. A., Cawthon, C., McNaughton, C. D., Rothman, R. L., Osborn, C. Y., & Kripalani, S. (2014). Psychometric properties of the brief health literacy screen in clinical practice. *Journal of General Internal Medicine, 29*(1), 119–126. https://doi.org/10.1007/s11606-013-2568-0

CHAPTER 12

The Big Challenge:
Spread and Scale

uccessful geriatric care models have been developed in response to the important needs of vulnerable older persons. However, as noted, most models reach only a small portion of those who could benefit from the care. Some models are difficult to disseminate and scale because of, for example, high costs of personnel or space. Each model must identify the older adults who could benefit from the model and, therefore, improve in care. The methodology of some models is difficult to reproduce in community hospitals with fewer resources. When an inventory is taken in any given health system, multiple models coexist and may confuse both staff and older adults. When getting started, it is important to assess the status and progress of 4Ms implementation. Team Action Planning (TAP) is recommended (IHI, 2018a). A central part of TAP is the effective use of action communities.

Becoming an Age-Friendly Health System entails reliably providing a set of four evidence-based elements of high-quality care, known as the "4Ms," to all older adults in your system. When implemented together, the 4Ms represent a broad shift by health systems to focus on the needs of older adults. To accelerate the adoption of the 4Ms across health systems, IHI developed an Action Community model to facilitate peer learning and active testing of evidence-based changes.

An Action Community is a network of teams from across different health systems around the country and world who come together to support their adoption of the 4Ms. Guided by expert faculty and an "all teach, all learn" model, teams participate in monthly webinars, attend a convening, and test specific changes to improve care for older adults (IHI, 2018a). The Action Community is designed as an "on-ramp" for hospital-based teams (e.g., emergency departments, intensive care units, general wards, medical-surgical units), ambulatory care teams (e.g., primary care, specialty care), and nursing home teams (e.g., post-acute and long-term care) to test and adopt age-friendly care.

To participate in the Action Community, health systems identify a clinical care setting to pilot-test the 4Ms; bring together an interdisciplinary team (ideally including an older adult and/or family caregiver); and identify a leader with authority over the selected care setting or population to support the team's activities and progress.

Teams involved in the Action Community join monthly team webinars that focus on understanding the steps for testing and implementing age-friendly care in their setting and illustrating 4Ms care in action through case examples from their peers. In addition, teams participate in peer-coaching webinars to share ideas, successes, and challenges related to specific topics; quarterly webinars for leaders and sponsors to support leaders in the scale-up of age-friendly care beyond the pilot site and throughout the health system; and an in-person (or virtual, when necessary) convening to build relation-ships and create momentum for committing to the practice of age-friendly care.

At the end of the 7-month Action Community, participating orga-nizations have implemented specific changes of the Age-Friendly Health Systems 4Ms framework in their unit, clinic, emergency department, or program. For the majority of the team, participation in an Action Community results in recognition as an Age-Friendly Health System Participant and Committed to Care Excellence by IHI and The John A. Hartford Foundation. To be recognized, health orga-nizations submit a description of how they are operationalizing the 4Ms in their setting, as well as monthly counts of the older adults reached by 4Ms care in their setting.

Building on the success of the Action Community model, IHI has developed template Action Community materials, training, and a model of support to engage partners in the Age-Friendly Health Systems movement in facilitating Action Communities with teams from their own network. Partner organizations that have facilitated an Action Community include the American Geriatrics Society, the American Hospital Association, the Healthcare Association of New York State, and the Michigan Hospital Association Keystone Center. IHI and these partners have facilitated nine Action Communities, and at least five more will launch in 2021 (IHI, 2021h).

Resistance

Resistance in any change process or with the introduction of any new approach is inevitable. Thus, it is important to identify the sources of resistance and determine how everyone can work together to address the resistance and assess how to overcome the unintended barriers to progress (IHI, 2021d). There is also fear that a project will be forced into place; that is where it is very important to reframe the ideas and explain how people can do what they want to do, while at the same time doing what you want them to do. This means working together to unearth shared values, focus on stories, craft a shared outcome, and make collective choices. Resistance should never be taken personally, and when someone answers "no," that does not mean "never." Making change a personal performance target can be an effective way of thinking about how to "fail forward," in which you can explain your way to improvement and understand that virtually all innovation, improvement, or acquisition of a new skill requires that there will be mistakes and lessons learned. Mistakes should be shared openly to determine how the next phase of the work will be successful.

Tool 1: Planning to Fail Forward

If/Then Planning:

1. State the goal.
2. Turn into if/then statement.
3. Develop an if/then plan.

Tool 2: Failure Modes

1. Identify a potential failure or risk.
2. Assess its likelihood of occurring (1–10).
3. Assess the severity if it occurs (1–10).
4. Generate a total score: likelihood × severity.
5. Determine mitigation strategies.

Figure 12.1. E. M. Rogers's Diffusion of Innovation, 1962

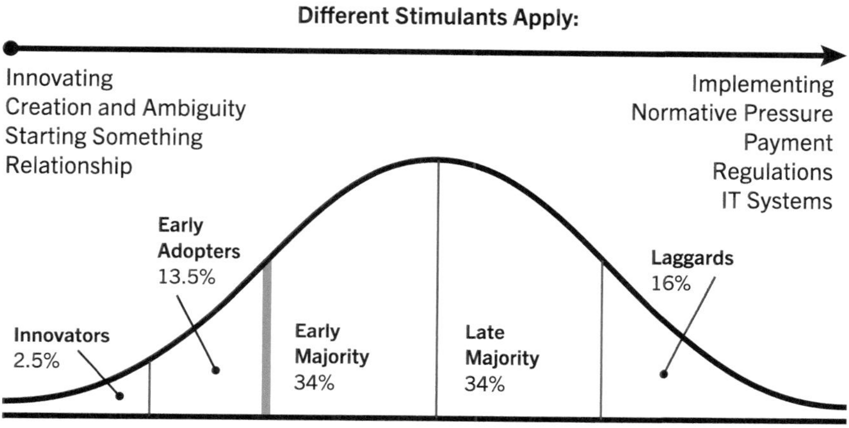

Different Stimulants Apply:

Innovating
Creation and Ambiguity
Starting Something
Relationship

Implementing
Normative Pressure
Payment
Regulations
IT Systems

Early Adopters
13.5%

Laggards
16%

Innovators
2.5%

Early Majority
34%

Late Majority
34%

Organizing = People, Power, and Change

Fundamental to organizing any change process is understanding the people involved, how to empower them, and being very clear on the change they want to see (IHI, 2021e).

- Who are our People?
- What Change do they want?
- How can they get the Power they need to achieve that change?

It should be noted that economic assets (money, materials, technology) diminish with use; moral assets (relationships, commitment, discretionary effort) grow with use. This is an uplifting message to share with the people with whom you are working so they understand that it is not simply a matter of more money but more commitment and joy in the outcome of the work.

Figure 12.2. *Organizing to Accelerate Quality Improvement at Scale*

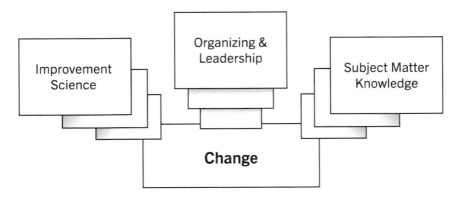

Organizing

In his organizing work, Ganz (2010) emphasizes the subjective agency of social-movement participants, whose values, intentions, and narratives constitute the essential material of analysis. Ganz begins with the famous three questions of Hillel the Elder: "If I am not for myself, who will be for me? But if I am only for myself, what am I? And if not now, when?" Ganz relates these questions to "the story of self," "the story of us," and "the story of now." Making the work clear and accessible to those you are inviting to the table is the first step, which will

- accelerate the adoption of quality improvements;
- build an equal-status contract around a shared purpose;
- be commitment-driven, not compliance-based;
- cultivate people's agency to act—increasing joy, job satisfaction, and improved health; and
- build capacity that serves as an ongoing resource for addressing other problems.

Mapping Stakeholders and Assets

Any one of us who has begun a project in our healthcare setting knows the challenge, potential resistance, and inertia that can come into play as we get underway. We have found that it is extremely important to think about how to map stakeholders and assets and to be transparent with all members participating to ensure that the community involved understands the goals and is fully participatory in the solutions (IHI, 2018b). Fundamental starting points include the following:

- creating a collaborative workspace
- collecting tools to facilitate collaboration
- brainstorming with stakeholders (e.g., individuals, institutions/ governments, organizations, sources of community pride, other capital)
- mapping stakeholders: who will care about the work? who will resist?
  - constituents
  - leadership
  - supporters
  - competition
  - opposition
- brainstorming and mapping stakeholders' values
- brainstorming and mapping stakeholders' interests
- brainstorming and mapping stakeholders' assets
  - primary asset: most-accessible assets are located in the neighborhood or community and controlled by those who are members of that neighborhood or community
  - secondary asset: located in the neighborhood or community, but controlled by individuals and/or organizations outside the neighborhood

- potential asset: least-accessible assets are located and controlled outside the neighborhood

Once you have created your map, you can use it to advance your project, keeping in mind that it is not a static device but rather a way to help discern values and distinguish between values and interests. Regular review will help you understand why it is important to do the work and understand what the assets you have to bring to bear for progress.

Relational Tactics

Any change in a system requires careful communication and an exquisite understanding of the relationships involved in the way that people think about change as well as how embedded they are to their current status quo (IHI, 2020). As you begin your spread-and-scale process of change, several things need to take place:

- one-on-one meetings to identify and recruit leaders and get to know your people
- unit meetings to build community around the effort
- leadership team meetings to build relationships among those leading the work
- prototype actions to build relationships among those taking action
- leadership training to introduce relationship building as a skill

A Plan for Intentional Spread

Intentional spread is at the heart of a strong and successful campaign. This means that the goal necessarily needs to be the development of initial internal success stories and that key stakeholders who understand the needs can bring them to the internal group. It is also important to have an intentional naming of the launch for the initiative.

Figure 12.3. How Will We Get There? (Massoud et al., 2006)

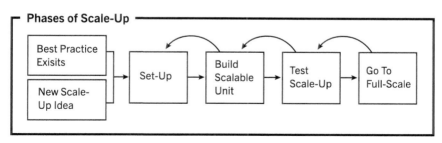

When you launch your Age-Friendly Health System, you need to work with your communications department in order to set a date for the launch, use your press kit that has been developed by IHI, and have a strong launch day (IHI, 2021b). Your local newspapers and radio stations should be invited to your launch day. About 80% of the work is available to you from IHI, and about 20% will need to be customized to your organization. Public celebrations are also very important and allow everyone to engage in meaningful change.

Assessing the Readiness of an Idea for Rapid Spread

The field of geriatrics has matured to the point where we have the evidence required to make the case for the 4Ms and clearly show why 4Ms care is better than the old way of supporting older adults (IHI, 2021a). In the past, if someone was not eating, clinicians used a feeding tube to ensure calories were acquired. If older people were incontinent, clinicians used protective devices and Foley catheters instead of working on bladder training. If older people were falling, clinicians would place them in protective restraints in order to keep them still so that they would not fall instead of enhancing their mobility. And finally, if older adults were delirious, clinicians used medication to silence their cries for help. Healthcare professionals have learned a great deal over the past five decades, and reviewing our past practices makes us cringe. Pointing out these changes can be very motivational not only for staff but for older patients and families as well as informal caregivers. As healthcare professionals, we know how to do the work, and it is up to us to make sure that the work is done reliably through an Age-Friendly Health Systems 4Ms approach.

When introducing the approach, it is important to explain the following:

- simplicity of the change: how easy the 4Ms model is to adopt
- testability: people can try the 4Ms model
- observability: people can see the 4Ms model in action before trying it
- flexibility: the extent to which individuals customize the 4Ms model to their context

Spread and Scale Framing

Table 12.1. *5× Scale-Up for Improving Care for Older Adults*

NUMBER OF INDIVIDUALS	SYSTEMIC ISSUES TO OVERCOME OR QUESTIONS TO ANSWER
5	Can we make these changes—within a practitioner's scope of practice? Solve role.
25	Can we test and regularize time, setting, and information? Solve measure, flow, scope in team.
125	Can we settle on standard practice and standard measures? Test information, payment, add sites.
625	Can we automate, and can we get paid? Solve many locations, subcategories, information, payment.
3,125	Can we change jobs, personnel, and patient expectations? Solve professional norms, standards.
15,625	Can we improve care for all older adults? Solve regulation, standards, payment, information, culture.

Using a Campaign Strategy to Test Scale-Up and Go to Full Scale

Originally adapted from the works of Marshall Ganz, Harvard University; modified by Kate B. Hilton, IHI

In organizing, a campaign is a way to mobilize time, resources, and energy to achieve an aim. In a campaign, we view time as an arrow instead of as a cycle (IHI, 2021g). Thinking of time as a cycle helps us maintain our routines, our annual budget, and our seasonal events. Thinking of time as an arrow focuses us on making change, on achieving specific outcomes, and on focusing our efforts. A campaign encompasses intense streams of activity beginning with a foundational period, building to a kickoff, then building to periodic peaks in which we achieve nested outcomes, and culminating with a final peak (our aim), which is followed by resolution. This creates momentum strategically by gathering more and more resources as we go.

Reaching a threshold that gives us new capacity is a campaign "peak." It is a threshold that we are able to cross as a result of mobilizing the most resources we can to achieve it. It is an unsustainable peak of effort—once we cross that peak, we can relax our effort briefly to study and move on to another PDSA cycle to reach our next peak. This way, we also make adjustments to our approach based on observable data as we go. A campaign is necessarily built around a series of peaks and PDSA cycles, culminating in a final peak when we have either achieved our overarching aim or not.

Campaigns call on three types of metrics for each "peak":

- aim achieved
- capacity built
- leaders developed

That is because we focus on building the leadership and capacity of our people, teams, health systems, and partners to work together to generate enough commitment to achieve our overarching aim to create Age-Friendly Health Systems. This means that we "chunk out" how we will achieve the 4Ms over time and identify milestones for when we will have created enough new capacity and developed enough power to undertake activities that we could not before. Each peak launches us forward toward our next peak.

As you consider capacity building aims, consider how you might employ relational tactics of one-to-one meetings, age-friendly team meetings, unit meetings, 4Ms improvement events, partner gatherings, and leadership trainings. Set clear targets around the number of people you set out to engage. How many people will you build relationships with through one-to-one meetings and by when? How many unit leaders and teams will you recruit across your health system, and how many community partners will you engage? What are your targets? We set targets so we can evaluate and learn from our success and failure.

Figure 12.4. *The Sequence of Improvement*

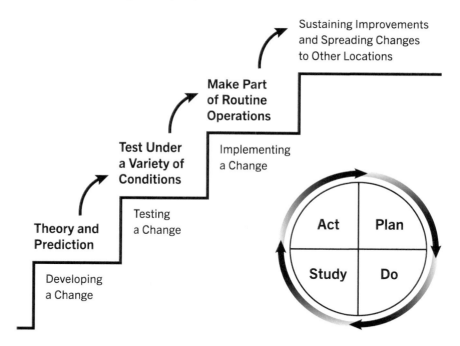

Many assume that innovative, evidence-based ideas will be easily adopted and implemented through education and changes in policies. Those tactics are essential but not sufficient. Spread of an innovation across a site of care or a health system occurs with intentional effort and specific activities.

Table 12.2. Testing Versus Implementation

TESTING	IMPLEMENTATION
Trying and adapting ideas on a small scale	A permanent change in how work is done
• Change is temporary • Variation is good • Learning what works in local system • Failure is valuable and welcome • "Coalition of the willing" • Old system remains in place	• Change is permanent • Standard work • Failure not expected • Everyone expected to adopt • Old system is no longer an option • Requires changes in support processes

Science of Improvement: Testing Changes

Plan-Do-Study-Act

- Initial PDSAs often *collect information* about how a process or system is working and prompt ideas for change.

- Early small-scale PDSAs focused on identifying and *testing useful changes and ideas.*

- Promising changes tested as a new *process design.* Refine, adapt, and test in all required conditions.

- *Implementation* installs fully tested prototype as new standard of work. Support functions adapted as required.

- *Spread*: Implemented model adopted and adapted in new facilities, sites, units, and teams.

Changes to Become Age-Friendly System-Wide

Figure 12.5. Macroenvironment Changes to Motivate Systems to Become Age-Friendly Health Systems

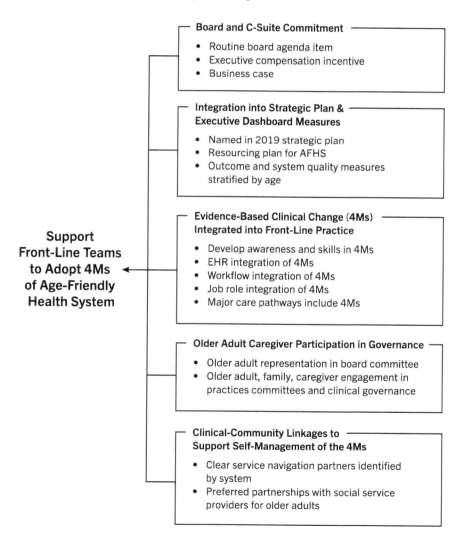

Board and C-Suite Commitment
- Routine board agenda item
- Executive compensation incentive
- Business case

Integration into Strategic Plan & Executive Dashboard Measures
- Named in 2019 strategic plan
- Resourcing plan for AFHS
- Outcome and system quality measures stratified by age

Evidence-Based Clinical Change (4Ms) Integrated into Front-Line Practice
- Develop awareness and skills in 4Ms
- EHR integration of 4Ms
- Workflow integration of 4Ms
- Job role integration of 4Ms
- Major care pathways include 4Ms

Older Adult Caregiver Participation in Governance
- Older adult representation in board committee
- Older adult, family, caregiver engagement in practices committees and clinical governance

Clinical-Community Linkages to Support Self-Management of the 4Ms
- Clear service navigation partners identified by system
- Preferred partnerships with social service providers for older adults

Support Front-Line Teams to Adopt 4Ms of Age-Friendly Health System

Strategize Forward

Now focus on your next peak. What measurable aim will you try to achieve with this peak? How will this peak be motivational for your people, units, community partners, age-friendly patients, and health systems? How will it reveal to your community its own resources, courage, and solidarity?

Brainstorm as many tactics for this peak as you can in 5 minutes. Try to use "Yes, and!" strategizing, rather than "No, but!" Build on your partners' ideas.

Imagine it. What will it look like? When will it take place? Where? Who will be involved? How many people? What will they be doing? What will they be wearing? What will you be doing? When?

Figure 12.6. Creating an Enabling Environment

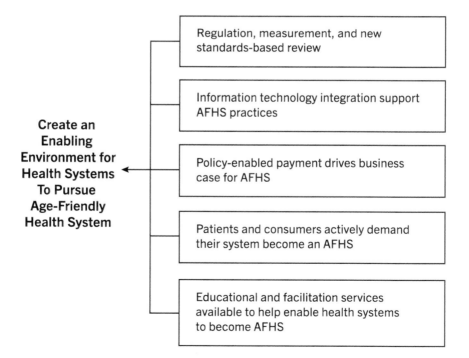

Crafting an Effective Narrative

Campaigns require an exquisite narrative that highlights specific moments, names, images, sounds, and smells from the movement. It needs to be communicated with authenticity so that people feel something from the stories they hear that makes them want to be even more effective and engage more fully. People like to hear a challenge, a choice, and an outcome. They like to understand the values of the work and how their choices demonstrate those values in regard to their work. Finally, the ability to show a transition in the story related to how we are doing now is critical in order to make the ask "Will you join us and stay with us?"

Table 12.3. *Steps to Becoming an Age-Friendly Health System*

Gather evidence of impact during piloting of the 4Ms	• Gather qualitative and quantitative data for every test of change, known as a PDSA cycle (even when you practice the 4Ms as a set with one older adult).
	• Recognize that the data can be broadly defined and encompassing—for example, a quote or a story from a care team member, an older adult, or a family caregiver.
	• Identify one team member as the gatherer of data or rotate the role between team members.
	• Remember that the data is for improvement, not research; try different measures and approaches to gathering and sharing data.
	• Start by tracking process measures and move on to outcome measures
	• Maintain clarity that the aim is to pilot 4Ms practices that lead to improved outcomes for older adults across age, race, and ethnicity.
	• All of this data will be the foundation to spread the 4Ms.
Set an aim for spread within, and across, your sites of care	• Begin with the end in mind; know from the start how far and by when you will spread the 4Ms.
	• Consider the utility of the 4Ms in service lines, practices, and units where older adults are cared for without geriatricians; where are those places in your system?

Get specific about which health system priorities are advanced by the 4Ms	• Review your health system's strategic priorities, and identify those that are advanced by the age-friendly process and outcome measures. • Write down what you think the 4Ms can do to advance the strategic priorities of your health system, and share with senior leaders. • Attend committee meetings and find out What Matters to leaders across your system; get clear on how the 4Ms can enable leaders of your system to achieve What Matters to them; tell that story.
Learn from, and act on, data stratified by race/ethnicity and age	• Use data to test the assumption that people of all races/ethnicities are positively impacted by your practice of the 4Ms. • Stratify age-friendly process and outcome measures by race/ethnicity and age in your pilot and in each step of spread. • Maintain clarity that the aim is to pilot and spread 4Ms practices that lead to improved outcomes for older adults across age, race, and ethnicity.
Calculate the financial impact of practicing the 4Ms	• One aspect of What Matters is financial well-being of your health system; there is a business case for practicing the 4Ms. • Calculate the return on investment of the 4Ms in your hospital and practices.
Celebrate and tell your stories	• Stories can drive change; make sure you and your leaders have enough to share. • Share stories by email with leaders, make brief videos, and share quotes. • Consider developing a communications plan in a table that identifies each of your stakeholders, how the 4Ms advance What Matters to them, and tactics for engaging and communicating.

Measuring Campaign Success

Campaigns are used to create something new, something that requires energy and coordination to combine our assets in new ways. A campaign is a concentrated, intense effort that has a clear beginning and end. After the campaign is over, it is clear whether or not we have achieved our specific, measurable aim (Massoud et al., 2006).

- people: individual leadership development
  - motivating others to action, building intentional relationships, collaborating, taking action, enabling others to lead
- power: capacity built
  - team capacity, community capacity, resources mobilized and deployed to generate more resources
- change: outcomes in the world
  - 4Ms, age-friendly systems, quality improvement

Figure 12.7. Mapping Campaign Success

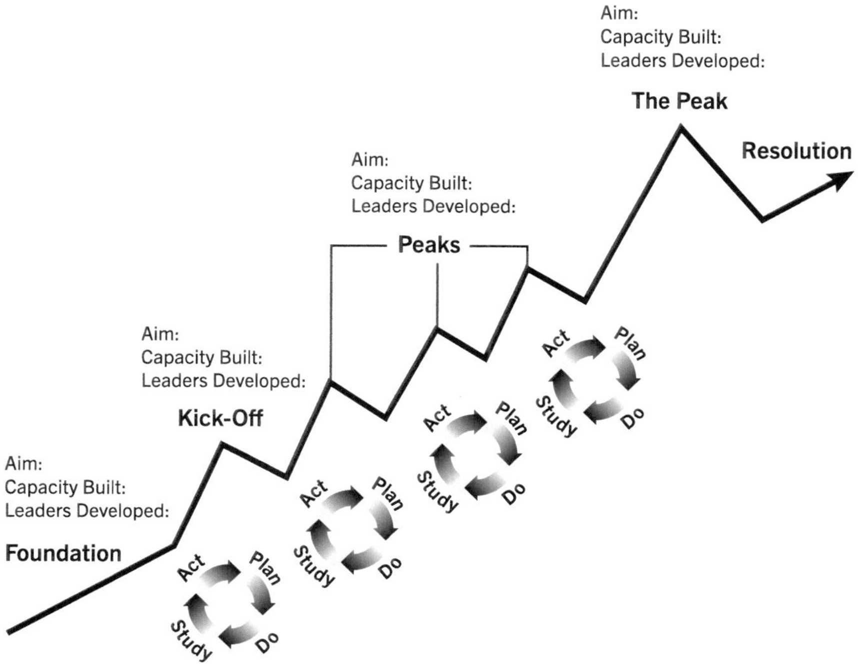

Essential Measure Sets

Essential measures are produced monthly and reviewed by senior leaders.

What Is Leadership?

Thousands of books have been written about leadership, and while there is no one definition, there are certain constructs that transcend the multiple definitions. In general, leadership is accepting responsibility for enabling others to achieve shared purpose in the face of uncertainty. *Leadership* need not mean that one person is captain of the ship but instead that there are multiple people who are leading as a team. This is also known as *distributed leadership* (IHI, 2021i).

Advantages of distributed leadership include the distribution of work to achieve aims and also breaking an audacious goal into achievable chunks across different teams and team leaders, with different entry points for people to join and participate. This also builds the capacity for sustainability as workforce leaders transition and ensure that that collective decision-making process has a memory across the organization. Further development of leaders helps create opportunities for those who are looking for an opportunity to show their leadership skills and participate deeply in a change process.

Coaching by more-senior leaders is a very effective way to ensure that there is a pipeline for leadership in your organization and solid relationships among in-between team leaders. The three conditions that enable a team's effectiveness include

- a real team: bounded, stable, and interdependent;
- a compelling purpose: clear, challenging, and consequential; and
- an enabling structure: diverse, interdependent roles, real teamwork, and norms of conduct.

Figure 12.8. Essential Measure Sets

AFHS Project Conceptual Goals

Measure	Best Care Possible	Experiences No Healthcare-Related Harms	Satisfied with Healthcare	Realizes Optimal Value
Hospital Essential Measures (stratified by age: 65–74; 75+)				
WM (TBD)	O			O
Falls with Injury		●		
30-Day All Cause Readmissions	O	O		O
HCAMPS[1]			●	
Delirium Rate	O	O		
% of Patients with Documented Healthcare Agent	O			O
Primary Care Essential Measures (stratified by age: 65–74; 75+)				
WM (TBD)	O			
ED Visits per 1000		O		O
CGCAMPS[2]			●	
Annual Wellness Visit	O			
% of Patients with Documented Healthcare Agent	O			O
Assisted Living (stratification pending futher discussion 9 Jan 2018)				
WM (TBD)	O			O
Falls with Injury		●		
30-Day All Cause Readmissions		O		O
Experience Survey[3]			●	
Use of Off-Label Anti-Psychotic Meds	O		O	
% of Patients with Documented Healthcare Agent	O			O

Moderate Relationship = O   Strong Relationships = ●

1 Composite scores in six domains and Questions 21 (rating of hospital) and 22 (willingness to recommend)
2 Composite questions ("Access," "Communication," "Care Coordination," and "Rating of Provider")
3 For example, the CoreQ survey questions for Assisted Living Residents, www.coreq.org

Table 12.4. High-Impact Leadership Behaviors

Person-centeredness	Be consistently person-centered in word and deed.
Front-line engagement	Be a regular, authentic presence at the front line and a visible champion of improvement.
Relentless focus	Remain focused on the vision and strategy.
Transparency	Require transparency about results, progress, aims, and defects.
Boundarylessness	Encourage and practice systems thinking and collaboration across boundaries.

Table 12.5. Critical Leader Roles During Prototyping

Age-friendly as a priority	Promote the team's work wherever and whenever you can: importance of this work to the organization's mission; positive results.
Create a sense of urgency	Visit the team, if only for 5 minutes, to learn what they are working on and to show your support.
Keep track	Set up monthly meetings with the leader of the team and request the most recent Monthly Team Progress Report in advance.
Remove barriers	At the monthly meetings, review their progress and determine what barriers they are facing that you can remove.

Distributed Leadership

The interdependent leadership model is often referred to as a "snow-flake." The leader at the center of this model has built a team of leaders around them who, in turn, develop teams of leaders around them, and so on.

In this model, leadership is bidirectional with interdependence, which requires mutual commitment.

Case Study

Distributed Leadership to Reach May 31, 2018, Aim

The Center for Healthy Aging (CHA) Care Team develops the 4Ms-focused *Age-Friendly Care* guide and provides training to assist seven Medicare Wellness Nurses to

- integrate the 4Ms into the Medicare Wellness Exams;
- identify appropriate referral sources when needs are identified; and
- document findings in EMR.

Figure 12.10. St. Vincent Medical Group Practices

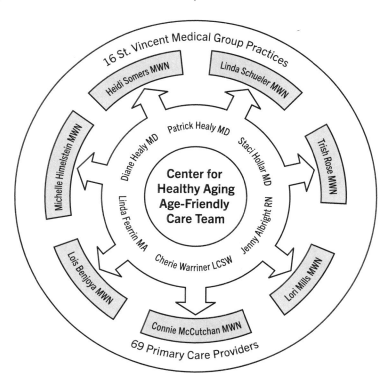

Distributed Leadership to Reach December 31, 2018, Aim

The CHA Care Team will build on learnings from phase one and utilize the 4Ms-focused *Age-Friendly Care* guide to provide training to 11 additional Medicare Wellness Nurses to

- integrate the 4Ms into the Medicare Wellness Exams;
- identify appropriate referral sources when needs are identified;
- document findings in EMR;
- provide age-friendly training to 18 St. Vincent nurse navigators and 14 St. Vincent Care Management Team members;
- provide age-friendly training to 50+ St. Vincent Case Managers;
- ensure CHA Care Team members integrate the 4Ms into care provided to patients at North Willow assisted living facility; and
- ensure CHA Care Team Nurse Practitioners integrate age-friendly care into their work at eight Senior Living Communities.

Foundational Supports

The most successful organizations will have the full support of their leadership and will be able to clearly delineate how the Age-Friendly Health Systems work reflects the culture and commitment of the organization. Not only clinical leaders but patients and families will understand why the work is important and will be able to articulate it when asked to do so. The highest priorities will include engaging with patients and families in order to specifically provide education and other resources so they can take an active role

Figure 12.11. St. Vincent Medical Group Practices

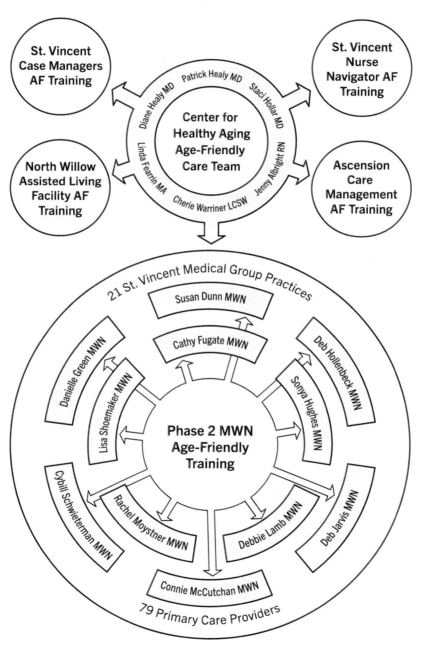

in their own care, building the infrastructure for population management and specifically supporting a substantial number of older adults with complex needs, and working to retain them in your process. The complex building of a sustainable infrastructure requires that everyone involved becomes a participant, a stakeholder, and an architect to that infrastructure. At IHI, we refer to the person who has executive authority and provides liaisons without their areas of the organizations as the sponsor. That sponsor is usually the Chief Executive Officer or the Chief Nursing Officer who has the authority to make changes and is provided resources to complete the work. That individual has a clear understanding of the strategic aims of the organization and can link the Age-Friendly Health Systems work to the mission, vision, and goals of the organization. The sponsor is not typically a day-to-day participant in team meetings but reviews the team's progress on a regular basis and helps with barriers and unexpected complexities.

Table 12.6. Roles of Teams, Leaders, and Infrastructure

	PROTOTYPE	SCALE-UP	CAMPAIGN
The team	Try, measure, try again	New teams adapt and adopt	Campaign team adapts and rolls out to all
The leaders	Resources, support, communicate, remove barriers	Charter and oversee spread process (resources, support, communicate, remove barriers)	Oversight (resources, support, communicate, remove barriers)
The infrastructure	Consider infrastructure needed	Build infrastructure to sustain and spread	Extend infrastructure to scale-up

How to Get Underway at Your Institution

Team Action Planning requires self-assessment and reflection. It starts with the 4Ms (IHI, 2021f).

Revisiting the 4Ms:

- What in the change package are we already doing?
  - Are all 4Ms change ideas present in our work in this care setting?
- What do we still need to do? What needs to be incorporated?
- How will we do it? (Who will do it?)
  - What are the barriers to and opportunities for incorporating the practices outlined in the change package? How will we address them?
- What will we be able to stop doing when the 4Ms are in practice? Which roles will stop activities? Who will notice that this has stopped?

Once you and your team have come to an appropriate agreement on these questions, the next step is to review your current efforts related to the 4Ms and determine the following.

Looking at Your Current 4Ms Interventions

- Are they scalable?
  - It is important to examine the attributes of your 4Ms interventions and determine their relative advantages, whether they are in their simplest form, whether they can be observed, and finally, if they are compatible with other interventions you have in place.
  - What is the infrastructure required to support full-scale implementation (e.g., data systems, IT, financial model,

communication systems, people, education and training, learning system and feedback loops to monitor progress and adjust)?

- What is the human capacity and capability needed to support the method being used to scale up?
- What is the belief and will of leaders and staff to support these changes?
- If not, how will we make them more so? (Who will do it?)
- How will we document results?
- What is our campaign strategy for scaling up?

Capturing feedback from staff is crucial for successful implementation. If staff perceive the work as valuable and responsive, they will participate much more readily. Regular check-ins to make sure that staff are still engaged and being listened to is also obviously important to the success of the campaign for spreading scale.

Workflow

Workflow is another critical component to spread and scale. Excessive or redundant steps that create a burden and reduce value need to be anticipated and eliminated. As you customize the workflow for your setting(s), consider the following for each step:

- Who does this step?
  - How will engagement be assured? What is the relational strategy?
- Where is this step conducted?
- When is it done?
- How should this step be done?
- How long should it take?
- Where is this step documented in the medical record?

Figure 12.12. Age-Friendly Strategies and Resources

Access
Access to affordable, equitable health, behavioral and social services

Value
The best care that adds value to lives

Partners
Embrace diversity of individuals and serve as partners in their health

Well-Being
Focus on well-being and partnership with community resources

Coordination
Seamless care propelled by teams, technology, innovation and data

Age-Friendly Strategies

Advocacy/Representation

- State Hospital Associations
- Regional Policy Boards
- Specialty Committees

The Value Initiative

Taskforce on Vulnerable Communities

Thought Leadership

- AHA Physician Alliance
- American Organization of Nurse Executives
- Strategic Leadership Groups
- Best practice case studies

On the CUSP: Stop CLABSI

Knowledge Exchange

- AHA Today
- Huddle for Care
- Trustee Magazine
- AHA Leadership Summit
- ACHI Conference
- Hospital Improvement Innovation Network
- AONE Annual Meeting
- AHA Annual Meeting

HIIN Change Packages

Agent of Change

- Boards of trustees, C-suite
- Physicians, nurses, and other care providers
- Institute for Diversity
- Association for Community Health Improvment
- State hospital association and public health department convenings
- Social media presence

A Playbook for Fostering Hospital-Community Partnerships to Build a Culture of Health

Foundational Elements

Leadership, culture, capability, care team training, caregiver engagement, infrastructure, information ecosystem

Co-producing the answers to the questions above with the stake-holders involved at each step is essential to ensure workflow patterns are enhanced and readily reflect value. It is always important to do regular PDSA cycles to check in on ways to continue improvement and demonstrate that every voice in the process is equally important.

Equity

As Age-Friendly Health Systems are scaled up, a critical issue to address is equity. Social determinants play a major role in health, leading to disparities in care that are particularly magnified for older adults with complex conditions. The lack of resources and barriers to access present a formidable obstacle to healthy aging. In Black and Hispanic communities, poverty rates are significantly higher. And the life expectancy of Black people has been historically much lower than those of white people in the US, a trend that persists to this day (Figure 12.13; The Institute for Health Metrics and Evaluation, 2015).

Figure 12.13. Life Expectancy of Black and White People in the US (1950–2010) (National Center for Health Statistics, 2019)

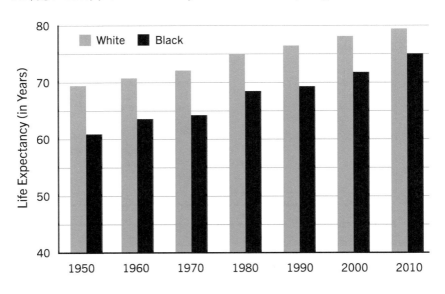

Race and ethnicity are not the only factors that lead to health disparities. Thus, it is essential to consider all socioeconomic aspects to provide holistic care to older adults.

Case Study

Rush University Medical Center, Chicago, Illinois

Adapted from Learning from the Pursuing Equity Initiative (IHI, 2021c).

One health system that has taken initiative to address the health disparities in its communities is Rush University Medical Center (RUMC). The life-expectancy gap between some of Chicago's most and least affluent neighborhoods is estimated at 16 years. To work toward decreasing this gap by 50% by 2030, RUMC has implemented various system-level strategies:

- In July 2017, Rush made health equity a strategic priority for the Rush University Health System (Rush). Being a catalyst for Community Health and Economic Vitality was identified as one of four transformative strategic priorities, and Dr. David Ansell was named Senior Vice President for Community Health Equity to lead these efforts.

- Engaged in explicit discussions about structural racism and economic investment with the senior leadership team and the system's board.

- Partnership with Information Services (IS), Knowledge Management, Quality Improvement, and Population Health Departments to form Rush's Ambulatory & Population Health

Data Governance Subcommittee, giving the Equity team a platform to bring Equity and social determinants of health (SDOH)-related data requests.

- Established infrastructure and governance for health equity work (SDOH Ops and Leadership Committee), as well as integration of health equity goals into the annual Performance Improvement Plan for the medical center.

- Built a racial health equity collaborative with other health systems and the community called West Side United to address the structural, economic, and political determinants of health in 10 Chicago West Side neighborhoods.

- Published the first *State of Health Equity Report* at Rush.

RUMC has also developed strategies to address social determinants of health needs (Screening Process Implementation):

- Established SDOH screening workflows and began implementing screening across Rush University Medical Group (RUMG) primary care, the ED, and inpatient units. Discussions are underway with Rush Oak Park and Rush Copley to screen for SDOH in the ED.

- Used PDSA cycles to test the screening workflow with multidisciplinary team members, including first-year medical students, medical assistants, social workers, patient care navigators, and residents.

- Developed formal partnerships with NowPow and other community partners to establish closed-loop referrals and provide relevant resources to patients with needs. NowPow is a women-owned and women-operated company that uses a digital platform and data analytics to link people known to have chronic health and social problems to community-based providers of the health and social services that have been prescribed for them.

- Hired a team of community health workers (CHWs) and a patient care navigator within the population health umbrella to provide timely communication and follow-up to patients who screen positive for SDOH.

- Developing a system-level quality and equity dashboard, with plans to implement by June 30, 2019.

- Developing an RUMG/RUMC SDOH Dashboard that displays progress on screening, intervention, and trends, with plans to implement by June 30, 2019.

- Partners in Rush's Information Services and Knowledge Management are in the process of developing a Health Equity data mart.

- Developing SDOH risk/predictive model with Knowledge Management, IS, and Rush Health.

Rush began its journey in screening for SDOH in September 2017, starting with the Rush University Medical Center (RUMC) Emergency Department (ED), and quickly expanding to other areas across the Rush system, including Rush University Primary Care, RUMC inpatient units, Rush Oak Park Hospital ED, as well as in the community. In May 2018, Rush began participating in a second collaborative with Health Leads called Collaborative to Advance Social Health Integration (CASHI) to expand its reach with SDOH screening in primary care and begin developing an evaluation framework.

As a major focus area for the IHI Pursuing Equity initiative, between July 2017 and March 2019, the Rush Pursuing Equity team, Social Work team, and Rush University Primary Care at RUMC undertook SDOH screening efforts through an office visit, social work visit, and patient telephone outreach. The following data reflect the results of these efforts (note that the data are not inclusive of primary care patients being screened in the ED or inpatient units):

- number of patients screened for SDOH: 1,944
- number of patients screening positive for one or more SDOH need: 547
- top three SDOH needs identified: utilities, food, and transportation
- number of patients screening positive for one or more SDOH need who then received After Visit Summary with NowPow resources/referrals: 139

Standard workflows for screening and referrals have been developed for primary care clinics and rolled out in three out of 13 clinics. The Rush Social Work and Community Health team is continuing to develop and spread standard workflows for screening and resources in primary care, the ED, and inpatient units so that all patients receive the resources and supports they need to thrive.

Rush recognized through this journey how pervasive structural racism is in our healthcare system, particularly in Chicago, and has worked to shed light on this topic across clinical settings. Making health equity a strategic priority was essential to advancing our efforts and identifying needed internal and community resources to address SDOH for patients in our system. We continue to collect and publish data on the community needs for our larger region and strive to develop a collaborative model with stakeholders to offer high-quality care to all patients who require it.

Additional Case Studies

The following cases highlight elements of a successful launch of an Age-Friendly Health System, with the anticipated pushback and barriers, and ways that they have been overcome.

Providence St. Joseph Health, Oregon Region

Figure 12.14. *Providence St. Joseph Health Spread and Scale*

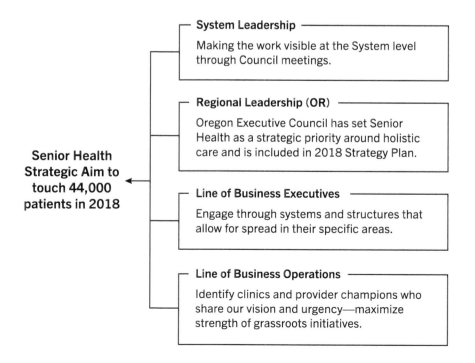

- Challenges:
  - System has already established strategic priorities, which do not include senior health as a population at present.
  - Adoption of standardized processes across our many clinics is not easily accomplished.
  - Optimizing Epic to improve tools for geriatric encounters is complicated because there are many different users and setups across the system.
- What will facilitate scale-up of age-friendly changes in our region?
  - Provide data, patient stories, and tested integrated work.
  - Engage financial and quality leaders involved in Population Health and Providence Health Plan 5-Star CMS for Medicare Advantage.
  - Develop tailored strategy options to best navigate our region across rural and urban settings that have different cultures and unique environments in which they provide care to seniors.

Kaiser Permanente Woodland Hills, Woodland Hills, California

- Challenges:
  - Addressing the capacity challenges in unit.
  - Collecting timely and manual data.
  - Distinguishing between competing priorities for support staff and services.
- What will facilitate scale-up of the age-friendly changes in our system?
  - "Medicare Acceleration Site" designation: As an "acceleration site," Woodland Hills will test tools, programs, and practices that have proven potential to accelerate performance improvement across Kaiser Permanente on specific measures of safety and experience.

- Accelerating Learning and Spread (XLS Model): This Spread and Scale methodology is proprietary to Kaiser Permanente.

Figure 12.15. Kaiser Permanente Woodland Hills Spread and Scale

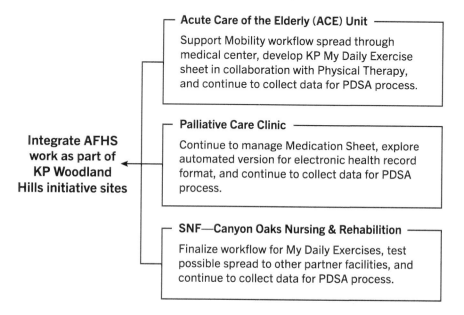

Integrate AFHS work as part of KP Woodland Hills initiative sites

Acute Care of the Elderly (ACE) Unit

Support Mobility workflow spread through medical center, develop KP My Daily Exercise sheet in collaboration with Physical Therapy, and continue to collect data for PDSA process.

Palliative Care Clinic

Continue to manage Medication Sheet, explore automated version for electronic health record format, and continue to collect data for PDSA process.

SNF—Canyon Oaks Nursing & Rehabilitation

Finalize workflow for My Daily Exercises, test possible spread to other partner facilities, and continue to collect data for PDSA process.

Anne Arundel Medical Center, Annapolis, Maryland

- Challenges:
  - There is a lack of knowledge on best practices for managing our older patients.
  - There is resistance to implement change as departments juggle multiple priorities.
  - Determining time to meet with staff to plan educational and practice changes.
  - Recognizing that the implementation of the 4Ms will vary by service line/department.

Figure 12.16. Anne Arundel Medical Center Spread and Scale

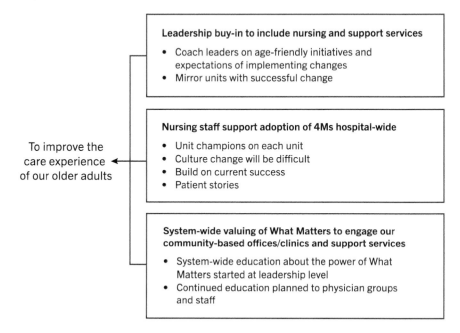

- What will facilitate scale-up of the age-friendly changes in our system?
  - resources: intense education of the PT / OT / Care Management / palliative care / social work to support and spread age-friendly work
  - system-wide development of Institute of Healthy Aging— approved through our Foundation for a $10 million campaign
  - system-wide education on the importance of What Matters and developing ways to communicate this information through the electronic record to all staff
  - ER involvement and education to promote completion of accurate medication history prior to or upon admission and additional pharmacy technician support

- primary medical offices to develop outreach program with our primary and specialty practice physician groups to assist in education

Recommendations and Summary

The scaling of geriatric models of care can be difficult due to many issues, such as inconsistent dissemination and high costs. However, it is essential to work toward spreading such models, which can benefit a greater portion of the population. This can be done by creating a campaign and strategies for advancing. Each health system is different and should work to target its own priorities and problems. Cases have exhibited different challenges, with competing priorities and lack of management support being foremost in the concerns. Potential suggestions for facilitating the scale-up of the age-friendly change included providing more evidence-based data, information dissemination across stakeholders, and regular communication amongst those involved on barriers and solutions. Recommendations for a successful launch and campaign are, in summary:

1. Map stakeholders and assets.
2. Establish measures for evaluating campaign progress and success.
3. Build a strong leadership, with impactful behaviors and foundational supports.
4. Construct a fitting narrative.
5. Assess the readiness of an idea for rapid spread.

References

Ganz, M. (2010). Leading change: Leadership, organization, and social movements. In N. Nohria & R. Khurana (Eds.), *Handbook of leadership theory and practice: A Harvard Business School centennial colloquium.* Harvard Business Press.

Institute for Health Improvement. (2018a). *Creating age-friendly health systems* [Workshop].

Institute for Health Improvement. (2018b). *Lesson 4 exercise: Mapping stakeholders and assets.* http://www.ihi.org/education/IHIOpenSchool/ Courses/Documents/ICAN/Lesson4Exercise_Final.doc

Institute for Health Improvement. (2020). *Scale-up of age-friendly health systems* [Sponsors call].

Institute for Health Improvement. (2021a). *Creating the enabling conditions for age-friendly care.*

Institute for Health Improvement. (2021b). *Getting ready for spread: Planning your system-wide spread.*

Institute for Health Improvement. (2021c). *Learning from the Pursuing Equity Initiative.*

Institute for Health Improvement. (2021d). *The mindset & skill: Embracing resistance & falling forward.*

Institute for Health Improvement. (2021e). *Organizing for health.*

Institute for Health Improvement. (2021f). Scale-up of age-friendly care webinar #5: Reaching more older adults with the evidence-based care through the 4Ms in your health system.

Institute for Health Improvement. (2021g). *Scale up: Tools, tactics, & action plans.*

Institute for Health Improvement. (2021h). *Spring 2021 age-friendly health systems action community: An invitation to join us.*

Institute for Health Improvement. (2021i). *Strategy & structure to scale age-friendly health systems.*

The Institute for Health Metrics and Evaluation. (2015). *Country profile: United States.*

Massoud, M. R., Nielsen, G. A., Nolan, K., Nolan, T., Schall, M. W., & Sevin, C. (2006). *A framework for spread: From local improvements to system-wide change* [White paper]. IHI Innovation Series. http://www.

ihi.org/resources/Pages/IHIWhitePapers/AFrameworkforSpreadWhite
Paper.aspx
National Center for Health Statistics. (2019). Health, United States, 2011.
CDC. www.cdc.gov/nchs/hus/contents2011.htm

CHAPTER 13

Role of Public Health in Age-Friendly Health Systems

What Is Healthy Aging?

Healthy aging encompasses a holistic approach to the whole person, ensuring longer, healthier, and more productive lives, and may be defined as

- promoting health, preventing injury, and managing chronic conditions;
- optimizing physical, cognitive, and mental health; and
- facilitating social engagement (Lehning & De Biasi, 2018).

It is an adaptive process in response to the challenges that can occur as we age, and a proactive process to reduce the likelihood, intensity, or impact of future challenges, such as disease, disability, social isolation, and loneliness. It calls for maximizing physical, mental, emotional, and social well-being, while recognizing that aging is often accompanied by chronic illnesses and functional limitations, including the exacerbation of lifelong conditions.

What Is a Public Health System?

A public health system is an extensive network of governmental and nongovernmental organizations that aim to prevent disease, promote life, and promote health through organized efforts and well-informed choices for communities and individuals. Public health focuses on physical, mental, and social well-being, including the environments that contribute to or detract from health, not merely the absence of disease.

Trust for America's Health Advancing an Age-Friendly Public Health System Grant With The John Hartford Foundation

Trust for America's Health (TFAH) is a nonpartisan public health policy, research, and advocacy organization that envisions a nation that values the health and well-being of all and where prevention and health equity are foundational to policymaking at all levels of society. TFAH is an essential partner in the development, spread, and scale of Age-Friendly Public Health Systems that intersects seamlessly with Age-Friendly Health Systems.

> **Vision**: To develop an integrated and seamless Age-Friendly Health System that links the provision of comprehensive medical care with the creation of health-promoting conditions and services in the communities where older adults live, work, shop, and socialize.

The public health system can play a critical role in achieving this vision by implementing its prevention activities with a healthy-aging lens, including focusing its attention on the needs of older adults that are associated with affordable and appropriate housing, access to nutritious food, social engagement, transportation, and safety as well as by providing educational information and promoting healthier individual behaviors, such as better nutrition and more physical activity. However, public health has not historically prioritized the older adult population.

Foundational Capabilities

There are nine foundational capabilities that the public health system could leverage to make healthy aging a core function. These are listed below, along with examples of possible applications of these capabilities to the health of older adults:

1. **Assessing (surveillance, epidemiology, and laboratory capacity)**: monitoring diseases—both infectious and chronic—among different sub-segments of older adults

2. **Developing policy to effectively promote and improve health**: implementing policies that address the lack of accessible healthy food options for older adults in low-income neighborhoods

3. **Using integrated data sets for assessment, surveillance, and evaluation to identify crucial health challenges, best practices, and better health**: linking public health and healthcare databases to identify and respond to the needs of older adults

4. **Communicating with the public and other audiences to disseminate and receive health-related information in an effective manner**: providing information regarding the importance of and sites to receive vaccinations for the prevention of shingles

5. **Mobilizing the community and forging partnerships to leverage resources (including funding)**: convening meetings that bring together organizations that provide services to older adults with housing experts to consider how to expand age-friendly housing options

6. **Building new models that integrate clinical and population health**: utilizing community health workers to visit at-risk older adults following hospitalization

7. **Cultivating leadership with the skills needed to build and sustain an effective health department and workforce**: training the public health workforce to understand and then skillfully address the health needs of older adults

8. **Demonstrating accountability for what governmental public health does directly and for those things that it oversees**: establishing training and accreditation opportunities for jobs such as community health workers conducting home visits

9. **Protecting the public in the event of an emergency or disaster, as well as responding to day-to-day challenges or threats**: identifying and registering people who are frail or disabled for future public health emergencies that require evacuation

Five Key Roles for Public Health

In 2017, TFAH, in partnership with The John Hartford Foundation, held a convening called A Public Health Framework to Support the Improvement of the Health and Well-Being of Older Adults. National, state, and local public health officials; aging experts, advocates, and service providers; and healthcare officials came together to discuss how public health could contribute to an "age-friendly" society and improve the health and well-being of older adults living in the United States. The result was a Framework for an Age-Friendly Public Health System that includes five roles for public health in the healthy-aging effort.

1. Connecting and Convening Multiple Sectors and Professions That Provide the Supports, Services, and Infrastructure to Promote Healthy Aging

A greater focus on prevention, such as falls prevention and initiatives to promote physical activity or brain health, can help forestall declines in health and well-being. A focus on policy, systems, and environmental change complements the efforts to address the needs of individual older adults by focusing on improvements that impact entire populations or communities.

One example that highlights this role is in promoting and supporting physical activity. There are numerous barriers to regular physical activity in later life, including restricted access to indoor and outdoor recreational facilities, concerns about neighborhood safety, limited individual knowledge about the benefits of exercise, and the absence of walkable neighborhood features (e.g., well-maintained sidewalks, raised crosswalks, speed bumps, and a variety of food and shopping destinations; Clark, 1999; Schutzer & Graves, 2004).

Public health could bring together the multiple actors that could alleviate these barriers, including law enforcement, public works, parks and recreation, city planning, local businesses, physicians, senior centers, and other community groups.

Another example is the need to address social isolation in later life. Social isolation can involve an objective separation from a social network, such as living alone, or more subjective feelings of loneliness (Golden et al., 2009).

Public health can work with community-based organizations, such as senior centers, community centers, and YMCAs, to address loneliness and social isolation by providing opportunities for social interaction and the development of new friendships. Public health professionals can also partner with "Villages," grassroots consumer-driven community-based organizations that aim to promote aging in place by combining services, participant engagement, and peer support (Village to Village Network, 2021).

2. Coordinating Existing Supports and Services to Avoid Duplication of Efforts, Identify Gaps, and Increase Access to Services and Supports

For example, many older adults do not receive preventive health services, such as those recommended by the US Preventive Services Task Force, including screenings, behavioral health monitoring and counseling, and immunizations (US Preventive Services Task Force, 2021).

Public health has been a key partner in the work of Vote & Vax, a national initiative that has received support from the CDC and the Robert Wood Johnson Foundation to provide flu vaccines in polling places. Bringing together multiple sectors, including public health, pharmacy, and nursing, Vote & Vax has demonstrated success in improving vaccination rates among those with access barriers to the more traditional vaccination sites of physician offices or pharmacies (Shenson et al., 2015).

3. Collecting Data to Assess Community Health Status (Including Inequities) and Aging Population Needs to Inform the Development of Interventions

Public health can help document population and community health status by collecting and analyzing data, including data from multiple sectors and sources.

One example is the Behavioral Risk Factor Surveillance System (BRFSS), administered by the CDC, which includes two modules that states can use to assess and track two issues critical to the health and well-being of older adults: the cognitive decline module and the caregiver module. Public health departments can advocate for wider implementation of these modules in states that have not yet adopted them and can analyze and disseminate the data in states that have.

As another example, public health can provide important information about older adults using hotspot analysis, a technique to examine the geographic distribution of populations, features, or events. Such data can be essential in mapping neighborhoods in which older adults are at a higher risk for a fall or have less access to a grocery store. This essential data can then be analyzed and disseminated to target audiences in easy-to-use fact sheets.

The Department of Health and Human Services' Office of the Assistant Secretary for Preparedness and Response developed the emPOWER Initiative through a partnership with the Centers for Medicare & Medicaid Services. The emPOWER Initiative provides federal data and mapping tools to local and state public health departments to help them identify vulnerable populations who rely upon electricity-dependent medical and assistive devices or certain healthcare services, such as dialysis machines, oxygen tanks, and home health services. The emPOWER Map is a public and interactive map that provides monthly de-identified Medicare data down to the zip-code level and an expanded set of near real-time hazard-tracking services. Together, this information provides enhanced situational awareness and actionable information for assisting areas and at-risk populations that may be impacted by severe weather, wildfires, earthquakes, and other disasters. Public health and emergency management officials, AAAs, and community planners can use emPOWER to better understand the types of resources that may be needed in an emergency.

The public health sector may also bring an asset-based approach to community assessment, documenting the collective resources of older adults, their families, and their communities. This aligns with the work of aging services and other providers to move away from an emphasis on deficits and toward a recognition of strengths, skills, and capacities.

4. Communicating and Disseminating Research Findings and Best Practices to Support Healthy Aging

A key component of this initiative is supporting applied research and translating evidence into practice for providers and policymakers. Public health can also assist with neurocognitive disorder public awareness campaigns around modifiable risk factors, signs of disease progression, strategies for addressing changes in behavior, and community supports. Public health can also support the development and implementation of evidence-based programs and evidence-informed policies.

Public health organizations may provide central locations for information on healthy aging, including best practices, toolkits, and research. The ready availability of such a site can assist other sectors and professions in their efforts to address the needs of older adults.

5. Complementing, Integrating, and Supplementing Existing Supports and Services, Particularly in Terms of Integrating Clinical and Population Health Approaches

The aging services network is beginning to recognize the value of community health workers (CHWs), a public health approach that has long been working with populations with limited access to formal health and social services. CHWs are trusted members of a community and conduct outreach, provide education, and serve as liaisons to formal systems of support. Preliminary research indicates the promise of CHWs for reducing healthcare costs, supporting transitions back home from the hospital, and connecting low-income senior housing residents to community services (De Biasi et al., 2020).

Public health can also complement existing programs for informal caregivers providing assistance to older adults with disabilities.

Public health can provide critical education and training on performing the tasks needed to support older care recipients—such as safely bathing or transferring from a bed to a chair—or address the behavioral changes associated with dementia.

Table 13.1. Health Department Steps to the
Age-Friendly Public Health Systems Framework

AGE-FRIENDLY PUBLIC HEALTH SYSTEMS FRAMEWORK	HEALTH DEPARTMENT ACTION STEPS
Connecting and convening	• Engage at least one new aging sector or other community partner in collaborative efforts to support older adult health • Enhance at least one existing relationship with an aging sector partner • Create or join a multi-sector coalition, committee, or council that addresses healthy aging • Engage in or lead policy, systems, and/or environmental change to improve older adult health and well-being (e.g., Age-Friendly Communities and Age-Friendly Health Systems) • Increase awareness of existing services and facilitate referrals to improve access
Coordinating	• Review and strengthen emergency preparedness plan to ensure it addresses the needs of vulnerable older adults
Collecting and disseminating data	• Collect, analyze, and disseminate local-level data • Review and strengthen the community health assessment to ensure it addresses older adult health needs • Identify a priority around older adult health in the community health improvement plan • Conduct an assessment to identify community programs that address older adult needs

Collecting and disseminating data *(continued)*	• Establish a mechanism for ongoing input of older adult residents to identify needs and inform the community health assessment process and policy development
Communicating	• Develop messaging or communication strategies and tools to engage additional partners and/or improve visibility of healthy-aging programs/services
Complementing and supplementing	• Implement at least one new education program or service targeted at older adults

In 2017, in partnership with TFAH, the Florida Department of Health worked with the Department of Elder Affairs to create the Aging in Florida profiles for all 67 counties in the state. Leveraging the new data available, Florida Network counties created infographics and other messaging to engage community partners around older adult health and well-being in their counties. TFAH and the Florida Department of Health identified 13 Age-Friendly Public Health Systems indicators and asked each Florida Network county to select four. In a significant show of engagement and enthusiasm for this work, many counties took action on all 13. These indicators track domains of work such as expanding emergency preparedness to include older adults and convening multi-sector stakeholders, among others. Under the Florida-based Age-Friendly Public Health Systems pilot, 37 counties (65% of the Florida older adult population) implemented the Age-Friendly Public Health Systems framework.

Barriers to Creating an Age-Friendly Public Health System

What have we learned thus far in advancing the idea of an Age-Friendly Public Health System? First and foremost, we have learned that public health has traditionally focused on maternal and child

Figure 13.1. Intersection Between Age-Friendly
Public Health and Age-Friendly Health System

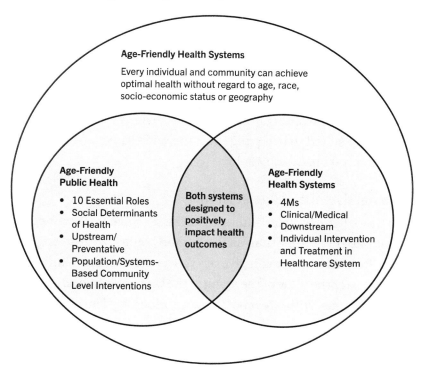

care but that, at this moment of demographic change, it is more important than ever to engage and fund the public health system in our country to also address the health needs of older adults, especially around the social determinants of health and disease prevention. How might we do that? There are three key elements.

1. The Need to Break Down Professional and Disciplinary Silos

Promoting a public health strategy for healthy aging requires a collective-impact approach that recognizes that the solutions to complex social problems do not emerge from the activities of a single individual, social service agency, or sector, but rather from the activities of multiple entities, including businesses, nonprofits, governments, and the general public (Kania & Kramer, 2011).

Forming and maintaining collaborations of diverse partners requires time, energy, dedication, and funding. Helping stakeholders who have not traditionally focused on older adults recognize the role that they can play to promote healthy aging across the life course will be an additional challenge. Those in the public health sector are often accustomed to convening and facilitating diverse collaborations and may be well suited to bring together the wide range of stakeholders needed to promote healthy aging.

2. The Persistence of Ageist Norms

In the United States, older adults are often seen primarily as needy or helpless patients rather than as full human beings, with strengths as well as limitations, who can give as well as receive. Such limited perceptions foster the view of the aging of the US population as a problem. At the same time, with a few notable exceptions, ageism also prevents the needs of older adults from becoming a priority at the local, state, and federal levels. In an effort to combat the deleterious effects of ageism, eight leading aging organizations (AARP, American Federation for Aging Research, American Geriatrics Society, American Society on Aging, Gerontological Society of America, Grantmakers in Aging, National Council on Aging, and National Hispanic Council on Aging) have partnered for the Reframing Aging Project. State and local public health departments can embrace the goals of the Reframing Aging Project by incorporating the needs and assets of the aging population into their own priorities, serving as a model for other sectors and professions to adopt an aging-in-all-policies-and-practices approach. Through assessment and research activities that complement the work of others, public health can highlight the ways older adults are assets to their families and communities and promote the message that the aging of the population is a success story and not a crisis.

3. A Need for More Funding From Both the Public and Private Sectors to Support Healthy Aging

As the number of older adults continues to grow in this country, the relative amount of public health and social service funding from the federal, state, and local levels is shrinking. Furthermore, funding is rarely available for the larger-scale collective-impact activities required to fully support healthy aging. Grants are often given to one specific agency to support one specific intervention for one specific health or social problem. Promoting healthy aging across diverse populations will likely require a substantial investment of financial and human resources. However, stakeholders can develop strategies to maximize existing resources and identify new sources of support. These include focusing on relatively low-cost policies and programs, enlisting the participation of multiple stakeholders, considering how existing policies and programs can meet the needs of older adults, and braiding together funding from multiple sectors.

Recommendations and Summary

Lessons learned from the Age-Friendly Public Health Systems initiative have demonstrated the positive effect of these public health roles:

- Connect and convene multiple sectors and professions that provide the supports, services, and infrastructures to promote healthy aging.
- Coordinate existing supports and services to avoid duplication of efforts, identify gaps, and increase access to services and supports.
- Collect data to assess community health status (including inequities) and aging population needs to inform the development of interventions.

- Communicate and disseminate research findings and best practices to support healthy aging.
- Complement, integrate, and supplement existing supports and services, particularly in terms of integrating clinical and population health approaches.

It is critical to integrate public health into Age-Friendly Health Systems, as it takes a holistic approach to the well-being of older adults beyond the management of disease. As mentioned above, the public health system is based on nine core capabilities that can be leveraged to improve older adult health and well-being: assessing through surveillance, epidemiology, and laboratory capacity; developing policy to effectively promote and improve health; using integrated data sets for assessment, surveillance, and evaluation to identify crucial health challenges, best practices, and better health; communicating with the public and other audiences to disseminate and receive health-related information in an effective manner; mobilizing the community and forging partnerships to leverage resources; building new models that integrate clinical and population health; cultivating leadership with the skills needed to build and sustain an effective health department and workforce; demonstrating accountability for what governmental public health does directly and for those that it oversees; and protecting the public in the event of an emergency or disaster, as well as responding to day-to-day challenges or threats.

References

Clark, D. O. (1999). Identifying psychological, physiological, and environmental barriers and facilitators to exercise among older low-income adults. *Journal of Clinical Geropsychology*, 5(1), 51–62. https://doi.org/10.1023/A:1022942913555

De Biasi, A., Wolfe, M., Carmody, J., Fulmer, T., & Auerbach, J. (2020). Creating an age-friendly public health system. *Innovation in Aging*, 4(1), 1–11. https://doi.org/10.1093/geroni/igz044

Golden, J., Conroy, R. M., Bruce, I., Denihan, A., Greene, E., Kirby, M., & Lawlor, B. A. (2009). Loneliness, social support networks, mood and wellbeing in community-dwelling elderly. *International Journal of Geriatric Psychiatry*, 24(7), 694–700. https://doi.org/10.1002/gps.2181

Kania, J., & Kramer, M. (2011). Collective impact. *Stanford Social Innovation Review*, 9(1), 36–41. https://ssir.org/articles/entry/collective_impact

Lehning, A. J., & De Biasi, A. (2018). *Creating an age-friendly public health system: Challenges, opportunities, and next steps*. Trust for America's Health. https://www.tfah.org/wp-content/uploads/2018/09/Age_Friendly_Public_Health_Convening_Report_FINAL__1___1_.pdf

Schutzer, K. A., & Graves, B. S. (2004). Barriers and motivations to exercise in older adults. *Preventive Medicine*, 39(5), 1056–1061. https://doi.org/10.1016/j.ypmed.2004.04.003

Shenson, D., Moore, R. T., Benson, W., & Anderson, L. A. (2015). Polling places, pharmacies, and public health: Vote & vax 2012. *American Journal of Public Health*, 105(6), e12–e15. https://doi.org/10.2105/AJPH.2015.302628

US Preventive Services Task Force. (2021). *A and B recommendations*. https://www.uspreventiveservicestaskforce.org/uspstf/recommendation-topics/uspstf-and-b-recommendations

Village to Village Network. (2021). *Village map*. http://www.vtvnetwork.org/content.aspx?page_id=1905&club_id=69101

What Recognition, Credentialing, and Accreditation Do We Need for Age-Friendly Health Systems?

Not everything that can be counted counts and
not everything that counts can be counted.

—attributed to Albert Einstein

The Age-Friendly Health Systems faculty have debated the merits of recognition, credentialing, and accreditation. We have found that recognition, special notice, or attention is very important at the local level and can serve as an inspiration to continue difficult work and engage in a community that is doing that same work. Recognition as an Age-Friendly Health System is gaining momentum and affirming hard work and positive outcomes. Credentialing, that is, warranting credit or confidence, is a higher level of order and is generally done by an external body that can judge the quality and progress of a given undertaking. Finally, accreditation, which is to recognize or vouch for as conforming with a standard, is yet a higher order of review also done by an external body and, in most cases, at the national level.

IHI provides recognition for clinical care settings that are working toward reliable practice of the 4Ms framework for all older adults in their care (IHI, 2021c). However, there is currently no official credentialing or accreditation for becoming an Age-Friendly Health System.

There are two levels of recognition by IHI Age-Friendly Health Systems:

- Age-Friendly Health Systems Participant
- Age-Friendly Health Systems Committed to Care Excellence for Older Adults

Age-Friendly Health Systems Participant

An **Age-Friendly Health Systems Participant** is recognized for being on the journey to becoming an Age-Friendly Health System and has submitted a description of how it is putting the 4Ms into practice.

To be recognized, complete the 4Ms Description survey (IHI, 2021a). The survey will ask you to describe how you plan to adopt the 4Ms in your setting of care. Refer to *Age-Friendly Health Systems: Guide to Using the 4Ms in the Care of Older Adults* to learn more about the 4Ms and how to put them into practice (IHI, 2020). IHI will then send you a Participant badge and a communications kit so you can celebrate this recognition in your local community. IHI may recognize your system's achievement on our website and via media releases.

Age-Friendly Health Systems Committed to Care Excellence

An **Age-Friendly Health System Committed to Care Excellence** is a recognition for being an exemplar in the movement based on 4Ms work that is aligned with *Age-Friendly Health Systems: A Guide to Using the 4Ms While Caring for Older Adults* and at least 3 months' count of older adults reached with evidence-based 4Ms care.

To gain this level of recognition, reach out to IHI at afhs@ihi.org to ensure your 4Ms work has remained aligned with *Age-Friendly Health Systems: A Guide to Using the 4Ms While Caring for Older Adults* and make adjustments as needed. IHI will also verify that you have shared at least three monthly counts of older adults benefiting from evidence-based 4Ms care. IHI will then send you a Committed to Care Excellence badge and a communications kit so you can celebrate this recognition in your local community. IHI may recognize your system's achievement on our website and via media releases. As an exemplar in the movement, IHI and partners may invite you to share your story and support other health systems.

Frequently Asked Questions

Will My Whole Health System Be Recognized as an Age-Friendly Health System?

IHI will recognize the individual hospitals and practices in your health system that meet the two levels of recognition outlined above. For example, if one of the hospitals in your health system submits to IHI its description of how it is putting the 4Ms into practice, that hospital will be recognized as an Age-Friendly Health System Participant. If your Medicare Wellness Nurses use the 4Ms and submit to IHI a description of how they are putting the 4Ms into practice, each of the practices where the Medicare Wellness Nurses conduct visits will be recognized as Age-Friendly Health System Participants.

Do I Have to Take Any Steps to Sustain My Recognition as an Age-Friendly Health System?

The Participant and Committed to Care Excellence recognitions will be valid for one year from the date you receive your badges from IHI (IHI, 2021b).

Credentialing and Accreditation

The Joint Commission is an independent, not-for-profit organization founded in 1951 that evaluates and accredits nearly 21,000 healthcare organizations in the US and 1,100 in 69 countries worldwide (The Joint Commission, 2021). The mission is to continuously improve healthcare for the public, in collaboration with other stakeholders, by evaluating healthcare organizations and inspiring them to excel in providing safe and effective care of the highest quality and value. The vision is for all people to always experience the safest, highest-quality, best-value healthcare across all settings.

It accredits organizations across the spectrum of healthcare, including hospitals, skilled nursing facilities, home care, and ambulatory care. There are Advanced Certification programs (credentialing) for selected clinical areas such as stroke, cardiac, joint replacement, and perinatal care, but to date, not for aging programs. On June 26–27, 2019, a technical expert panel was convened in The Joint Commission Board Room. The purpose was to identify specific, evidence-based, generalizable interventions to improve quality, safety, and outcomes for older patients that can be used to create foundational requirements for an Age-Friendly Hospital certification program. This work continues as we document the evidence required for this program.

Figure 14.1. The Joint Commission Golden Circle

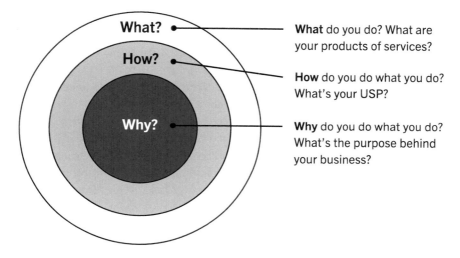

What **do you do? What are your products of services?**

How **do you do what you do? What's your USP?**

Why **do you do what you do? What's the purpose behind your business?**

Recommendations and Summary

There is value to the public when recognition, credentialing, and accreditation programs measure and reflect the reliability and quality of a system responsible for the care of older adults. This book has laid out the case for creating Age-Friendly Health Systems, described approaches to the implementation of the 4Ms model, discussed measurement and documentation strategies, and shared inspiring cases from the Age-Friendly Health Systems community, which is doing the work and seeing the exciting possibilities and positive outcomes. Our purpose has been to provide a guide that will make your journey easier and engage you in this exciting work. You will help us continuously improve, and we welcome all the ways you will participate in the IHI model of "all teach, all learn." The older adults we serve will be our best teachers if we listen and use What Matters to ensure person-centered, age-friendly care.

References

Institute for Healthcare Improvement. (2020). *Age-friendly health systems: Guide to using the 4Ms in the care of older adults.* http://www.ihi. org/Engage/Initiatives/Age-Friendly-Health-Systems/Documents/ IHIAgeFriendlyHealthSystems_GuidetoUsing4MsCare.pdf

Institute for Healthcare Improvement. (2021a). *Age-friendly health systems: 4Ms care description.* https://www.surveymonkey.com/r/Z2SGZNJ

Institute for Healthcare Improvement. (2021b). *Age-friendly health systems frequently asked questions.* http://www.ihi.org/Engage/Initiatives/Age-Friendly-Health-Systems/Pages/Frequently-Asked-Questions.aspx

Institute for Healthcare Improvement. (2021c). *Age-friendly health systems recognition.* http://www.ihi.org/Engage/Initiatives/Age-Friendly-Health-Systems/Pages/Recognition.aspx

The Joint Commission. (2021). *Joint Commission FAQs.* https://www. jointcommission.org/about-us/facts-about-the-joint-commission/ joint-commission-faqs/

Conclusion

We are in an era of demographic transformation, one that should be celebrated as well as acknowledged for the change it brings to healthcare for all older adults. Embracing an Age-Friendly Health System means that all of us commit to using the science and evidence that provides the best possible care in a reliable way for every older adult, no matter who provides that care or in what setting the care is provided. Clinicians, families, and society want to do the right thing, and through this Age-Friendly Health Systems social movement, we intend to continuously provide the best content for the best age-friendly outcomes. We wish you success and joy in your work.

Detailed Information on What Matters Process and Outcome Measures

Process Measure—Document What Matters

Hospital Setting

Measure name	Documentation of What Matters
Measure description	Percentage of patients with documentation of What Matters conversations (calculated as numerator / denominator × 100)
Site	Inpatient unit
Population measured	Patients 65 years or older
Measurement period	Weekly or monthly
	Weekly measurement will support faster testing and learning cycles but has consequently higher measurement burden and may not be feasible.
Numerator	*Inclusion*: Patients in the denominator with documentation of What Matters, per the unit's definition of What Matters. Your process should allow patients to decline to engage in What Matters conversations—an older adult who declines to answer and has "declined to answer" documented should be included in the numerator.
	Exclusions: None

Denominator	*Inclusion*: Patients with length of stay (LOS) greater than or equal to day present on the unit between 12:01 a.m. on the first day of the measurement period and 11:59 p.m. on the last day of the measurement period
	Exclusions: None
Method details	Asking What Matters is defined by the unit for the patients it serves. At a minimum, asking What Matters involves (a) querying the medical record for existing documentation of goals and preferences and (b) engaging patients in discussion of What Matters to them as defined by the unit.
	Documentation standard is defined by the unit for the patients it serves; standard describes the information that is recorded and the method of recording that information.
	If an automated report is possible, calculate denominator and numerator.
	If a complete manual tally is possible, calculate denominator and numerator.
	If neither an automated report nor a complete tally is possible, sample records at the end of the measurement period, and calculate numerator and denominator. You can apply a stopping rule to reduce measurement effort.

Primary Care Setting

Measure name	Documentation of What Matters
Measure description	Percentage of patients with documentation of What Matters conversations (calculated as numerator / denominator × 100)
Site	Primary care
Population measured	Patients 65 years or older
Measurement period	Monthly
Numerator	*Inclusion*: Patients in the numerator with documentation of What Matters within 12 months of the most recent office visit, home visit, or telemedicine visit in the measurement month, per the primary care unit's definition of What Matters. Your process should allow patients to decline to engage in What Matters conversations—an older adult who declines to answer and has "declined to answer" documented should be included in the numerator.

Exclusions: None |
| **Denominator** | Inclusion: All patients in the population considered to be patients of the primary care practice (e.g., patients assigned to a care team panel and seen by the practice within the past three years) who have an office visit, home visit, or telemedicine visit with the practice during the measurement period

Exclusions: None |
| **Method details** | Asking What Matters is defined by the primary care practice for the patients it serves. At a minimum, asking What Matters involves (a) querying the medical record for existing documentation of goals and preferences and (b) engaging patients in discussion of What Matters to them as defined by the unit.

Documentation standard is defined by the primary care practice for the patients it serves; standard describes the information that is recorded and the method of recording that information.

If an automated report is possible, calculate denominator and numerator.

If a complete manual tally is possible, calculate denominator and numerator.

If neither an automated report nor a complete tally is possible, sample records at the end of the measurement period and calculate numerator and denominator. You can apply a stopping rule to reduce measurement effort. |

Outcome Measure: Care Concordance With What Matters

Hospital Setting

Measure name	Care concordance with What Matters
Measure description	Percentage collaboRATE top-box score
Site	Inpatient unit
Population measured	Patients 65 years or older
Measurement period	Weekly or monthly Weekly measurement will support faster testing and learning cycles but has consequently higher measurement burden and may not be feasible.
Numerator	Inclusion: Count of surveys with top-box answers to all three questions ("all-or-nothing" score) Exclusions: None
Denominator	Count of complete surveys returned from patients Inclusion: Patients with LOS greater than or equal to 1 day present on the unit between 12:01 a.m. on the first day of the measurement period and 11:59 p.m. on the last day of the measurement period. For patients who are unable to respond to the questions due to cognitive impairment, use the proxy version of collaboRATE. Exclusions: None
Method details	Collect a minimum of 25 completed surveys to compute a top-box percentage (see http://www.glynelwyn.com/scoring-collaboRATE.html). Recognize that if respondent confidentiality cannot be ensured, scores may be biased upward. To support informed analysis and interpretation, units should track total number of patients approached to obtain the completed number of surveys. Paper/manual data tools will work for initial testing but may not scale to additional units. Organizations will need to develop information technology to allow patients to respond to the questions and to summarize the measurement with low effort.

Primary Care Setting

Measure name	Care concordance with What Matters
Measure description	Percentage collaboRATE top-box score
Site	Primary care practice
Population measured	Patients 65 years or older
Measurement period	Weekly or monthly
	Weekly measurement will support faster testing and learning cycles but has consequently higher measurement burden and may not be feasible.
Numerator	Inclusion: Count of surveys with top-box answers to all three questions ("all-or-nothing" score)
	Exclusions: None
Denominator	Number of surveys completed
	Inclusion: Patients in the population seen for any reason by the primary care practice during the measurement period
	Exclusions: None
Method details	Collect a minimum of 25 completed surveys to compute a top-box percentage (see http://www.glynelwyn.com/scoring-collaboRATE.html).
	Recognize that if respondent confidentiality cannot be ensured, scores may be biased upward.
	To support informed analysis and interpretation, practices should track total number of patients approached to obtain the completed number of surveys.
	Paper/manual data tools will work for initial testing but may not scale to additional practices. Organizations will need to develop information technology to allow patients to respond to the questions and to summarize the measurement with low effort.

Resources to Support What Matters Conversations With Older Adults

Online Tools

- **Decision Worksheets** (Health Decision Sciences Center, Massachusetts General Hospital): Worksheets for diabetes, depression, high blood pressure, high cholesterol, and acute low-back pain, as well as guides for using the treatment worksheets during visits

- **Geritalk**: Communication skills training for geriatrics and palliative medicine fellows

- **Hebrew Senior Life—Vitality 360 Program**: Comprehensive wellness and exercise program offered at Orchard Cove (part of Hebrew Senior Life)

- **How's Your Health? Patient Checkup Survey**: Tool for assessing patient self-confidence in health management

- **Patient Priorities Care**: Resources to support aligning care with what matters most to patients. The "Specific Ask (Matters Most) Conversation Guide" and the Patient Priorities identification conversation guide help identify the values, outcome goals, and care preferences for older adults with multiple chronic conditions.

- **Person-Centred Health and Care Programme (Healthcare Improvement Scotland)**: Practical guidelines for person-centered healthcare
  - **Preference Based Living** and the **Preference for Everyday Living Inventory**: Tools and resources for assessing individual preferences for "social contact, personal development, leisure activities, living environment, and daily routine," both at home and in nursing homes, including the Preferences for Everyday Living Inventory (PELI)

- **Project Implicit** (Harvard University): Tests for identifying social attitudes and implicit associations

- **Shared Decision-Making National Resource Center** (Mayo Clinic): Tools and resources for clinicians to use in practicing shared decision-making with patients, including patient decision aids, trainings, and workshops

- **Stanford Medicine Bucket List Planner**: Tool for reflecting on core values and goals through "bucket list" planning

- **Stanford School of Medicine Ethnogeriatrics Ethno Med Website**: Resources for providing high-quality geriatrics care to a multicultural population

- **STEPS Forward**: An online physician education module that guides physicians through how to discuss end-of-life decisions with patients and caregivers

- *Transforming Patient Experience: The Essential Guide* (NHS Institute for Innovation and Improvement; Archived): Results from the UK National Health Service (NHS) on developing an evidence base on what matters to patients

Blog Posts

- "Why 'What Matters to You?' Matters Around the World." Bisognano, M. *Institute for Healthcare Improvement Blog.* February 24, 2017.

- "Asking (and Listening to) Pediatric Patients." Kassam-Adams, N. *Health Care Toolbox Blog.* May 16, 2016.

- "Asking Pediatric Patients, 'What Matters to You?'" Pickard Sullivan, L. *Institute for Healthcare Improvement Blog.* March 18, 2016.

Conversation Guides

- *Conversation Ready* (IHI White Paper): Framework to help healthcare organizations become "Conversation Ready" (i.e., reliably support clinicians and patients in having end-of-life conversations, documenting these conversations, and providing concordant care)

- **How to Talk to Your Doctor** (The Conversation Project): Conversation guide for individuals to use when having conversations to articulate end-of-life goals and care preferences

- *Your Conversation Starter Guide for Caregivers of People With Alzheimer's or Other Forms of Dementia* (IHI, The Conversation Project): Conversation guide for end-of-life care goals and preferences, with specific considerations for caregivers of individuals with different forms of cognitive impairment

- *Serious Illness Conversation Guide* (Ariadne Labs): Conversation guide for clinicians that outlines steps for having conversations with seriously ill patients about their goals and values

Books

- *Doorway thoughts: Cross-cultural health care for older adults* (Vols. 1, 2, and 3). The Ethnogeriatrics Steering Committee of the American Geriatrics Society. (2008). Jones & Bartlett Learning.

- Hospice/palliative care: Concepts of disease and dying. Cruz-Oliver, D. (2016). In L. Cummings-Vaughn & D. M. Cruz-Oliver (Eds.), *Ethnogeriatrics: Healthcare needs of diverse populations*, 159–178. Springer Press.

- *Humble inquiry: The gentle art of asking instead of telling.* Schein, E. H. (2013). Berrett-Koehler.

Audio/Video

- "WIHI: Realizing 'What Matters' (to Patients and Families)" (Podcast)

- *What Matters to Me* from Yorkhill Children's Hospital (Video)

Commercial Tools and Trainings

- **PatientWisdom**: Online digital platform for connecting patients and clinicians

- **VitalTalk**: Online faculty development courses on improving communication skills

- **Motivational Interviewing Network of Trainers (MINT)**: Online network of trainers for motivational interviewing, including a library of resources and event and training listings

- **Cake App**: Mobile app with end-of-life preference and planning tools

- **PREPARE for Your Care**: Online tools for advance care planning and advance directives

- **Massachusetts General Hospital Health Decisions Science Center**: Multidisciplinary research group that provides tools and trainings on shared decision-making and informed medical decision-making, including decision worksheets

A Multicultural Tool for Getting to Know You and What Matters to You

This tool was developed by the Stanford Inreach for Successful Aging (iSAGE) for Diverse Older Adults.

1. **What matters most to you?** (Examples: being at home, gardening, going to church, playing with my grandchildren)

2. **Who are the people in your life you hold dear or care about?** (Examples: my friend Tom, my niece Maria)

Name	Relationship	When did you last see this person?

3. **Name three treasured moments in your life.** (Examples: meeting the love of my life, birth of my daughter, my graduation, getting my first car)

4. **Name three life experiences you would like to have or
    tasks you would like to complete in the next 6 months.**
    (Examples: travel to Europe, fishing trip, family reunion,
    50th wedding anniversary)

5. **Name three activities you enjoy doing regularly.**
    (Examples: walking, reading, cooking, hiking, dancing)

Activity	When was the last time you did this activity?	What assistance do you need to do this? (If no assistance needed, say none.)
1.		
2.		
3.		

6. **Describe what a good day looks like for you.** (Example:
    I wake up at 7:00 a.m. and do not have *any* pain. I have a
    hot breakfast with my family, then go for a walk and meet
    my friends. In the evening, I watch football while eating
    chocolate ice cream.)

7. **In what languages are the TV programs you usually
    watch?** (Examples: English, Spanish, Cantonese)

8. **How confident are you with filling out medical forms by
    yourself? Do you need help?** (Yes/No)

1 (Not confident)	2	3	4	5 (Very confident)

9. Who/what provides you with strength and hope?
   (Examples: going to church, meditation)

10. Do you have a community that supports you? Who are they and how do they help?

Examples of What Matters Conversations

Example: Newly Retired Man With Diabetes

Peter is 68 years old and has been managing his type 2 diabetes and moderate hypertension for the past two years. Peter is getting ready to retire and wants to spend more time gardening and traveling around the country in an RV with his wife. His primary care physician (PCP) has prescribed multiple medications to control his hypertension as well as regular appointments to monitor Peter's blood glucose, which has been difficult to get under control despite dietary changes.

At an annual wellness visit, the PCP asks about goals and preferences around Peter's retirement. Peter is nervous about bringing it up but mentions that he often feels lightheaded from the hypertension medication and, as a result, is not able to garden as much each day as he would like. Peter also mentions that the weekly doctor's appointments his doctor has requested will affect his ability to go on longer trips. It's important to him that his diabetes and hypertension are well managed, but he worries that this management is making his life less enjoyable. This creates an opportunity for Peter and his PCP to have a conversation about how to reconcile his physician's goals around hypertension and diabetes management with Peter's goals for doing what he enjoys.

Example: New Diagnosis

Last week, Carol, age 81, was diagnosed with colon cancer. Four days after her diagnosis visit, a nurse navigator called Carol to schedule an appointment to talk about What Matters to her and treatment options. The nurse navigator set up an hour-long appointment and arranged for Carol to meet her in a small conference room rather than an exam room. The nurse navigator starts the conversation by asking Carol specific questions about her health preferences and goals. He then broadens the conversation to talk to Carol about what her hopes, fears, and concerns are for her health as well as how her health could impact her ability to do what she enjoys. Carol notes that she is not afraid of dying, but she is afraid of missing out on important time and events with her family, and it is important to her that she be able to spend as much time with them as possible. Carol tells the navigator that she wants to start treatment soon but also wants to be able to attend her granddaughter's wedding in 2 months.

The nurse navigator shares this information with Carol's oncologist, who then sits down with Carol to talk about options for the timing of chemotherapy so that Carol will be able to see her granddaughter get married. Carol and the oncologist also discuss how different treatment options may affect her prognosis, her ability to stay at home, and other aspects that may impact her ability to spend time with her family and attend important events. As Carol begins her course of treatment, the nurse navigator checks in with her monthly by phone about how her treatment is going and whether any of her preferences have changed. At the beginning of every appointment, Carol's oncologist reviews notes in the EHR from pre-vious visits and calls with the nurse navigator and takes 5 minutes at the beginning of the appointment to follow up with Carol on any changes or updates.

Process Walkthrough

Know the 4Ms in Your Health System

There are two key drivers to age-friendly care: knowing about the 4Ms for each older adult in your care ("assess") and incorporating the 4Ms into the plan of care ("act on"). The aim in an Age-Friendly Health System is to reliably assess and act on the 4Ms with all older adults. Just about all systems are integrating some of the 4Ms into care, some of the time, with some older adults, in some place in their systems. The work now is to understand where that is happening and build on that good work so that all 4Ms occur reliably for all older adults in all care settings.

How do you already assess and act on each of the 4Ms in your setting? One way is to spend time in your unit, your practice, or your hospital observing the care. As you do, note your observations to the questions below as you learn more about how the 4Ms are already in practice in your system.

- What are current activities and services related to each of the 4Ms? What processes, tools, and resources to support the 4Ms do we already have in place here or elsewhere in the system?

- Where is the prompt or documentation available in the electronic health record or elsewhere for all clinicians and the care team? Is there a place to see the 4Ms (individually or together) across team members? Across settings?

- What experience do your team members have with the 4Ms? What assets do you already have on the team? What challenges have they faced? How have they overcome them?

- What internal or community-based resources do you commonly refer to and for which of the 4Ms? For which of the 4Ms do you need additional internal and/or community-based resources?

- Do your current 4Ms activities and services appear to be having a positive impact on older adults and/or family caregivers? Do you have a way to hear about the older adults' experience?

- Do your current 4Ms activities and services appear to be having a positive impact on the clinicians and staff?

- Which languages do the older adults and their family caregivers speak? Read?

- Do the health literacy levels, language skills, and cultural preferences of your patients match the assets of your team and the resources provided by your health system?

- What works well?

- What could be improved?

4Ms Age-Friendly Care Description Worksheets

Hospital Setting

Please document below your description of age-friendly (or 4Ms) care as your team currently describes it. To be considered age-friendly, you must explicitly engage or screen/assess people aged 65 and older for all 4Ms (What Matters, Medication, Mentation, Mobility), document 4Ms information, and act on the 4Ms accordingly.

Health System Name:
Key Contact:
Name of Hospital:
Site of Care:
- ☐ Hospital-wide
- ☐ Specialty unit (e.g., ACE)
- ☐ General medical/surgical unit
- ☐ Other

If specialty unit or other, please describe:

	WHAT MATTERS	MEDICATION	MENTATION	MOBILITY
Aim	Know and align care with each older adult's specific health outcome goals and care preferences, including, but not limited to, end-of-life care and across settings of care	If medication is necessary, use age-friendly medication that does not interfere with What Matters to the older adult, Mobility, or Mentation across settings of care	Prevent, identify, treat, and manage delirium across settings of care	Ensure that each older adult moves safely every day to maintain function and do What Matters
Engage/Screen/ Assess *Please check the boxes to indicate items used in your care or fill in the blanks if you check "other."*	List the question(s) you ask to know and align care with each older adult's specific outcome goals and care preferences: *One or more What Matters question(s) must be listed. Question(s) cannot focus only on end-of-life forms.*	Check the medications you screen for regularly: ☐ benzodiazepines ☐ opioids ☐ highly anticholinergic medications (e.g., diphenhydramine) ☐ all prescription and over-the-counter sedatives and sleep medications ☐ muscle relaxants ☐ tricyclic antidepressants ☐ antipsychotics ☐ other: _____ *Minimum requirement: At least one of the first seven boxes must be checked.*	Check the tool used to screen for delirium: ☐ UB-2 ☐ CAM ☐ 3D-CAM ☐ CAM-ICU ☐ bCAM ☐ Nu-DESC ☐ other: _____ *Minimum requirement: At least one of the first six boxes must be checked. If only "Other" is checked, will review.*	Check the tool used to screen for mobility limitations: ☐ TUG ☐ Get Up and Go ☐ JH-HLM ☐ POMA ☐ refer to physical therapy (PT) ☐ other: _____ *Minimum requirement: One box must be checked. If only "Other" is checked, will review.*

Frequency	□ once per stay □ daily □ other: _____ *Minimum frequency is once per stay.*	□ once per stay □ daily □ other: _____ *Minimum frequency is once per stay.*	□ every 12 hours □ other: _____ *Minimum frequency is every 12 hours.*	□ once per stay □ daily □ other: _____ *Minimum frequency is once per stay.*
Documentation *Please check the "EHR" (electronic health record) box or fill in the blank for "other."*	□ EHR □ other: _____ *One box must be checked; preferred option is EHR. If "Other," will review to ensure documentation method is accessible to other care team members for use during the hospital stay.*	□ EHR □ other: _____ *One box must be checked; preferred option is EHR. If "Other," will review to ensure documentation method is accessible to other care team members for use during the hospital stay.*	□ EHR □ other: _____ *One box must be checked; preferred option is EHR. If "Other," will review to ensure documentation method can capture assessment to trigger appropriate action.*	□ EHR □ other: _____ *One box must be checked; preferred option is EHR. If "Other," will review to ensure documentation method can capture assessment to trigger appropriate action.*

Act On *Please describe how you use the information obtained from Engage/Screen/Assess to design and provide care. Refer to pathways or procedures that are meaningful to your staff in the "other" field.*	☐ align the care plan with What Matters most ☐ other: _____ *Minimum requirement: First box must be checked.*	☐ deprescribe (includes both dose reduction and medication discontinuation) ☐ pharmacy consult ☐ other: _____ *Minimum requirement: At least one box must be checked.*	☐ Delirium prevention and management protocol including, but not limited to: ☐ ensure sufficient oral hydration ☐ orient older adult to time, place, and situation on every nursing shift ☐ ensure older adult has their personal adaptive equipment (e.g., glasses, hearing aids, dentures, walkers) ☐ prevent sleep interruptions; use nonpharmacological interventions to support sleep ☐ avoid high-risk medications ☐ other: _____ *Minimum requirement: First five boxes must be checked.*	☐ ambulate three times a day ☐ out of bed or leave room for meals ☐ PT intervention (balance, gait, strength, gait training, exercise program) ☐ avoid restraints ☐ remove catheters and other tethering devices ☐ avoid high-risk medications ☐ other: _____ *Minimum requirement: Must check first box and at least one other box.*
Primary Responsibility *Indicate which care team member has primary responsibility for the older adult.*	☐ nurse ☐ clinical assistant ☐ social worker ☐ MD ☐ pharmacist ☐ other: _____ *Minimum requirement: One role must be selected.*	☐ nurse ☐ clinical assistant ☐ social worker ☐ MD ☐ pharmacist ☐ other: _____ *Minimum requirement: One role must be selected.*	☐ nurse ☐ clinical assistant ☐ social worker ☐ MD ☐ pharmacist ☐ other: _____ *Minimum requirement: One role must be selected.*	☐ nurse ☐ clinical assistant ☐ social worker ☐ MD ☐ pharmacist ☐ other: _____ *Minimum requirement: One role must be selected.*

Ambulatory Care Setting

Please document below your description of age-friendly (4Ms) care as your team currently describes it. To be considered age-friendly, you must explicitly engage or screen/assess people aged 65 and older for all 4Ms (What Matters, Medication, Mentation, Mobility), document 4Ms information, and act on the 4Ms accordingly.

Health System Name:
Key Contact:
Site of Care:
☐ Primary care practice
☐ Specialty practice (e.g., geriatric service)
☐ Other
If specialty practice or other, please describe:

	WHAT MATTERS	MEDICATION	MENTATION: DEMENTIA	MENTATION: DEPRESSION	MOBILITY
Aim	Know and align care with each older adult's specific health-outcome goals and care preferences including, but not limited to, end-of-life care and across settings of care	If medication is necessary, use age-friendly medication that does not interfere with What Matters to the older adult, Mobility, or Mentation across settings of care	Prevent, identify, treat, and manage dementia across settings of care	Prevent, identify, treat, and manage depression across settings of care	Ensure that each older adult moves safely every day to maintain function and do What Matters most
Engage/Screen/Assess *Please check the boxes to indicate items used in your care or fill in the blanks if you check "other."*	List the question(s) you ask to know and align care with each older adult's specific outcome goals and care preferences *One or more What Matters question(s) must be listed. Question(s) cannot focus only on end-of-life forms.*	Check the medications you screen for regularly: ☐ benzodiazepines ☐ opioids ☐ highly anticholinergic medications (e.g., diphenhydramine) ☐ all prescription and over-the-counter sedatives and sleep medications ☐ muscle relaxants ☐ tricyclic antidepressants ☐ antipsychotics ☐ other: ____ *Minimum requirement: At least one of the first seven boxes must be checked.*	Check the tool used to screen for dementia: ☐ Mini-Cog ☐ SLUMS ☐ MoCA ☐ other: ____ *Minimum requirement: At least one of the first three boxes must be checked. If only "Other" is checked, will review.*	Check the tool used to screen for depression: ☐ PHQ-2 ☐ PHQ-9 ☐ GDS–short form ☐ GDS ☐ other: ____ *Minimum requirement: At least one of the first four boxes must be checked. If only "Other" is checked, will review.*	Check the tool used to screen for mobility limitations: ☐ TUG ☐ Get Up and Go ☐ JH-HLM ☐ POMA ☐ refer to physical therapy (PT) ☐ other: ____ *Minimum requirement: One box must be checked. If only "Other" is checked, will review.*

Optional: Check the tool used for functional assessment:
- □ Barthel Index of ADLs (in Epic)
- □ Lawton IADLs
- □ Katz ADL
- □ other: _____

Frequency	□ annually □ other: ___ *Minimum frequency is annually.*	□ annually □ at a change of medication □ other: ___ *Minimum frequency is annually.*	□ annually □ other: ___ *Minimum frequency is annually.*	□ annually □ other: ___ *Minimum frequency is annually.*	□ annually □ other: ___ *Minimum frequency is annually.*
Documentation *Please check the "EHR" box (electronic health record) or fill in the blank for "other."*	□ EHR □ other: ___ *One box must be checked; preferred option is "EHR." If "Other," will review to ensure documentation method is accessible to other care team members for use during care.*	□ EHR □ other: ___ *One box must be checked; preferred option is "EHR." If "Other," will review to ensure documentation method is accessible to other care team members for use during care.*	□ EHR □ other: ___ *One box must be checked; preferred option is "EHR." If "Other," will review to ensure documentation method can capture assessment to trigger appropriate action.*	□ EHR □ other: ___ *One box must be checked; preferred option is "EHR." If "Other," will review to ensure documentation method can capture assessment to trigger appropriate action.*	□ EHR □ other: ___ *One box must be checked; preferred option is "EHR." If "Other," will review to ensure documentation method can capture mobility status in a way that other care team members can use.*

Act On					
Please describe how you use the information obtained from Engage/Screen/Assess to design and provide care. Refer to pathways or procedures that are meaningful to your staff in the "other" field.	□ align the care plan with What Matters most □ other: _____ *Minimum requirement: First box must be checked.*	□ educate older adult and family caregivers □ deprescribe (includes both dose reduction and medication discontinuation) □ refer to: _____ □ other: _____ *Minimum requirement: At least one box must be checked.*	□ share results with older adult □ provide educational materials to older adult and family caregivers □ refer to community organization for education and/or support □ refer to: _____ □ other: _____ *Minimum requirement: Must check first box and at least one other box.*	□ educate older adult and family caregivers □ prescribe antidepressant □ refer to: _____ □ other: _____ *Minimum requirement: At least one of the first three boxes must be checked.*	□ multifactorial fall prevention protocol (e.g., STEADI) □ educate older adult and family caregivers □ manage impairments that reduce mobility (e.g., pain, balance, gait, strength) □ ensure safe home environment for mobility □ identify and set a daily mobility goal with older adult that supports What Matters; review and support progress toward the goal □ avoid high-risk medications □ refer to PT □ other: _____ *Minimum requirement: Must check the first box or at least three of the remaining boxes.*

Primary Responsibility *Indicate which care team member has primary responsibility for the older adult.*	☐ nurse ☐ clinical assistant ☐ social worker ☐ MD ☐ pharmacist ☐ other: _____ *Minimum requirement: One role must be selected.*	☐ nurse ☐ clinical assistant ☐ social worker ☐ MD ☐ pharmacist ☐ other: _____ *Minimum requirement: One role must be selected.*	☐ nurse ☐ clinical assistant ☐ social worker ☐ MD ☐ pharmacist ☐ other: _____ *Minimum requirement: One role must be selected.*	☐ nurse ☐ clinical assistant ☐ social worker ☐ MD ☐ pharmacist ☐ other: _____ *Minimum requirement: One role must be selected.*	☐ nurse ☐ clinical assistant ☐ social worker ☐ MD ☐ pharmacist ☐ other: _____ *Minimum requirement: One role must be selected.*

Key Actions and Getting Started with Age-Friendly Care

Hospital-Based Care

Assess: Know about the 4Ms for each older adult in your care

KEY ACTIONS	GETTING STARTED	TIPS AND RESOURCES
Ask the older adult What Matters	If you do not have existing questions to start this conversation, try the following, and adapt as needed: *"What do you most want to focus on while you are in the hospital / emergency department for _____ [fill in health problem] so that you can do _____ [fill in desired activity] more often or more easily?"* (Naik et al., 2018; Tinetti et al., 2016) For older adults with advanced or serious illness, consider: *"What are your most important goals if your health situation worsens?"*	**Tips** • This action focuses clinical encounters, decision-making, and care planning on What Matters most to the older adults. • Consider segmenting your population by healthy older adults, those with chronic conditions, those with serious illness, and individuals at the end of life. How you ask What Matters of each segment may differ. • Consider starting these conversations with *who* matters to the patient. Then ask the patient what their plans are related to life milestones, travel plans, birthdays, and so on in the next 6 months to emphasize "I matter too." Once "who matters" and "I matter too" are discussed, then *what matters* becomes much easier to discuss. The What Matters Most letter template (Stanford Letter Project) can guide this discussion. • Responsibility for asking What Matters can rest with any member of the care team; however, one person needs to be identified as responsible to ensure it is reliably done. • You may decide to include family caregivers in a discussion about What Matters; however, it is important to also ask the older adult individually. • Ask people with dementia What Matters. Ask people with delirium What Matters at a time when they are suffering least from delirium symptoms.

Ask the older adult What Matters *(continued)*		**Additional Resources** • *What Matters to Older Adults? A Toolkit for Health Systems to Design Better Care With Older Adults* • The Conversation Project and *Conversation Ready* • Patient Priorities Care • *Serious Illness Conversation Guide* • Stanford Letter Project • *"What Matters to You?" Instructional Video and A Guide to Having Conversations About What Matters* (BC Patient Safety & Quality Council)
Document What Matters	Documentation can be on paper, on a whiteboard, or in the electronic health record (EHR), where it is accessible to the whole care team across settings.	**Tips** • Convert whiteboards to What Matters boards and include information about the older adults (e.g., what they like to be called, favorite foods, favorite activities, what concerns or upsets them, what soothes them, assistive devices, and family caregiver names and phone numbers). Identify who on the care team is responsible for ensuring they are updated. • Consider documentation of What Matters to the older adult on paper that they can bring to appointments and other sites of care. • Identify where health and healthcare goals and priorities can be captured in your EHR and available across care teams and settings. • Review What Matters documentation across older adult patients to ensure it is specific to each person (i.e., watch for generic answers or the same answer across all patients, which suggests a deeper discussion of What Matters is warranted). **Additional Resources** • *"What Matters to You?" Instructional Video and A Guide to Having Conversations About What Matters* (BC Patient Safety & Quality Council)

Review for high-risk medication use	Specifically, look for these: • benzodiazepines • opioids • highly anticholinergic medications (e.g., diphenhydramine) • all prescription and over-the-counter sedatives and sleep medications • muscle relaxants • tricyclic antidepressants • antipsychotics (Hill-Taylor et al., 2013)	**Tips** • If you select to limit the number of medications to focus on, identify those most frequently dispensed in your hospital or unit, or those for whom there is a champion to deprescribe. **Additional Resources** • American Geriatrics Society 2019 Updated AGS Beers Criteria for Potentially Inappropriate Medication Use in Older Adults • AGS 2019 Beers Criteria Pocketcard • *Reducing Inappropriate Medication Use by Implementing Deprescribing Guidelines*
Screen for delirium at least every 12 hours	If you do not have an existing tool, try using Ultra-Brief 2-Item Screener (UB-2; Fick et al., 2018).	**Tips** • Decide on the tool that best fits your care team culture. • Be aware that low prevalence rates of delirium before the 4Ms are in place may indicate inaccurate use of a screening or assessment tool. • It is critical to use any tool only as instructed and to do ongoing training (yearly competency) to make sure it is being used correctly. • Ask questions in a way that emphasizes the older adult's strengths (e.g., "Please tell me the day of the week" rather than "Do you know what day it is today?"). • Educate family caregivers on the signs of delirium and enlist their support to alert the care team to any changes as soon as they notice them. Ask them if their loved one seems "like themselves." • Document mental status in the chart to measure changes shift-to-shift.

Screen for delirium at least every 12 hours *(continued)*

Tips *(continued)*
- Until ruled out, consider a change in mental status to be delirium and raise awareness among care team and family caregivers about the risk of delirium superimposed on dementia.
- *Note:* Delirium has an underlying cause and is preventable and treatable in most cases. Care teams need to do the following:
  - Remove or treat underlying cause(s) if it occurs
  - Restore or maintain function and mobility
  - Understand delirium behaviors
  - Prevent delirium complications

Additional Resources
- Confusion Assessment Method (CAM) and its variations: 3D-CAM for medical-surgical units, CAM-ICU for intensive care units, bCAM for emergency departments
- Nursing Delirium Screening Scale (Nu-DESC)
- Hospital Elder Life Program (HELP)
- www.idelirium.org

Screen for mobility limitations

If you do not have an existing tool, try using the Timed Up & Go (TUG) Test.

Tips
- Recognize that older adults may be embarrassed or worried about having their mobility screened.
- Underscore that a mobility screen allows the care team to know the strengths of the older adult.

Additional Resources
- Get Up and Go and demonstration video
- Johns Hopkins—Highest Level of Mobility (JH-HLM) Scale
- Tinetti Performance-Oriented Mobility Assessment (POMA)

Act On: Incorporate the 4Ms into the plan of care

KEY ACTIONS	GETTING STARTED	TIPS AND RESOURCES
Align the care plan with What Matters	Incorporate What Matters into the goal-oriented plan of care and align the care plan with the older adult's goals and preferences (i.e., What Matters).	**Tips** • Health outcome goals are the activities that matter most to an individual, such as babysitting a grandchild, walking with friends in the morning, or continuing to work as a teacher. Healthcare preferences include the medications, healthcare visits, testing, and self-management tasks that an individual is able and willing to do. • When you focus on the patient's priorities, Medication, Mentation, and Mobility usually come up so the patient can do more of What Matters. • Consider how care while in the hospital can be modified to align with What Matters. • Consider What Matters to the older adult when deciding where they will be discharged. • Use What Matters to develop the care plan and navigate trade-offs. For example, you may say, "There are several things we could do, but knowing what matters most to you, I suggest we…" • Use the patient's priorities (not just diseases) in communicating, decision-making, and assessing benefits. • Use collaborative negotiations; agree there is no best answer, and brainstorm alternatives together. For example, you may say, "I know you don't like the CPAP mask, but are you willing to try it for 2 weeks to see if it helps you be less tired, so you can get back to volunteering, which you said was most important to you?" • Care options likely involve input from many disciplines (e.g., physical therapy, social work, community organizations).

Align the care plan with What Matters (continued)	**Additional Resources**
	• *What Matters to Older Adults? A Toolkit for Health Systems to Design Better Care With Older Adults* • *Patient Priorities Care* • *Serious Illness Conversation Guide* • *"What Matters to You?" Instructional Video and A Guide to Having Conversations About What Matters* (BC Patient Safety & Quality Council)

| Deprescribe or do not prescribe high-risk medications* | Specifically avoid or deprescribe the high-risk medications listed below.
• benzodiazepines
• opioids
• highly anticholinergic medications (e.g., diphenhydramine)
• all prescription and over-the-counter sedatives and sleep medications
• muscle relaxants
• tricyclic antidepressants
• antipsychotics (Lumish et al., 2018; Reuben et al., 2017)

If the older adult takes one or more of these medications, discuss any concerns the patient may have, assess for adverse effects, and discuss deprescribing with the older adult. | **Tips**
• These medications, individually and in combination, may interfere with What Matters, Mentation, and safe Mobility of older adults because they increase the risk of confusion, delirium, unsteadiness, and falls (O'Mahony et al., 2015).
• Deprescribing includes both dose reduction and medication discontinuation.
• Deprescribing is a positive, patient-centered approach requiring informed patient consent, shared decision-making, close monitoring, and compassionate support.
• When possible, avoid prescribing these high-risk medications (prevention); consider changing order sets in the EHR to change prescribing patterns (e.g., adjust/reduce doses, change medications available).
• Your institution should have delirium and fall prevention and management protocols that include guidance to avoid high-risk medications.
• Offer nonpharmacological options to support sleep and manage pain.
• Upon discharge, do not assume all medications should be sustained. Remove medications the older adult can stop taking upon discharge. |

Deprescribe or do not prescribe high-risk medications* *(continued)*	**Tips** *(continued)*
	• Include a medication list printout as part of standard check-out steps and ensure that the older adult and family caregivers understand what their medications are for, how to take them, why they are taking them, and how to monitor whether they are helping or possibly causing adverse effects.
	• Inform the patient's ambulatory clinicians of medication changes.
	• Consult pharmacy.
	• When instituting an age-friendly approach to medications:
	• Identify who on your team is going to be the champion of this "M." The champion may not be a pharmacist, but it is vital to have a pharmacist or physician, as well as the patient, work on the plan.
	• Review your setting's or system's data, if possible, to identify medications that may be high risk (e.g., anticoagulants, insulin, opioids) or potentially inappropriate medications (e.g., anticholinergics).
	• Determine your goal(s) with respect to the medication(s) identified in the previous step.
	• Conduct a series of PDSA cycles to achieve your goal(s).
	Additional Resources
	• deprescribing.org
	• *Reducing Inappropriate Medication Use by Implementing Deprescribing Guidelines*
	• "Alternative medications for medications included in the use of high-risk medications in the elderly and potentially harmful drug-disease interactions in the elderly quality measures"
	• HealthinAging.org (expert health information for older adults and caregivers about critical issues we all face as we age)
	• *Crosswalk: Evidence-Based Leadership Council Programs and the 4Ms*

Ensure sufficient oral hydration*	Identify a target amount of oral hydration appropriate for the older adult and monitor to confirm it is met.	**Tips** • Ensure water and other patient-preferred non-caffeinated fluids are available at the bedside and accessible to the older adult. • The focus here is on oral hydration so that the patient is not on an IV that may interfere with Mobility. • Your institution should have a delirium prevention and management protocol that includes oral hydration. • Replace pitchers with water bottles with straws for easier use by older adults.
Orient older adults to time, place, and situation*	Make sure day and date are updated on the whiteboard. Provide an accurate clock with a large face visible to older adults. Consider the use of tools such as an "All About Me" board or poster/card that shows what makes the older adults calm and happy, who is important to them, names of pets, etc. Make newspapers and other periodicals available in the patient's room. Invite family caregivers to bring familiar and orienting items from home (e.g., family pictures).	**Tips** • For older adults with dementia, consider gentle reorientation or the use of orienting cues; avoid repeated testing about the orientation if the older adult appears agitated (Marcantonio, 2017). • Conduct orientation during every nursing shift. • Your institution should have a delirium prevention and management protocol that includes orientation. • Identify person-centered environmental and personal approaches to orienting the older adult.

Ensure older adults have their personal adaptive equipment*	Incorporate routine intake and documentation of the older adult's personal adaptive equipment. At the beginning of each shift, check for sensory aids and offer to clean them. If needed, offer the older adults a listening device or hearing amplifier from the unit.	**Tips** • This includes equipment such as glasses, hearing aids, dentures, and walkers. • Your institution should have a delirium prevention and management protocol that includes this action. • Note use of personal adaptive equipment on the whiteboard. • Confirm need for personal adaptive equipment with family caregivers.
Prevent sleep interruptions; use non-pharmacological interventions to support sleep*	Avoid overnight vital checks and blood draws unless absolutely necessary. Create and use sleep kits (Hshieh et al., 2015). Sleep kits include items such as a small CD player and CD to play relaxing music, lotion for a back rub or hand massage, non-caffeinated tea, lavender, sleep hygiene educational cards (that, for example, outline actions such as no caffeine after 11 a.m. or promote physical activity). These can be placed in a box on the unit to use in patient rooms as needed.	**Tips** • Nonpharmacological sleep aids include earplugs, sleeping masks, muscle relaxation such as hand massage, posture and relaxation training, white noise and music, and educational strategies. • Your institution should have a delirium prevention and management protocol that includes nonpharmacological sleep support. • Make a sleep kit available for order in the EHR. • Engage family caregivers to support sleep with methods that are familiar to the older adult.

Ensure early, frequent, and safe mobility* (Larson, 2017)

Ambulate three times a day.

Set and meet a daily mobility goal with each older adult.

Get patients out of bed or have them leave the room for meals.

Tips

- Assess and manage impairments that reduce mobility. For example:
  - manage pain
  - assess impairments in strength, balance, or gait
  - remove catheters, IV lines, telemetry, and other tethering devices as soon as possible
  - avoid restraints
  - avoid sedatives and drugs that immobilize the older adult
  - refer to physical therapy; have physical therapy interventions to help with balance, gait, strength, gait training, or an exercise program if needed
- Your institution should have a delirium prevention and management protocol that includes mobility.
- Engage the older adult and family caregivers directly by offering exercises that can be done in bed (e.g., put appropriate exercises on a placemat that remains in the room).

Additional Resources

- Hospital Elder Life Program (HELP) Mobility Change Package and Toolkit

*These activities are also key to preventing delirium and falls.

Ambulatory/Primary Care

Assess: Know about the 4Ms for each older adult in your care

KEY ACTIONS	GETTING STARTED	TIPS AND RESOURCES
Ask the older adult What Matters	If you do not have existing questions to start this conversation, try the following, and adapt as needed: *"What is the one thing about your health or healthcare you most want to focus on related to_____ [fill in health problem OR the healthcare task] so that you can do_____ [fill in desired activity] more often or more easily?" (Naik et al., 2018; Tinetti et al., 2016)* For older adults with advanced or serious illness, consider: *"What are your most important goals if your health situation worsens?"*	**Tips** • This action focuses clinical encounters, decision-making, and care planning on What Matters most to older adults. • Consider segmenting your population by healthy older adults, those with chronic conditions, those with serious illness, and individuals at the end of life. How you ask What Matters of each segment may differ. • Consider starting these conversations with *who* matters to the patient. Then ask the patient what their plans are related to life milestones, travel plans, birthdays, and so on in the next 6 months to emphasize "I matter too." Once "who matters" and "I matter too" are discussed, then *what* matters becomes much easier to discuss. The What Matters Most letter template (Stanford Letter Project) can guide this discussion. • Responsibility for asking What Matters can rest with any member of the care team; however, one person needs to be identified as responsible to ensure it is reliably done. • You may decide to include family caregivers in a discussion about What Matters; however, it is important to also ask the older adult individually. • Ask people with dementia What Matters. • Integrate asking What Matters into Welcome to Medicare and the Medicare Annual Wellness Visit. • You may include What Matters questions in pre-visit paperwork and verify the answers during the visit.

Ask the older adult What Matters (continued)		**Additional Resources** • *What Matters to Older Adults? A Toolkit for Health Systems to Design Better Care With Older Adults* • The Conversation Project and *Conversation Ready* • Patient Priorities Care • *Serious Illness Conversation Guide* • Stanford Letter Project • *"What Matters to You?" Instructional Video and A Guide to Having Conversations About What Matters* (BC Patient Safety & Quality Council) • "End-of-Life Care Conversations: Medicare Reimbursement FAQs"
Document What Matters	Documentation can be on paper or in the electronic health record (EHR) where it is accessible to the whole care team across settings	**Tips** • Identify where health and healthcare goals and priorities can be captured in your EHR and available across care teams and settings. • Consider documenting What Matters to the older adult on paper that they can bring to appointments and other sites of care. • Invite older adults to enter What Matters to them on your patient portal. **Additional Resources** • My Story for Family Caregivers • Community Library for your EHR • *"What Matters to You?" Instructional Video and A Guide to Having Conversations About What Matters* (BC Patient Safety & Quality Council)

| Review for high-risk medication use | Specifically, look for these:
• benzodiazepines
• opioids
• highly anticholinergic medications (e.g, diphenhydramine)
• all prescription and over-the-counter sedatives and sleep medications
• muscle relaxants
• tricyclic antidepressants
• antipsychotics (Hill-Taylor et al., 2013) | **Tips**
• Consider this review a medication risk assessment and be sure to include over-the-counter medications at least annually.
• Engage the older adult and family caregiver in providing all medications (including over-the-counter medicines) for review.
• Medicare beneficiaries may be eligible for an annual comprehensive medication review.
• Medication reconciliation, part of the Medicare Annual Wellness Visit, may be an important step in identifying high-risk medications.

Additional Resources
• American Geriatrics Society 2019 Updated AGS Beers Criteria for Potentially Inappropriate Medication Use in Older Adults
• AGS 2019 Beers Criteria Pocketcard
• *Reducing Inappropriate Medication Use by Implementing Deprescribing Guidelines*
• Medicare Interactive, Annual Wellness Visit
• CDC Medication Personal Action Plan
• CDC Personal Medicines List |
| Screen for dementia/ cognitive impairment | If you do not have an existing tool, try using the Mini-Cog | **Tips**
• Normalize cognitive screening for patients. For example, say, "I'm going to assess your cognitive health like we check your blood pressure or your heart and lungs."
• Emphasize an older adult's strengths when screening and document them so that all providers have a baseline cognitive screen.
• If they have a sudden change (over the course of a day or weeks) in cognition, consider and rule out delirium.
• Screening for cognitive impairment is part of Welcome to Medicare and the Medicare Annual Wellness Visit.

Additional Resources
• Saint Louis University Mental Status (SLUMS) Exam
• Montreal Cognitive Assessment (MoCA) |

Screen for depression	If you do not have an existing tool, try using the Patient Health Questionnaire-2 (PHQ-2).	**Tips** • Screen if there is a concern for depression. • Screening for depression is part of Welcome to Medicare and the Medicare Annual Wellness Visit. **Additional Resources** • Patient Health Questionnaire-9 (PHQ-9) • Geriatric Depression Scale (GDS) and GDS: Short Form

Screen for mobility limitations	If you do not have an existing tool, try using the Timed Up & Go (TUG) Test.	**Tips**
		• Recognize that older adults may be embarrassed or worried about having their mobility screened.
		• Underscore that a mobility screen allows the care team to know the strengths of the older adult.
		• Screening for mobility is part of Welcome to Medicare and the Medicare Annual Wellness Visit.
		• Consider engaging the full care team in assessing mobility. Does the person walk into the waiting room? Are they able to stand up from the waiting room chair when called? Can they walk to the exam room?
		• Consider also conducting a functional assessment. Common tools include:
		  • Barthel Index of ADLs (in Epic)
		  • The Lawton Instrumental Activities of Daily Living (IADL) Scale
		  • Katz Index of Independence in Activities of Daily Living (ADL)
		
		Additional Resources
		• Get Up and Go and demonstration video
		• Johns Hopkins—Highest Level of Mobility (JH-HLM) Scale
		• Performance-Oriented Mobility Assessment (POMA)

Act On: Incorporate the 4Ms into the plan of care

KEY ACTIONS	GETTING STARTED	TIPS AND RESOURCES
Align the care plan with What Matters	Incorporate What Matters into the goal-oriented plan of care and align the care plan with the older adult's goals and preferences (i.e., What Matters).	**Tips** • Health outcome goals are the activities that matter most to an individual, such as babysitting a grandchild, walking with friends in the morning, or continuing to work as a teacher. Healthcare preferences include the medications, healthcare visits, testing, and self-management tasks that an individual is able and willing to do. • When you focus on the patient's priorities, Medication, Mentation (cognition and depression), and Mobility usually come up so the patient can do more of What Matters. • Use What Matters to develop the care plan and navigate trade-offs. For example, you may say, "There are several things we could do, but knowing what matters most to you, I suggest we…" • Use the patient's priorities (not just diseases) in communicating, decision-making, and assessing benefits. • Use collaborative negotiations; agree there is no best answer and brainstorm alternatives together. For example, you may say, "I know you don't like the CPAP mask, but are you willing to try it for 2 weeks to see if it helps you be less tired, so you can get back to volunteering, which you said was most important to you?" • Care options likely involve input from many disciplines (e.g., physical therapy, social work, community organizations). **Additional Resources** • *What Matters to Older Adults? A Toolkit for Health Systems to Design Better Care With Older Adults* • *Patient Priorities Care* • *Serious Illness Conversation Guide* • *"What Matters to You?" Instructional Video and A Guide to Having Conversations About What Matters* (BC Patient Safety & Quality Council)

Deprescribe or do not prescribe high-risk medications*	Specifically avoid or deprescribe the high-risk medications listed below:	Tips

	• benzodiazepines
	• opioids
	• highly anticholinergic medications (e.g., diphenhydramine)
	• all prescription and over-the-counter sedatives and sleep medications
	• muscle relaxants
	• tricyclic antidepressants
	• antipsychotics (Lumish et al., 2018; Reuben et al., 2017)
	
	If the older adult takes one or more of these medications, discuss any concerns the patient may have, assess for adverse effects, and discuss deprescribing with the older adult.
		• These medications, individually and in combination, may interfere with What Matters, Mentation, and safe Mobility of older adults because they increase the risk of confusion, delirium, unsteadiness, and falls (O'Mahony et al., 2015).
		• Deprescribing includes both dose reduction and medication discontinuation.
		• Deprescribing is a positive, patient-centered approach requiring informed patient consent, shared decision-making, close monitoring, and compassionate support.
		• When possible, avoid prescribing these high-risk medications (prevention).
		• Consider changing order sets in the EHR to change prescribing patterns (e.g., adjust/reduce doses or change medications available).
		• Provide ongoing patient/caregiver education about potentially high-risk medications through all care settings (e.g., outpatient pharmacy) to help improve safe medication use and informed decision-making.
		• Consider community resources to support pain management with non-pharmacological interventions, including referral to community-based resources.
		• Communicate changes in medications across clinicians and settings of care, and with the primary pharmacy working with the older adult.
		• When instituting an age-friendly approach to medications:
		  • Identify who on your team is going to be the champion of this "M." The champion may not be a pharmacist, but it is vital to have a pharmacist or physician, as well as the patient, work on the plan.
		  • Review your setting's or system's data, if possible, to identify medications that may be high risk (e.g., anticoagulants, insulin, opioids) or potentially inappropriate medications (e.g., anticholinergics).
		  • Determine your goal(s) with respect to the medication(s) identified in the previous step.
		  • Conduct a series of PDSA cycles to achieve your goal(s).

Deprescribe or do not prescribe high-risk medications* *(continued)*	**Additional Resources** • deprescribing.org • Reducing Inappropriate Medication Use by Implementing Deprescribing Guidelines • "Alternative medications for medications included in the use of high-risk medications in the elderly and potentially harmful drug-disease interactions in the elderly quality measures" • HealthinAging.org (expert health information for older adults and caregivers about critical issues we all face as we age) • Crosswalk: Evidence-Based Leadership Council Programs and the 4Ms
Consider further evaluation and manage manifestations of dementia or refer to geriatrics, psychiatry, or neurology	Share the results with the older adult and caregiver. Assess for modifiable contributors to cognitive impairment. Consider further diagnostic evaluation if appropriate. Follow current guidelines for treatment of dementia and resulting behavioral manifestations or refer to geriatrics, psychiatry, or neurology for management of dementia-related issues. Provide educational materials to the older adult and family caregiver. Refer the older adult, family, and other caregivers to supportive resources, such as the Alzheimer's Association. **Tips** • Know about and refer older adults and their caregivers to local community-based organizations and resources to support them with education and/or support. • Include family caregivers. They provide a source of information and support. To identify these individuals, ask the older adult, "Who would you go for help?" and recommend they bring that person to the next visit. • Consider also assessing and managing caregiver burden. • Ensure follow-through on any referrals. • If a memory disturbance is found, avoid medications that will make cognitive health worse. • If there is a diagnosis of dementia, include it on the problem list. If not, include cognitive impairment. • Do not prescribe medications that can exacerbate cognitive impairment, such as benzodiazepines and anticholinergics. • Older adults with dementia will be at high risk of delirium, especially if hospitalized, so educate family and providers on delirium prevention. **Additional Resources** • Alzheimer's Association • Local Area Agency on Aging • Community Resource Finder • Zarit Burden Interview (for caregivers)

| Identify and manage factors contributing to depression | Identify and manage factors that contribute to depressive symptoms, including sensory limitations (vision, hearing), social isolation, losses of aging (job, income, societal roles), bereavement, and medications.

Consider the need for counseling and/or pharmacological treatment of depression or refer to a mental health provider if appropriate. | **Tips**
• Educate the patient and caregiver about depression in older adults
• Recognize social isolation as a risk factor for depression and identify community-based resources that support social connections.

Additional Resources
• Local Area Agency on Aging
• *Crosswalk: Evidence-Based Leadership Council Programs and the 4Ms* |
| Ensure safe mobility (Larson, 2017) | Assess and manage impairments that reduce mobility; such as:
• pain
• impairments in strength, balance, or gait
• hazards in home (e.g., stairs, loose carpet or rugs, loose or broken handrails)
• high-risk medications

Refer to physical therapy.

Support older adults, families, and other caregivers to create a home environment that is safe for mobility.

Support older adults to identify and set a daily mobility goal that supports What Matters.

Review and support progress toward the mobility goal in subsequent interactions. | **Tips**
• Have a multifactorial fall prevention protocol (e.g., STEADI) that includes:
  • educating the patient/family
  • managing impairments that reduce mobility (e.g., pain, balance, gait, strength)
  • ensuring a safe home environment for mobility
  • identifying and setting a daily mobility goal with the patient that supports What Matters, and then reviewing and supporting progress toward the mobility goal
  • avoiding high-risk medications
  • referring to physical therapy

Additional Resources
• Stopping Elderly Accidents, Deaths & Injuries (STEADI)
• CDC My Mobility Plan |

*These activities are also key to preventing delirium and falls.

References

Fick, D. M., Inouye, S. K., McDermott, C., Zhou, W., Ngo, L., Gallagher, J., McDowell, J., Penrod, J., Siuta, J., Covaleski, T., & Marcantonio, E. R. (2018). Pilot study of a two-step delirium detection protocol administered by certified nursing assistants, physicians, and registered nurses. *Journal of Gerontological Nursing*, 44(5), 18–24. https://doi. org/10.3928/00989134-20180302-01

Hill-Taylor, B., Sketris, I., Hayden, J., Byrne, S., O'Sullivan, D., & Christie, R. (2013). Application of the STOPP/START criteria: A systematic review of the prevalence of potentially inappropriate prescribing in older adults, and evidence of clinical, humanistic and economic impact. *Journal of Clinical Pharmacy and Therapeutics*, 38(5), 360–372. https://doi. org/10.1111/jcpt.12059

Hshieh, T. T., Yue, J., Oh, E., Puelle, M., Dowal, S., Travison, T., & Inouye, S. K. (2015). Effectiveness of multicomponent nonpharmacological delirium interventions: A meta-analysis. *JAMA Internal Medicine*, 175(4), 512–520. https://doi.org/10.1001/jamainternmed.2014.7779

Larson, E. B. (2017). Evidence supports action to prevent injurious falls in older adults. *JAMA*, 318(17), 1659–1660. https://doi.org/10.1001/ jama.2017.15098

Lumish, R., Goga, J. K., & Brandt, N. J. (2018). Optimizing pain management through opioid deprescribing. *Journal of Gerontological Nursing*, 44(1), 9–14. https://doi.org/10.3928/00989134-20171213-04

Marcantonio, E. R. (2017). Delirium in hospitalized older adults. *New England Journal of Medicine*, 377(15), 1456–1466. https://doi.org/10.1056/ NEJMcp1605501

Naik, A. D., Dindo, L. N., Van Liew, J. R., Hundt, N. E., Vo, L., Hernandez-Bigos, K., Esterson, J., Geda, M., Rosen, J., Blaum, C. S., & Tinetti, M. E. (2018). Development of a clinically feasible process for identifying individual health priorities. *Journal of the American Geriatrics Society*, 66(10), 1872–1879. https://doi.org/10.1111/jgs.15437

O'Mahony, D., O'Sullivan, D., Byrne, S., O'Connor, M. N., Ryan, C., & Gallagher, P. (2015). STOPP/START criteria for potentially inappropriate prescribing in older people: Version 2. *Age and Ageing*, 44(2), 213–218. https://doi.org/10.1093/ageing/afu145

Reuben, D. B., Gazarian, P., Alexander, N., Araujo, K., Baker, D., Bean, J. F., Boult, C., Charpentier, P., Duncan, P., Latham, N., Leipzig, R. M.,

Quintiliani, L. M., Storer, T., & McMahon, S. (2017). The strategies to reduce injuries and develop confidence in elders intervention: Falls risk factor assessment and management, patient engagement, and nurse co-management. *Journal of the American Geriatrics Society*, 65(12), 2733–2739. https://doi.org/10.1111/jgs.15121

Tinetti, M. E., Esterson, J., Ferris, R., Posner, P., & Blaum, C. S. (2016). Patient priority-directed decision making and care for older adults with multiple chronic conditions. *Clinics in Geriatric Medicine*, 32(2), 261–275. https://doi.org/10.1016/j.cger.2016.01.012

Age-Friendly Care Workflow Examples

Hospital-Based Care Workflows: Core Functions

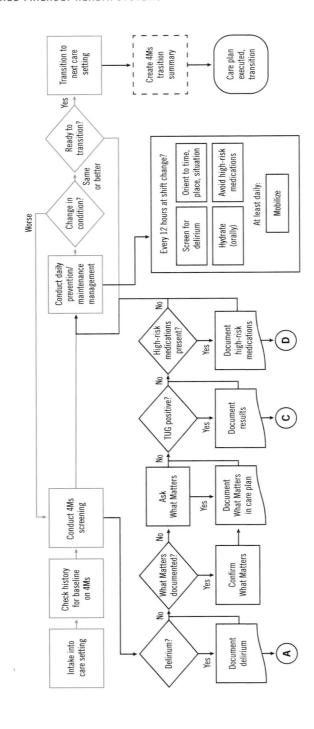

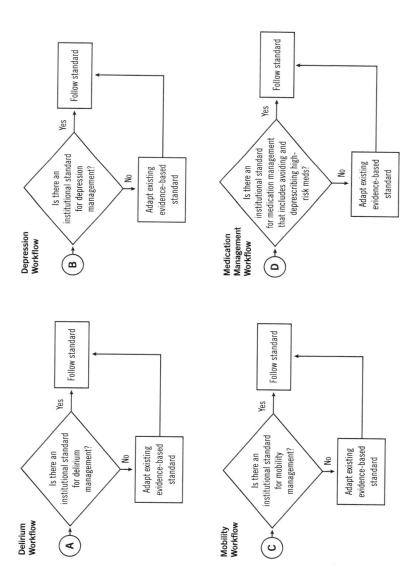

Delirium Workflow

A → Is there an institutional standard for delirium management?
- Yes → Follow standard
- No → Adapt existing evidence-based standard → Follow standard

Depression Workflow

B → Is there an institutional standard for depression management?
- Yes → Follow standard
- No → Adapt existing evidence-based standard → Follow standard

Mobility Workflow

C → Is there an institutional standard for mobility management?
- Yes → Follow standard
- No → Adapt existing evidence-based standard → Follow standard

Medication Management Workflow

D → Is there an institutional standard for medication management that includes avoiding and deprescribing high-risk meds?
- Yes → Follow standard
- No → Adapt existing evidence-based standard → Follow standard

Ambulatory/Primary Care Workflows

Ambulatory/Primary Care Workflows: Core Functions for New Patient, Annual Visit, or Change in Health Status

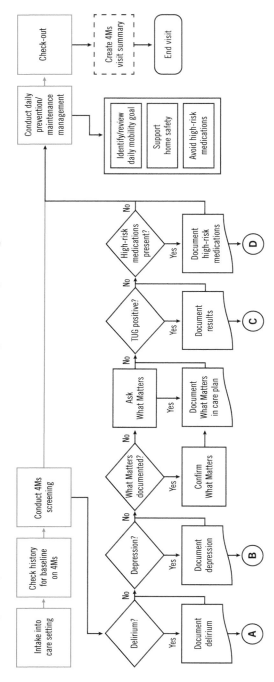

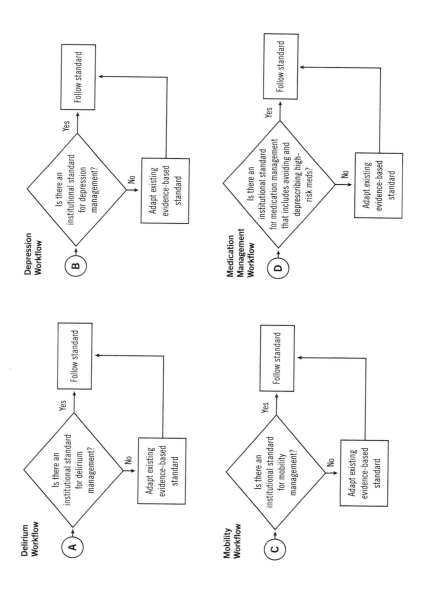

Delirium Workflow

A → Is there an institutional standard for delirium management?
- Yes → Follow standard
- No → Adapt existing evidence-based standard → Follow standard

Depression Workflow

B → Is there an institutional standard for depression management?
- Yes → Follow standard
- No → Adapt existing evidence-based standard → Follow standard

Mobility Workflow

C → Is there an institutional standard for mobility management?
- Yes → Follow standard
- No → Adapt existing evidence-based standard → Follow standard

Medication Management Workflow

D → Is there an institutional standard for medication management that includes avoiding and deprescribing high-risk meds?
- Yes → Follow standard
- No → Adapt existing evidence-based standard → Follow standard

Implementing Reliable 4Ms: Age-Friendly Care

The goal is to reliably integrate the 4Ms into the way you provide care for every older adult, in every setting, every time. How will you know that 4Ms care, as described by your site, is reliably in place?

The best way is to observe the work directly, using the 4Ms Age-Friendly Care Description Worksheet as an observation guide. Another way is to review patient records to confirm the completeness of 4Ms documentation and alignment of care team actions with information obtained in assessment. Note that you need only a handful of patient records to tell you that your 4Ms performance is not at a high level (say, 95% or higher). For example, if you see three instances of incomplete 4Ms care in a random sample of 10 records, you have strong evidence that your system is not performing in a way that 95% or more of your patients are experiencing 4Ms care.

If IHI visited your care setting, we also would look for several kinds of evidence that your site has the foundation for reliable 4Ms care, including:

- If we asked five staff members, they would use the same explanation for why your site does the 4Ms work.

- If we asked five staff members, they would use the same explanation for how your site does the 4Ms work.
- Staff at your site will have documentation for the 4Ms work; they can access your 4Ms care description and additional standard supporting operating procedures, flowcharts, and/or checklists.
- Training/orientation introduces new staff to the 4Ms work.
- Job descriptions outline elements of the 4Ms work as appropriate to the role.
- Performance evaluation refers to the 4Ms work.

IHI would also expect to learn about regular observation of 4Ms work by site supervisors and leaders who seek to understand and work with staff to remove barriers to reliable 4Ms care.

Additional Measurement Guidance and Recommendations

The tables below provide additional guidance for counting the number of patients receiving age-friendly (4Ms) care.

Hospital Site of Care

Measure name	Number of patients who receive age-friendly (4Ms) care
Measure description	Number of patients 65+ who receive 4Ms care as described by the hospital
Site	Hospital
Population measured	Adult patients 65+
Measurement period	Monthly
Count	*Inclusion*: Patients 65+ with LOS greater than or equal to 1 day present on the unit between 12:01 a.m. on the first day of the measurement period and 11:59 p.m. on the last day of the measurement period who receive the unit's description of 4Ms care *Exclusions*: None
Measure notes	The measure may be applied to units within a system as well as the entire system. See the 4Ms Care Description sheet to describe 4Ms care for your unit. To be considered age-friendly (4Ms) care, you must engage or screen all patients 65+ for all 4Ms, document the results, and act on them as appropriate. If total count is not possible, you can sample (e.g., audit 20 patient charts) and estimate the total number of patients receiving 4Ms care / 20 × total number of patients cared for in the measurement period. If you are sampling, please note that when sharing data. Once you have established 4Ms care as the standard of care on your unit, validated by regular observation and process review, you can estimate the number of patients receiving 4Ms care as the number of patients cared for by the unit. You do not need to filter the number of patients by unique MRN.

Ambulatory/Primary Care Site of Care

Measure name	Number of patients who receive age-friendly (4Ms) care
Measure description	Number of patients 65+ who receive 4Ms care as described by the measuring unit
Site	Ambulatory
Population measured	Adult patients 65+
Measurement period	Monthly
Count	Inclusion: All patients 65+ in the population considered to be patients of the ambulatory or primary care practice (e.g., patient assigned to a care team panel and seen by the practice within the past three years) who have an office visit, home visit, or telemedicine visit with the practice during the measurement period and who receive 4Ms care as described by the site Exclusions: None
Measure notes	The measure may be applied to units within a system as well as the entire system. See the 4Ms Care Description sheet to describe 4Ms care for your unit. To be considered age-friendly (4Ms) care, you must engage or screen all patients 65+ for all 4Ms, document the results, and act on them as appropriate. Note that the 4Ms care screening in primary care may be defined as screening within the previous 12 months. If a total count is not possible, you can sample (e.g., audit 20 patient charts) and estimate the total as the number of patients receiving 4Ms care / 20 × total number of patients cared for in the measurement period. If you are sampling, please note that when sharing data. Once you have established 4Ms care as the standard of care on your unit, validated by regular observation and process review, you can estimate the number of patients receiving 4Ms care as the number of patients cared for by the unit. You do not need to filter the number of patients by unique MRN.

Example PDSA Cycles for Age-Friendly Care

Example: Testing What Matters Engagement with Hospitalized Older Adult Patients

PLAN-DO-STUDY-ACT RECORD

Name of Health System: *Camden University Medical Center*
Name of Person Completing Form: *Erin Rush, RN*
Date: *March 29, 2019*

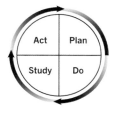

Change Idea to: ___ develop, or _X_ test, or ___ implement

Description:
Cycle 1: Test a What Matters engagement with a hospitalized patient.

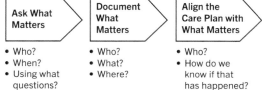

Ask What Matters	Document What Matters	Align the Care Plan with What Matters
• Who? • When? • Using what questions?	• Who? • What? • Where?	• Who? • How do we know if that has happened?

PLAN

Questions: What do we want to know?

• *Can physicians incorporate What Matters engagements into rounds with older adult patients?*

• *Will physicians learn something useful from this What Matters engagement relevant to care planning?*

Predictions: What do we think will happen?

• *Physicians can incorporate What Matters engagements into rounds with older adult patients.*

• *Physicians can learn something useful from What Matters engagements relevant to care planning.*

Plan for the change or test: Who, What, When, Where. What are we going to do to make our test happen?

List the tasks necessary to complete this test (what)	Person responsible	When	Where
Orient Dr. M (hospitalist) to this test	*Erin*	*Monday Morning*	*4 South*
Select older adult patient for test	*Erin & Dr. M*	*Monday Morning*	*4 South*
Ask older adult patient, "What's important to you in the next few days as you recover from your illness?"	*Dr. M*	*Monday*	*TBD*
Debrief test and complete PDSA cycle	*Erin & Dr. M*	*Tuesday Morning*	*4 South*

Plan for data collection: Who, What, When, Where. How will we compare predictions to actual?

Erin and Dr. M to meet the next day to debrief test, capture what happened, impressions, how that compared to predictions, next steps.

DO

Carry out the change or test; collect data and begin analysis; describe the test/what happened.

- *Dr. M asked 1, and then 4 more, older patients—went beyond testing with just 1 patient!*
- *Some answers were very health/condition related (e.g., a patient with shortness of breath/cough stated, "I just want my cough to be better and to be able to breathe.").*
- *Other answers were more life related, for example:*
  - *A patient being treated for stroke, who is a performance artist, shared a video of performance and indicated what matters is to be able to return to performing.*
  - *A patient with multiple falls wants to be able to stand to cook again.*

STUDY

Complete analysis of data; summarize what was learned; compare what happened to predictions above.

- *Asking a single question is not sufficient. Need the opportunity for follow-up questions and listening. For example: A patient with congestive heart failure and arthritis has an immediate goal to reduce swelling in her legs. Further probing revealed a desire to stay in her home and be able to cook to avoid delivered salty foods and to avoid rehospitalization. Possible solution: Prescription for homemaker assistance.*
- *Dr. M regularly engages patients with What Matters in an outpatient setting. New for inpatient rounds, but feasible to include.*
- *Worthwhile if there is time for follow-up (not just one question and one answer in 30 seconds).*
- *No patients responded with goals or needs that could not be addressed somehow in the care plan.*
- *Asking a What Matters question feels awkward. Need to build a relationship first before asking an "intimate" question. For example, asking on the second day of rounding feels better than asking on the first day.*
- *Asking a What Matters question helped Dr. M bond with the patients.*
- *There was a lack of clarity on what to do with the information learned from the What Matters engagement (e.g., how to document, how to share).*
- *Still have a concern about not knowing what to do if a patient expresses a need or goal beyond the specific health condition or issues that the physician (Dr. M) is trained to address.*

ACT

Are we ready to make a change? Plan for the next cycle.

Test again. Questions to explore through more testing include:

- *Is it better to ask the What Matters question at the beginning or end of the encounter?*
- *How can we get at What Matters for our patients with cognitive impairment?*
- *Where is the best place to document the information from the What Matters engagement?*
  - *Whiteboard: "Anyone" can use the whiteboard. Can this be done effectively?*
  - *Epic documentation agreement (meetings underway with Epic team to discuss options).*
- *Are the daily multidisciplinary rounds/huddles the best place to discuss what's learned from What Matters engagements?*
  - *Do we need to coordinate our engagement about What Matters? Nursing, care management, and physicians all could be asking variants of What Matters.*
- *Could the nurse or case manager have a What Matters conversation and document it so that it is available for physicians to reference in a consult visit or rounding?*

Example: Testing a 4Ms Screening for Older Adults in Primary Care

PLAN-DO-STUDY-ACT RECORD

Name of Health System: *Name*
Name of Person Completing Form: *Name*
Date: *Date*

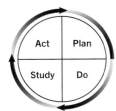

Change Idea to: ___ develop, or _X_ test, or ___ implement

Description:

Cycle 1: Test a 4Ms "screening set" with one older adult patient in your care.

- *What Matters:*
  - *Ask, "What makes life worth living?"; "What would make tomorrow a really great day for you?"; "What concerns you most when you think about your health and health care in the future?"*
  - *Confirm the presence of a healthcare proxy (proxy's name, contact information)*
- *Medication:*
  - *Identify use of high-risk medications*
- *Mentation:*
  - *Administer the Mini-Cog*
  - *Administer the PHQ-2*
- *Mobility:*
  - *Conduct the TUG Test*

PLAN

Questions: What do we want to know? [Add or edit questions below, as needed.]

1. *Can we conduct all 4Ms items (above) on intake for one older adult patient?*
2. *How long does it take?*
3. *How does it feel for the staff conducting the assessment? (e.g., What went well? What could be improved?)*
4. *How does it feel for the patient/family receiving the assessment? (e.g., What went well? What could be improved?)*
5. *What are we learning from conducting this 4Ms screening set? Did we learn anything about this patient that will improve our care, service, and/or processes?*

Predictions: What do we think will happen? [Edit the draft answers below, as needed.]

1. *Yes*
2. *10 minutes*
3. *Staff will give at least two ideas/identify two issues with the 4Ms screening set*
4. *Patient/family will give at least one idea/issue with the screening set use*
5. *Staff will get at least one insight/"aha" regarding care for the patient from the screening set*

Plan for the change or test: Who, What, When, Where. What are we going to do to make our test happen? [Edit the draft tasks below, as needed.]

List the tasks necessary to complete this test (what)	Person responsible	When	Where
1. Select an older adult patient with whom we are likely to be able to conduct this test in the next 3 days. Identify a patient who we might "easily" engage on all items of the 4Ms screening set.			
2. Select a staff person who will conduct the test and brief her/him.			
3. Decide on what you will say to invite the patient/family to participate in testing the 4Ms screening set. For example, "We are testing ways to know our patients better to develop the right care plan. Would you be willing to test a set of questions today and give your opinion about this experience?"			

Plan for data collection: Who, What, When, Where. How will we compare predictions to actual? [Adapt or edit the sample data collection form below, as needed.]

Fill in data collection plan (Who, What, When, Where) [example below]:

4Ms Screening Set Test: Name of Health System						
4Ms Screening Set Test: Name of Contact Person						
	Patient 1	Patient 2	Patient 3	Patient 4	Patient 5	Patient 6
Date						
What Matters						
Asked: What makes life worth living? (yes/no)	Y / N	Y / N	Y / N	Y / N	Y / N	Y / N
Asked: What would make tomorrow a really great day for you? (yes/no)	Y / N	Y / N	Y / N	Y / N	Y / N	Y / N
Asked: What concerns you most when you think about your health and healthcare in the future? (yes/no)	Y / N	Y / N	Y / N	Y / N	Y / N	Y / N
Has heathcare agent? (yes/no/didn't review)	Y / N / DR	Y / N / DR	Y / N / DR	Y / N / DR	Y / N / DR	Y / N / DR
Medication						
Identified use of high-risk medication (yes/no/didn't review)	Y / N / DR	Y / N / DR	Y / N / DR	Y / N / DR	Y / N / DR	Y / N / DR
Mentation						
Administered the Mini-Cog (yes/no)	Y / N	Y / N	Y / N	Y / N	Y / N	Y / N
Administered the PHQ-2 (yes/no)	Y / N	Y / N	Y / N	Y / N	Y / N	Y / N
Mobility						
Conducted TUG Test (yes/no)	Y / N	Y / N	Y / N	Y / N	Y / N	Y / N
Amount of time to complete						
Staff feedback						
Patient/family feedback						
Other notes and/or questions that came up from this test						

DO

Carry out the change or test; collect data and begin analysis; describe the test/what happened.
Fill in during or after conducting the test.

STUDY

Complete analysis of data; summarize what was learned;
compare what happened to predictions above.
Fill in during or after conducting the test.

ACT

Are we ready to make a change? Plan for the next cycle.
Fill in during or after conducting the test. Will you adopt, adapt, abandon, or run the test again?
For example, *PDSA cycle 2: Conduct test again with 5 patients making the following adjustments...*

Example: Ambulatory/Primary Care Multiple PDSA Cycles

4MS Screening Set

1. Test screening set with 1 patient
2. Complete PHQ-2 when check-in, test with 3 patients
3. Adapt What Matter question, test with 5 patients
4. Provide patient education, update EHR, test with 10 patients

TUG

1. Test TUG with 1 patient
2. Put line, stopwatch, worksheet in all rooms, test with 5 patients
3. Note exceptions to TUG in standard procedure, test with all Dr. Smith's patients
4. Update EHR

Example: Hospital-Based Care Multiple PDSA Cycles

4MS Screening Set (Ask and document What Matters; review high-risk meds; UB-2 every 12 hours; TUG)

1. Test screening set with 1 patient (all screenings done?)
2. Test set with 1 RN's patients for 1 day (all screenings done?)
3. Test with alll RNs on unit for 1 patient for 1 day (all screenings done?)
4. Test set with all RNs on unit for all patients for 1 day (all screenings done?)

UB2

1. Train 1 tech on UB-2, test with 1 patient
2. Include UB-2 with vital signs, test with 5 patients
3. Create triggers to admin 3D-CAM within 2 hours of positive screen
4. Train additional staff, test with all patients for 1 week
5. Update EHR

Measuring the Impact of 4Ms Age-Friendly Care

We highly recommend you create and monitor an age-friendly measurement dashboard to understand the impact of your efforts. This can be accomplished in two ways:

- segment an existing dashboard by age and monitor performance for older adults (aged 65 years and older); or
- focus on a small set of basic outcome measures for older adults.

The tables below list the outcome measures that IHI identified to help health systems understand the impact of 4Ms age-friendly care. These measures are not designed to compare or rank health systems in "age-friendliness." We seek to outline measures that are "good enough" to establish baseline performance and are sensitive to improvements while paying attention to feasibility for health systems with a range of skills and capacity in measurement.

BASIC OUTCOME MEASURES	HOSPITAL SETTING	AMBULATORY/PRIMARY CARE SETTING
30-day readmissions	X	
Emergency department utilization		X
Consumer Assessment of Healthcare Providers and Systems (CAHPS) survey questions	HCAHPS	CG-CAHPS
Length of stay	X	

ADVANCED OUTCOME MEASURES	HOSPITAL SETTING	AMBULATORY/PRIMARY CARE SETTING
Delirium	X	N/A
collaboRATE (or similar tool adopted by your site to measure goal-concordant care)	X	X

Additional Stratification: Race and Ethnicity

We recognize the persistence of important differences in treatment and health outcomes associated with race, ethnicity, and other social factors. Health equity requires that health systems stratify key performance measures by these factors to reveal disparities and provoke action to eliminate them. For Age-Friendly Health Systems, we encourage stratifying outcome measures for older adults using the Office of Management and Budget core race and ethnicity factors to identify disparities in patient care and experience.

IHI Age-Friendly Health Systems Inpatient ROI Calculator Instructions

At this stage, the Excel spreadsheet calculator is optimized for PC use. While it will work with the Apple OS, some features work more slowly.

The Inpatient ROI Calculator is designed for hospital clinicians and financial executives to assess the business case for providing an age-friendly approach to care using the 4Ms Framework of an Age-Friendly Health System (referred to as simply "4Ms" throughout these instructions). The user inserts the values for the 4Ms framework's inputs and the calculator's algorithm reports the financial results—the outputs. The calculator expresses the financial returns both in terms of net income and in the form of a percentage—the ROI. The source of the ROI for the 4Ms in this setting is the avoidance of medical expenses that the 4Ms have the capacity to avert by reducing iatrogenic events such as delirium, falls, infections, and so on.

How to Use the Excel Spreadsheet Calculator

The Excel spreadsheet calculator has two tabs: "Calculator" and "Sensitivity Analysis." Make sure you begin with the first tab, as the second tab requires the completion of the first. The second tab is optional (see an explanation at the end of these instructions).

The user progresses through five discrete steps, entering data inputs in the designated cells, leading to a "Results" section. Click on the numbered buttons sequentially to go to the corresponding section. (If you wish, you can explore the second tab, but only after you complete these five steps.)

How to Enter Inputs

The cells that require user inputs are identified by spinner buttons—up and down arrows. The user selects the appropriate value of the variable by clicking until the best estimate appears in the cell. *Do not type in the numbers directly; use only the arrows to select the desired number.*

"Help" Guidance

If you are uncertain as to what you are supposed to enter or what an output means, simply click on the cell with the caption next to that cell. You will then see a question mark (?), and when you click on it, a "help" note appears that explains its meaning.

Step 1: Specifications

First, decide the service line (e.g., coronary artery bypass surgery, orthopedics, Acute Care for the Elderly [or ACE] unit) for which you are inputting data, if not for the entire hospital. (The Scenario tool enables you to make comparisons of the financial returns across service lines.)

Next, choose whether to include utilization changes resulting from your hospital-based 4Ms effort that occur after discharge in post-acute care (PAC) facilities, such as a rehabilitation center or a skilled nursing facility. There is evidence that delirium and pressure sores increase PAC costs. If your organization does not have financial responsibility for post-acute care, it is suggested that you do not check that box since the changes here do not affect the 4Ms business case for the hospital.

Step 2: Population

Insert basic information that establishes the scale of the 4Ms program. First, enter the number of annual admissions. Be sure to insert a total number that corresponds to the chosen service line. Next, decide on the number of years, called the Amortization Period, over which you wish to spread any one-time-only or launch costs. If there are no startup costs, ignore this entry. If there are any launch costs, spread these over the number of years the 4Ms program will be in existence; the cost should not all be borne in the first year. Rather, amortize this cost by apportioning an annual amount to each year of the 4Ms program's life. There is no rule here as to how many years to stipulate. Once you select the number of years, divide the total launch expense by the chosen amortization period and then add the result to other annual fixed expenses.

Step 3: 4Ms Costs

The calculator performs an incremental analysis of what the 4Ms add to cost and what benefits they bring in terms of medical expense avoidance. The next set of entries accordingly allows the calculation of the incremental costs, if any, of incorporating the 4Ms into a usual care delivery system. These entries should reflect only those costs *over and above* usual care. These entries are *not* to reflect the total costs of the service line. The cost entries required are for fixed and variable expenses.

4MS PROGRAM LAUNCH COSTS

The launch costs do not recur annually. For example, the initial launch of the 4Ms program may require a retrofitting of the unit (i.e., adding a feature or otherwise modifying an existing space to have it conform to the needs of age-friendly care), a modification of the IT system, or an educational program for staff. You can set this cost to zero for established programs. Based on the amortization period you have already chosen, this expense will be spread evenly across the previously specified number of years.

Fixed Costs. There may be some 4Ms costs that are incurred each year but do not vary with the number of admissions. For example, there may be a lease expense for additional space to accommodate an exercise program. If it is a true fixed cost, then the expense will not change wit1hin a reasonable range of admissions and, therefore, of patients served. Another fixed cost is any added staff (nurses, medical assistants, etc.) associated with the 4Ms program. While staffing costs would be fixed within a range of admissions, this cost would increase when the staff capacity was reached and other staff needed to be added. It is advisable to consider staffing as a fixed cost within that plausible range of scale—that is, reflect on the incremental staffing needs for a 4Ms model of care for a plausible range of admissions centered around your entry above for annual admissions.

Variable Costs. Certain costs may rise continuously as the scale of the 4Ms program grows. These are called variable costs. An obvious example is the cost of age-friendly supplies provided to each patient (e.g., an easy-to-grip water pitcher to promote hydration). In the calculator, enter only the added cost of the age-friendly supplies relative to usual care. The calculator will then show the annual total cost of the 4Ms program.

Step 4: Estimates/Values

You may consider up to three hospital-acquired conditions that may be affected by implementation of the 4Ms. In the calculator, two conditions are named: delirium and hospital-acquired pressure ulcers (HAPUs). You can replace either of these conditions with other iatrogenic events by typing over these labels in the spreadsheet. There is also a third, blank option, where you may insert falls, infections, or any other hospital-acquired condition (HAC).

The instructions for this section use delirium as an example. The instructions apply equally to other conditions.

INCIDENCE

For each HAC, enter the incidence your facility has experienced or might be expected to experience under usual care. Later, you will have the opportunity to estimate the impact of an age-friendly model of care on this incidence figure. For delirium, it is often impossible to distinguish between prevalent (pre-admission) and incident (arising after admission) delirium. Incident delirium is expressed as a percentage of those individuals admitted who will develop the condition or who have a latent condition that becomes fully expressed while in the hospital. That is the percentage to enter here.

4MS PROGRAM EFFECTIVENESS

These are crucial entries. The 4Ms are expected to reduce the incidence of HACs. Enter the reduction in incidence that is expected, based on what the evidence has shown the effectiveness to be. Suppose that under usual care, the incidence of delirium amounts to 20% of all admissions. Suppose further that, with an age-friendly model of care, incidence drops to 15% of all admissions. That would translate to a program effectiveness of 25%, and the spinner should be set at 25%. (The 5-percentage-point reduction divided by 20 percentage points equals a 25% reduction.)

TYPE OF STAY

The entries here refer to the length of stay (LOS) and the cost per day under two types of stay.

"Normal" refers to the LOS and the cost per day in the absence of a given condition. For example, "normal" refers to the LOS for a patient who is negative for delirium. The other type of stay is called "Extended due to condition," which refers to a hospital-acquired condition. You will then record the consequences: the added number of days and any change in the cost per day when the condition occurs.

It might be reasonably expected that the HAC prolongs the LOS, in which case you will insert the added number of days caused by the acquisition of the condition.

The average cost per day may rise or fall when the stay is longer. Many hospitals believe that delirium's complications raise the average daily cost; others may find that the additional days are less expensive than the days prior to the acquisition of the condition. Thus, you can select a lower or a higher cost averaged over the entire prolonged stay.

If you elected to include the financial consequences of the 4Ms for post-acute care (PAC), then a similar set of entries for PAC needs to be inserted. The entries there refer to the changes that might be expected in a PAC stay in terms of LOS and daily cost when the HAC was present prior to hospital discharge.

Step 5: Cost Offset From Coding and Revenue for HAC

This section considers the possibility that additional payments will be made to the hospital (e.g., by CMS) if a case of delirium is detected and coded, and payment is received. Under Medicare fee-for-service, hospitals are entitled to bill for hospital-acquired delirium but not for pressure sores. To the extent that the hospital's cost of addressing delirium is reimbursed, even partially, you need to consider this reimbursement. The reimbursement offsets a portion of the cost burden of delirium to the hospital. Therefore, coding and the revenue affect the ROI from prevention and must be accounted for.

In order to calculate the amount of revenue needed to offset the cost per case of delirium, you will need to provide two pieces of information in the Excel spreadsheet:

- Revenue per case detected (code modification). CMS allows a code modification for delirium. There are several possible

Current Procedural Terminology (CPT) delirium-related codes, each of which offers a different fee that can be billed.

- Detection and coding effectiveness (percentage of cases detected). While there may be eligibility for a code modification for a case of delirium, often cases go undetected and, therefore, billing is not done. This entry is designed to reflect the share of all delirium cases that are detected and billed for.

Once this final step has been taken, the calculator has all the information required to provide the financial results from the provision of the 4Ms model of care in the hospital.

Results

This section summarizes the financial results of providing the 4Ms model of care.

"Net benefit" means the cost avoidance from reducing the number of all HACs minus the expense of the 4Ms program. There is another way of expressing the financial return: ROI, a percentage, is calculated by dividing the net benefit of the 4Ms program by its cost.

"Time reclaimed by the older adult" is another result that is reported. While not directly part of the 4Ms business case, this metric is a central and significant one to calculate and report. It's at the heart of an Age-Friendly Health System and pertains specifically to the What Matters element. Time not spent in the hospital and the PAC facility is certainly part of What Matters to the patient.

Based on your entries, the calculator will have tracked the impact of the 4Ms on rates of HACs and on the prolonged stays associated with them. The "time reclaimed by the older adult" figure covers the entire population that benefited from the 4Ms. Several factors in the model influence the result for "time reclaimed by the older adult": the number of admissions, the incidence of HACs, the effectiveness of the 4Ms program in preventing HACs, and the number of days the HACs add to inpatient and post-acute stays.

Optional Tools

Below, three optional tools within the Excel spreadsheet calculator are described: Find Levels (Target ROI), Scenarios, and Sensitivity Analysis.

FIND LEVELS (TARGET ROI)

The calculator computes the ROI based on your inputs. But you can use the Find Levels feature to determine the magnitudes of key variables that will result in a specific Target ROI. For example, if you are aiming to be cost-neutral, then you would insert 0% as the Target ROI, and the calculator will inform you of the levels of delirium prevention effectiveness required to achieve that goal. You can also see the maximum 4Ms program cost that can be expended while still achieving the ROI goal. These calculations can assist in setting goals for your 4Ms program.

Note: Make sure that after you insert the Target ROI, you click the button that says "Find Levels" in order to see the result.

SCENARIOS

You can save one set of entries in order to compare results with a second set of entries based on different assumptions. For example, you may wish to compare a conservative set of assumptions with a more optimistic one or to compare results for one service line with another. You can do both with the Scenarios tool.

To use this tool, first complete a set of entries. When finished, click on the "Scenarios" button. Select "Save Scenario," and the tool will allow you to recall this scenario later. Be sure to name the scenario saved. Then, when you wish to examine an alternative scenario, enter a different set of numbers corresponding to it; save and name that alternative scenario. When you click on the "Scenarios" button again, you will see the "Compare Scenarios" option, which will show you a side-by-side comparison of the results for the selected scenarios.

SENSITIVITY ANALYSIS

This tool is found on the second tab in the Excel spreadsheet and may be *used only after the first tab ("Calculator") has been completed.* This sensitivity analysis is a Monte Carlo simulation (a technique used to understand the impact of risk and uncertainty in forecasting the ROI). It permits an investigation into the probable range of estimates for the ROI. The tool is useful since there will be uncertainty regarding the exact values of the key inputs. In that context, it is wise to report a reasonable range rather than single estimates.

To run the simulation, follow these steps:

1. Select the independent variables from the menu on the left side that you believe are most subject to uncertainty. Remember that you have already inserted values for all the independent variables to get to this point. These entries will automatically appear in the middle column, labeled "Most Likely," if you click on the button labeled "Use Current Values."

2. Determine the degree of variability you want the simulation to consider by clicking on either "Make 90%–110% of Most Likely" or "Make 80%–120% of Most Likely." Choose the broader range if there is greater uncertainty regarding the central values in the middle column.

3. Click on the number of simulations to run. If you selected only a couple of variables to have subject to uncertainty,

you might select 200 runs, which can be completed quickly. The more runs you choose, the more accurate the results, although the time required to run the simulation is longer.

4. Now inspect the results appearing in the table on the right side. It will show the parameters of the distribution—minimum, maximum, span, average, and standard deviation—for the key result areas: Net Benefit, ROI, and Time Reclaimed by the Older Adult. A graphical portrayal of the ROI range should also appear along with the range for the extent of Costs Avoided.

5. If you return now to the first Excel tab, called "Calculator," you will see in the right-hand corner the Simulation Results summarized there as well.

IHI Age-Friendly Health Systems
Outpatient ROI Calculator Instructions
Note: At this stage, the Excel spreadsheet calculator is optimized for PC use. While it will work with the Apple OS, some features work more slowly.

The Outpatient ROI Calculator is to be used by clinicians and financial staff in outpatient settings to determine the financial return to a medical group from the provision of Medicare Annual Wellness Visits (AWVs), as part of their overall assessment of the business case for providing an age-friendly approach to care using the 4Ms Framework of an Age-Friendly Health System. The user inserts the values for the inputs, and the calculator's algorithm reports the financial results. A key feature of the calculator is that it examines not only the net income from the visits but also assesses the net income from advance care plans (ACPs) and prevention screenings driven by those visits.

Separate calculations for an age-friendly AWV (i.e., the AWV explicitly focuses on the 4Ms framework as the orientation for the visit) and for a "usual" AWV are possible. If you populate the entries in the column labeled "Usual AWV," you can explore the comparison. If you wish to consider only the age-friendly AWV, you can ignore the second column. In that case, you will be able to measure the ROI for the age-friendly AWV but unable to compare it to alternative versions.

How to Use the Excel Spreadsheet Calculator

NAVIGATION

The user progresses through three discrete steps, placing inputs in the designated cells, and then moves on to a fourth section, which provides the financial results. Click on the numbered buttons sequentially to go to the corresponding section and make your entries.

ENTERING INPUTS

The cells that require user input are identified by spinner buttons—up and down arrows. The user selects the appropriate value of the variable by clicking until the best estimate appears in the cell. *Do not type in the numbers directly; use only the arrows to select the desired number.*

"HELP" GUIDANCE

If you are uncertain as to what you are supposed to enter or what an output means, simply click on the cell with the caption next to that cell. You will then see a question mark (?), and when you click on it, a "help" note appears that explains its meaning.

Section 1: Population and Fees. The user inserts basic information regarding the total number of beneficiaries eligible to receive the AWV, the proportion of that number that elects to receive it, and the revenue per AWV. The number of beneficiaries provides the potential scale of the AWV program. Not all who are eligible will elect it. The higher the proportion that accepts the opportunity, the more attractive the ROI.

For the revenue (fee), the user enters the expected average fee the medical group expects to receive for an AWV. Since the fee for the initial visit differs from that for subsequent ones (i.e., the fee is higher for the initial visit), the user needs to insert a weighted average across all visits. Section 1, when complete, provides all the information required for the calculator to project total revenues from the AWVs.

Section 2: Annual Wellness Visit Costs. The calculator needs information about the costs of providing the AWVs. Total costs comprise those that do not vary with the number of visits, called fixed costs, and those that do vary. Examples of fixed costs might be any IT (re)configuration and training expenses. The costs that do vary with volume are the time-based costs of clinicians. Clinician costs depend on the annual salary, including benefits; the productivity of the clinician, expressed in the number of visits performed per day; and the number of weeks worked annually. Clinicians are generally nurses, nurse practitioners, or physicians.

When this information is entered into the spreadsheet, the total cost of providing all the projected visits along with the cost per visit is automatically calculated. Since the revenues are already established in Section 1, the calculator reports the net income stemming directly from the AWVs.

Section 3: Utilization of Advance Care Plans and Screenings. Section 2 reports the net income generated directly from the AWVs. However, there is a potential secondary, indirect source of ROI in the form of enhanced revenues from more ACPs and screenings that take place as a result of the AWVs. The evidence is very clear that the AWVs lead to more of these encounters. The user is presented with fields for the ACP and for three screenings, two of which are named. The user can input other screenings in place of the two named ones by typing over the names. The third screening is intentionally unspecified, and the user can choose another screening. The calculator can only consider three, so the user should select those screenings that are most common or most profitable, or a combination of both.

The net income from the additional encounters driven by the AWVs should be incorporated into the ROI for the AWVs. To make that calculation, the user must first estimate what the uptake for each of these encounters would have been without the AWVs. After all, ACPs and screenings would occur, albeit in smaller numbers, even in the absence of the AWVs.

After inserting the baseline incidence (without the AWV), the user must estimate the incidence (presumably higher) of these encounters when the AWV has been provided. The user can choose to consider whether the AWV when performed in an age-friendly manner drives these subsequent encounters to a different degree in comparison with a usual AWV. Alternatively, the "Usual AWV" column can be ignored.

The other data required to finalize the ROI calculation are the net income margins for each of the subsequent encounter types. The net income margins are entered in terms of dollars per encounter. The estimates of these margins are made by subtracting the estimated variable cost of each encounter from its corresponding fee. (Of course, if there is no margin on any of these, there is no indirect financial benefit from additional encounters.)

With the incremental incidence levels and the profit margins entered, the ROI for the AWVs has now captured *all* of the financial benefits—combining direct benefits from the AWVs along with the indirect benefits from subsequent encounters.

Section 4: Summary of Results. The user does not need to make any entries in this final section of the spreadsheet. The summary displays the financial return from the AWVs expressed as both an annual net income figure and as an ROI. The ROI is a percentage, defined as the AWV net income divided by its annual cost. If the user has chosen to compare two versions of the AWV—age-friendly versus usual—the comparative results will be displayed. It is possible that the age-friendly AWV will outperform the usual AWV if it leads to more subsequent encounters and does so at little, if any, additional cost.

ADDITIONAL TOOLS

Below, two optional tools within the Excel spreadsheet calculator are described: Decision Tree and Scenarios.

Decision Tree. To see a visual representation of the results, the user can click on the button labeled "Switch to Tree." If two versions of the AWV have been modeled, the tree identifies the more financially advantageous one by highlighting it in green. To switch back to the tabular form, click on "Switch to Model."

Scenarios. You can save one set of entries in order to compare results with a second set of entries based on different assumptions. For example, you may wish to compare a conservative set of assumptions with a more optimistic one or to compare results for one service line with another. You can do both with the Scenarios tool.

To use this tool, first complete a set of entries and, when finished, click on "Scenarios." Select "Save Scenario," and the calculator will allow recall of this scenario later. Be sure to name the saved scenario. Then, when you wish to examine an alternative scenario, enter a different set of numbers corresponding to that scenario. Make sure to save and name that scenario. When you click on the "Scenario" button again, you will see the "Compare Scenarios" option—displaying a side-by-side comparison of the results for the two scenarios.

Index

A

Accountability
  ACHIEVE project and, 258t, 262
  public health systems and, 312, 322
Accreditation of Age-Friendly Health
  Systems, 328–329
ACHIEVE project, 255, 257t–258t, 262
Action Community model, 268–269
Actions for Delirium Assessment
  Prevention and Treatment
  (ADAPT), 217–221
Activities of daily living (ADLs), 26, 112
Act On
  care concordance, 382t–385t
  for Medication management, 231–232,
    241–242, 241f
  Mentation assessments using, 243
  Mentation documented using,
    233–234
  Mobility assessment using, 235,
    244–245
  patient assessments using, 228–243
Acupuncture, 96t
Adaptive equipment, 234, 237, 376t
Adaptive systems, properties of, xix
Administrators, roles of, 150t. *See also*
  Leadership
Advance care plans (ACPs), 213–214, 230,
  239f
Advancing Caregiver Training (ACT), 96t
Adverse events. *See also* Fall prevention
  comorbidities and rates of, 254

  medications and, 64–69
  prevention by 4Ms, 217f
Affordable Care Act, 211
After Visit Summaries, 236, 237, 243, 250,
  300
Age, data stratification by, 222, 284f
Age-Friendly Health Systems
  accreditation of, 325–330
  ambulatory care worksheets,
    362t–365t
  the approach to, 5–6
  barriers to, 318–321
  business cases for, 201–224, 203f,
    204f, 208f
  Committed to Care Excellence, 327
  costs of, 209
  creation of, 3
  credentialing of, 328–329
  effectiveness of, 208
  equity in, 296–297
  health department steps to
    framework of, 317t–318t, 319f
  hospital care settings, 357–360
  impacts of, 409–410
  implementation of, 209, 395–396
  key actions, 367–387
  key drivers for, 161f, 226f
  movement toward, xxiii–xxiv
  participants, 326
  PDSA cycles in, 401–407
  public health's role in, 309–323
  recognition for, 325–330

Age-Friendly Health Systems *(continued)*
  resources for, 295f
  returns on investment, 206
  revenue generation from, 209–210
  steps toward becoming, 283t–284t
  summary of key actions, 152t–153t
  system-wide change, 281f–284f
  workflow examples, 155f, 389–393
  worksheets, 357–365
Age-Friendly Public Health Systems,
  321–322
Ageism biases, 98–99, 110, 138, 320
Aging populations, 1, 2, xix. *See also* Older
  adults
Agitation, delirium and, 102
Alarm fatigue, 137
Altered elimination, 116t
Altered levels of consciousness, 98
Alzheimer's dementia management,
  93–94
Ambulation, hospitalization and, 123. *See
  also* Mobility
Ambulatory care settings
  4Ms in, 175t, 238–245, 378t–381t
  Action Communities and, 268–269
  Age-Friendly Care worksheets,
    362t–365t
  Age-Friendly Health Systems and,
    152t
  assessment of 4Ms in, 163t–164t
  CG-CAHPS measures, 182t–183t
  collaboRATE scores, 184t–185t
  core function workflow, 392f–393f
  dementia screening in, 193t
  depression screening in, 194t–195t
  measures for, 172t, 191t–192t, 399t
  Mobility screening in, 195t–196t
  process measure overviews, 185t
  PSDA tools in, 407
  rate of ED visits, 181t–182t
  review compliance, 246–248
American Geriatrics Society (AGS), 69
American Hospital Association (AHA),
  3, xx
Androgens, Beers Criteria, 77t
Anne Arundel Medical Center,
    Annapolis MD, 5–6, 132–133,
    303–305, 304f

Annual Wellness Visits (AWVs). *See also*
  Wellness visits
  age-friendly, 209–210
  Cerner in, 239f
  financial returns from, 212–213
  outpatient case study, 211–216
  PowerForms, 244f
  preventive care and, 214–215
  returns on investment, 215, 215t
  revenue from, 205–206
  screening rates and, 215t
Antiarrhythmic agents, 197t
Anticholinergic agents, 71t–72t
Anticholinergic medications, 196–198,
  196t–197t
Antidepressants, 75t, 103–104, 197t
Antiemetic agents, 197t
Antiepileptic agents, 119
Antihistamines, 71t, 196t–197t
Anti-infective agents, 72t
Antimuscarinic agents, 197t
Antiparkinsonian agents, 71t, 197t
Antipsychotic agents, 65–67, 75t, 197t
Antispasmodic agents, 72t, 197t
Antithrombotic agents, 72t
Anxiety, management of, 66
Area agencies on aging (AAAs), 237
Aromatherapy, 96t
Ascension Medical Group (AMG), 5–6,
  211–216, 291f
Assessments
  4M processes for, 157, 161t–162t, 293–294
  documentation of, 226–230, 227f, 228f
  domains of, 261t–262t
  ERA approach and, 113t
  hospital care settings, 368t–371t
  Medication, 230–232
  Mentation, 232–233
  public health systems and, 311
  standardized, 261t–262t
Assets
  mapping of, 273–275
  stakeholder, 273–274
Assisted living settings, 291f
  4M care in, 290
  admissions from, 98
  care transitions and, 255
  essential measures, 287f

Assistive devices, 127, 135f, 237, 315, 369t
At-risk contracting, 209
Autonomy, patient, 44, 46

B
Barbiturates, 76t
Barry, Michael, 9
Bedside Mobility Assessment Tool
  (BMAT), 123, 127
Bedtime Readiness flowsheet, 234–235
Beers Criteria, 69–70, 71t–83t
Behavioral and psychological symptoms
  of dementia (BPSD), 95f
Behavioral Risk Factor Surveillance
  System (BRFSS), 315–316
Benzodiazepine receptor agonist
  hypnotics, 77t
Benzodiazepines, 76t, 119, 198t
Best-practice interventions, geriatric, 3
Blanchfield Army Community Hospital
  (BACH), Fort Campbell, KY, 29
Blog posts, 343
BPSD (behavioral and psychological
  symptoms of dementia), 95f
Brainstorming, 273–275, 282
BRFSS (Behavioral Risk Factor
  Surveillance System), 315–316
Business cases, 201–224
  case studies, 210–221
  enabling environments and, 282f
  inpatient studies, 216–221
  steps, 203–207

C
Cake App, 345
Cambridge Health Alliance, Cambridge,
  MA, 31–32
Campaigns
  distributed leadership and, 292t
  effective narrative in, 283–284
  mapping success of, 285f
  measures of success, 284–286
  metrics for, 278
  strategies used in, 277–280
Canada, quality improvement efforts, 27
Capacity building
  campaign success and, 285
  change and, 272

strategies, 278–279
Cardiovascular agents, 73t–74t, 83t–84t,
  197t
Care concordance, 20–21, 180t–181t,
  338–339, 372t–377t, 382t–385t
Caregivers
  ACHIEVE project and, 257t, 258t
  activities of daily living and, 26
  assessment tools, 262t
  care team roles of, 149t
  dementia management and, 96t
  education on 4Ms, 154
  fall prevention and, 122
  macroenvironment changes and, 281f
  open-ended questions for, 157
  questions about medications, 89
  transitions of care and, 256t
  wellness visits and, 148
  at What Matters conversations, 51
Care management using Cerner, 238f
Care managers, system list for, 237f
Care models, challenges of, 267–307
Care plans
  4Ms incorporated in, 162t–163t
  care transitions and, 256t
  customized, 9–10
  design of, 151–154
  ERA approach and, 113t
  fall prevention and, 121–122
  incorporation of 4Ms, 164t–165t
  individualized, 3
  Mobility assessment and, 123
  for older adults, 16–18
  patient confusion and, 118f
  using EHRs, 15, 236f
Care preferences, assessment tools, 261t
Care settings for older adults, 148–149.
  See also Ambulatory care settings;
  Hospital care settings; Primary
  care settings
Care teams
  aims of, 151
  member roles, 149t–150t
  patient engagement and, 131
  qualitative measures, 199–200
  roles of, 292t
  set-up for, 149–150
  sharing information with, 57

Care teams *(continued)*
   stresses on, 199–200
   St. Vincent Medical Group, 291f
   What Matters conservations and,
     52–53
Care touchpoints, 42–43, 42t
Case management training, 291f
Catholic Health Association, 3, xx
Centers for Disease Control and
     Prevention (CDC)
   BRFSS and, 315
   "Check for Safety" tool, 236, 249–250
   opioid guidelines, 198
   public health services and, 313
   Vax & Vote and, 314
Centers for Medicare & Medicaid
     Services (CMS)
   Annual Wellness Visits and, 211–216
   at-risk contracting, 209
   Hospital-Acquired Conditions
     Initiative, 110
   Medicare beneficiary rates, 253
   MedPAC Report, 253
   quality improvement services,
     205–206
Central nervous system agents, 75t–77t
Cerner electronic medical records. *See also*
     Electronic health records (EHRs)
   4M using, 238f
   ambulatory reports, 246f–247f
   care management using, 238f
   Depart Process, 237f
   discharge planning on, 236f
   Dynamic Documentation, 240f
   follow-up scheduling using, 237f
   Interdisciplinary Plan of Care, 229f
   Medication alerts on, 242f
   Medication reconciliation using, 232f
   Mentation assessments using, 233f,
     242f, 243
   Mentation documentation using, 235f
   Mobility assessment using, 244f
   patient assessments using, 228f
   PowerNote using, 230f, 240f
   What Matters and, 230f
CER (rule) records, 238f
Change. *See also* Improvements
   Age-Friendly System Wide, 281f–284f

campaign metrics, 278
campaign strategies, 277–280
efficacy of, 128–131
failure modes, 270
flexibility of, 276
foundational supports, 290–292
geriatric care and, 276–277
If/Then planning, 270
interdisciplinary care teams and,
     124–125
launch of initiatives, 274–275
leadership involvement in, 129, 137
measurable, 282
observability of, 276
organizing for, 271–272
phases of, 275f
relational tactics, 274
resistance to, 269–271
simplicity of, 276
spread of, 274–275, 276–277, 283t
testability of, 276
testing versus implementation, 280,
     280t
urgency of, 129
Chaplains, 47, 150t
Chart reviews, 158–159
"Check for Safety" tool, 236
Chronic diseases
   healthy aging and, 309–310
   in older adults, 1
   What Matters conversations, 42t
Chronic kidney disease, 86t
Clinician and Group Consumer
     Assessment of Healthcare
     Providers and Systems Survey
     (CG-CAHPS), 25
Clinicians
   biases of, 45
   care team roles of, 150t
Code status documentation, 230
Cognitive impairment
   Beers Criteria on drugs in, 85t
   delirium and, 97, 101t
   depression and, 94
   screening for, 53–54, 380t
Cognitive rehabilitation, 96t
Cognitive status
   testing, 99

What Matters conversations and, 43–44
Cognitive training, 96t
CollaboRATE tool, 21–23, 180t–181t, 184t–185t
  alternatives to use of, 23–25
  outcomes measures, 410t
Collaboration
  with caregivers, 2–3
  care management, 2–3
  patient and family participation in, 27
  stakeholders and, 273–275
Collaborative to Advance Social Health Integration (CASHI), 300
Committed to Care Excellence badges, 327
Communication
  care touchpoints, 42–43
  care transitions and, 256t, 262
  change initiatives and, 275
  effective narratives, 283–284
  MinuteClinic innovations for, 35
  nonverbal, 46
  past trauma and, 46
  public health systems and, 312, 317t–318t
  of research findings, 316
Communities of health workers (CHWs), 299
Community advisors, 31–32
Community health workers (CHWs), 316–318
Community mobilization, public health and, 312
Community resources, care plans and, 18
Comorbidities, outcomes and, 254
Confusion
  fall risk and, 116t, 117, 117f
  HIIRRM scoring, 125f–127f
Confusion Assessment Method (CAM), 97t, 98, 105t
Consumer Assessment of Healthcare Providers and Systems Clinical Group Survey (CG-CAHPS), 182t–183t, 247f, 410t
Consumer Assessment of Healthcare Providers and Systems Survey (CAHPS), 205–206

Continuum of care. *See also* Transitions of care
  4M documentation across, 226
  ACHIEVE project and, 258t
  care transitions and, 256t
  transitional care model and, 259–262
Conversation Ready, 10, 343
COVID-19 pandemic, 2, 127
Credentialing of Age-Friendly Health Systems, 328–329
Cultural change. *See* Change
Cultural diversity
  level of acculturation and, 46
  multicultural tools, 347–349
  patient preferences, 147t
  What Matters case study, 31–32
  What Matters conversations and, 44–46
Cultural identity, preferred terms for, 45

D
Daily Cares flowsheet, 234
Dana-Farber Cancer Institute, Boston, MA, 33
Dartmouth Institute for Health Policy & Clinical Practice, 21
Data
  for improvement, 172–185
  stratification of, 222, 284f, 410
Data analysts, roles of, 150t
Data collection
  community health status and, 315–316
  public health systems and, 311, 317t–318t
  returns on investment and, 223
Decision-making
  autonomy in, 46
  family caregivers and, 27, 46
  gender and, 46
  mobilization, 134f
  participation in, 27
  patient education and, 16–17
  What Matters and, 12, 33
Decision Worksheets, 341
Dehydration. *See also* Hydration assessment, 375t
  delirium risk and, 101t

Dehydration *(continued)*
documentation of, 233–234
plans of care and, 162t
Delirium, 97–101
assessment of, 97–101, 97t, 164t, 261t
Beers Criteria on drugs in, 84t
diagnoses of, 179t–180t
essential measures, 287f
outcome measures, 172t, 179t–180t, 410t
per-patient costs of, 219t
prevention of, 99–101, 216–221
screening for, 102, 188t–189t, 218, 232–233, 370t–371t
treatment of, 99–101, 101t
Delirium superimposed on dementia (DSD), 97
Delirium Superimposed on Dementia Algorithm, 97t, 98–99
Dementia
Age-Friendly Care worksheets, 362t–365t
Beers Criteria on drugs in, 85t
care plans in, 165t
causes of, 94
disruptive behavior in, 66–67
factors related to, 95f
hospitalization and, 94–96
orientation of patients, 162t
outcomes and, 94–95
reduction of symptoms of, 96t
referrals, 384t
screening for, 102, 105t, 193t, 380t
symptoms of, 94, 95f
What Matters conversations and, 44
Your Conversation Starter Guide, 344
Deprescribing, 87. *See also* Medication
care plans and, 164t
medications, 383t–384t
Deprescribingnetwork.ca, 65, 67
Depression, 102–104
Age-Friendly Care worksheets, 362t–365t
assessment of, 103, 385t
assessment of 4Ms in, 164t
care plans in, 165t
cognitive impairment and, 94
fall risk and, 116t

recognition of, 102–103
screening for, 105t, 194t–195t, 243, 381t
treatments for, 103–104
Desiccated thyroid, 77t
Dicks, Robert S., 217
Dignity, PFCC goals for, 27–28
Discharge planning, 236f, 237f
Disorganized thinking, 98
Disruptive behavior, 66
Dizziness, fall risk and, 116t
Documentation. *See also* Specific conditions
of advance care plans (ACPs), 213–214, 230
assessment of 4Ms in, 164t
of delirium screening, 232–233
electronic medical records, 225–251
getting started, 19–20
Medication reconciliation, 231f, 232f
MinuteClinic innovations for, 35–36
Mobility measures and, 137–139
of MOLST, 230
of POLST, 230
quality improvement methods for, 20
target goals for, 20
of What Matters conversations, 43, 47, 57, 240f
of What Matters measures, 18–20, 18t, 190t–191t
of the What Matters process, 12–16, 13t–14t, 186t–187t, 335–337, 379t
write-in templates, 48
Drug-drug interactions, 63
Duodenal ulcers, 86t
Dynamic Documentation (DynDoc), 230f, 240f

E
Edgman-Levitan, Susan, 9
EHRs. *See* Electronic health records (EHRs)
Electroconvulsive therapy (ECT), 104
Electronic health records (EHRs). *See also* Cerner; Epic electronic health records
After Visit Summary on, 236–238
approaches to Medication using, 88f

benefits of, 15–16
customization of, 15–16
ERA approach and, 113t
fall prevention and, 115–118
inpatient settings, 245–246
MinuteClinic innovations for, 35–36
Mobility measures and, 115–118,
   137–139
outpatient primary care using, 238
patient-facing portals, 15
patient volume reports, 159–160
pros and cons, 13t–14t
role in aging populations, 225–251
transitions of care using, 236–238
What Matters documentation in, 12,
   13t–14t
Embarrassment, patient, 50–51
Emergency departments (ED)
adverse drug events seen in, 64
essential measures, 287f
outcomes measures, 410t
patient reports, 247f
rate of visits, 181t–182t
visits as an outcome measure, 172t
visits by older adults, 2
What Matters conversations, 42–43
EmPOWER Initiative, 315–316
Endocrine system agents, 77t–79t
End-of-life care, 10
Environment
care settings, 148–149
dementia management and, 96t
enabling, 282f
fall prevention and, 115
macroenvironment changes, 281f
Epic electronic health records, 15–16. *See
   also* Cerner electronic medical
   records; Electronic health records
   (EHRs)
Advance Care Planning activity, 239f
beginning, 226f
Best Practice Advisory, 229f
care management using, 237f
CER records on, 238f
clarity reports, 247f–248f
delirium screening using, 233f
discharge planning using, 237f
dotphrase, 240f

long-term reports, 247f–248f
Medication management using, 231f,
   241f
Mentation assessments using, 235f,
   242f, 243
Mobility assessments using, 236f,
   244f, 245f
for patient reports, 246f
Reporting Workbench reports, 246f,
   247f
SmartData Element, 240f
SmartLink created using, 229f
SmartPhrase created using, 229f
What Matters documentation using,
   227f–228f
Willow alternative alert reporting,
   246f, 247f
Epic™ App Orchard™, 115–116
ERA approach, 111, 112–121, 113t–114t
Ergoloid mesylates, 77t
Estrogens, 78t
Evidence-based interventions
4M piloting and, 283t
4Ms and, 5, 268
fall prevention and, 110
returns on investment and, 223
Excel spreadsheets, 411–424

F
Failures, preoccupation with, 131
Fall prevention
Beers Criteria on drugs in, 85t
care plans and, 121–122
confusion scoring and, 125f–127f
EHRs and, 115–118
essential measures, 287f
Hendrich II Fall Risk Model and,
   115–119, 116t, 120f, 126f
prevention of, 2
public health systems and, 313
risk assessment, 118–122
safe mobility and, 109–110, 131
Family advisors, 32
Family caregivers
age of, 26
collaboration with, 2–3
decision-making and, 27, 46
patient autonomy and, 46

Family caregivers *(continued)*
support by, 25–26
at What Matters conversations, 51
Family councils, 25–26
Finance representatives, 150t
Flexibility of change, 276
Fluid restriction, documentation of, 234
Flu vaccines, 313
Formality, patient preferences, 45
4Ms (What Matters, Medication,
Mentation, and Mobility), xix,
xx. *See also* Age-Friendly Health
Systems; Specific care settings
in ambulatory care, 238–245
approach to, 5–6
business case for, 216–221
care consistent with, 150–151
chart review processes, 158–159
current health system settings, 148
financial impacts of, 284f
framework for, 4–5
measures, 171–200
piloting, 283t
Plan-Do-Study-Act (PSDA) tools,
160–165, 160f
process walkthrough, 355–356
reliability of care using, 156–160
standards of care and, 145–169
summary of key actions, 152t–153t,
154–156
supporting actions, 153–154
testing of, 5–6
Fractures, 85t
Function assessment tools, 261t
Funding, support for healthy aging, 321

G
Gastric ulcers, 86t
Gastrointestinal agents, 79t–80t, 86t
Gender, decision-making and, 46
Genitourinary agents, 82t
Geriatric Depression Scale (GDS), 103
Geriatric Depression Scale: Short Form
(GDS-15), 103
Geriatric models of care, 305
Geritalk, 341
Growth hormone, 78t

H
Hackensack Meridian Health, 123–128
Hartford Hospital, Hartford, Connecticut,
210, 216–221
Health care equity, 173
Health care inequities, 173
Health care utilization, 2
Health literacy levels, 147t, 261t. *See also*
Patient education
Health literacy tools, 55
Health status changes, 42t, 44
Healthy aging, description of, 309–310
Hearing impairment, 101t
Heart failure, 83t
Hebrew Senior Life - Vitality 360
Program, 341
Hendrich II Fall Risk Model (HIIFRM),
115–119, 116t
4Ms framework with, 120f
confusion scoring, 125f–127f
multidisciplinary teams and, 125
rollout plan, 126f
validation of, 119
HIIFRM. *See* Hendrich II Fall Risk Model
(HIIFRM)
Home Alone findings, 26
Hospital-Acquired Conditions Initiative
(CMS), 110
Hospital care settings
4M measures, 174t
4M workflow, 155f
Age-Friendly Care worksheets,
357–360
Age-Friendly Health Systems, 152t
assessments, 368t–371t
core function workflow, 390f–391f
delirium screening measures,
188t–189t
essential measures, 287f
HCAHPS measures, 177t–178t
lengths of stay, 172t, 178t, 202,
218–220, 245, 410t
measures, 398t
measures overview for, 172t
Mobility screening, 189t–190t
outcome measures, 176t–177t,
179t–180t
process measure overviews, 185t

process measures, 186t–187t
targeted medications, 187t–188t
What Matters documentation,
    335–336
Hospital Consumer Assessment of
    Healthcare Providers and Systems
    (HCAHPS)
    collaboRATE tool and, 22
    nurse communication scores, 24
    outcomes measures, 177t–178t
    overall experience scores, 24
    reports, 245
Hospital Elder Life Program (HELP), 101,
    218
Hospitalization
    ambulation, 123
    bed rest and, 123
    cost of, 254
    dementia and, 94–96
    depression and, 94
    falls and, 109–110
    immobilization and, 111–112
How's Your Health? Patient Checkup
    Survey, 341
How to Talk to Your Doctor, 344
Hurdle rates, 206
Hydration
    assessment of, 375t
    delirium risk and, 101t
    documentation of, 233–234 (See also
        Dehydration)
    plans of care and, 162t

I
Identities, What Matters conversations
    and, 44–46
Immigrants, acculturation of, 46
Immobilization
    deconditioning and, 129
    delirium risk and, 101t
    harm caused by, 129
    hospitalization and, 111–112
Improvements. See also Change
    data for, 172–185
    science of, 280
    sequences in, 279f
    spread of, xix
    testing versus implementation, 280t

Inattention, delirium and, 98
Indomethacin, 81t
Information sharing, PFCC goals for,
    27–28
Innovations, 271f, xviii
Inpatient visits, What Matters
    conversations, 42t
Institute for Healthcare Improvement
    (IHI), 3, 10, xix–xx, xxiii–xxiv
Institutionalization, 2, 112
Insulin, 79t
Integrated Patient-, Family-, Public-, and
    Community-Centered Care, 28t
Interdisciplinary care teams
    culture change and, 124–125
    fall prevention and, 124–125
    patient care plans and, 17
    review of 4Ms, 154
Interdisciplinary Plans of Care, 229f
Interpreters, assistance from, 46

J
John A. Hartford Foundation, xix–xx, xxiii
    Action Community results, 269
    goals for Age-Friendly Health
        Systems, 3
    MinuteClinic grant from, 34
    TFAH and, 310–311, 313
Johns Hopkins Fall Risk Assessment Tool
    (JHFRAT), 119–120
Johns Hopkins Medicine, 135f
Joint Commission, 328–329, 329f

K
Kaiser Permanente Woodland Hills,
    California, 5–6, 302–303, 303f
Kidney issues, 86t

L
Language, patient preferences, 45–46,
    147t
Leadership
    business case presentation to,
        202–207
    campaign success and, 279, 285
    care team roles of, 149t
    culture change and, 129–130, 137
    distributed, 286, 288–290

Leadership *(continued)*
 foundational supports, 290–292
 high-impact behaviors, 288t
 macroenvironment changes and, 281f
 nature of, 286–288
 prototyping and, 288t
 Providence St. Joseph case study, 301f
 public health systems and, 312
 roles of, 292
Lengths of stay (LOSs)
 4Ms and, 216–221
 cost savings and, 202
 delirium screening and, 218–220
 hospital sites of care, 178t
 outcome measures, 172t, 410t
 reports, 245
Life context, 48–49
Life expectancy, race/ethnicity and, 296f
Life-stage changes, 42t
Light therapy, 96t
Listening skills, 55
Long-term services and supports (LTSS),
 255

M
Mammography, 29
Massachusetts General Hospital Health
 Decisions Science Center, 345
MCG Health System, Augusta, GA, 30–31
Medical assistants, 47
Medical Orders for Life-Sustaining
 Treatment (MOLST), 230
Medicare Payment Advisory Commission
 (MedPAC) Report, 253
Medicare Wellness Nurses (MWNs),
 211–216
Medication, 63–92
 ACHIEVE project and, 257t
 adverse events, 64–69
 Age-Friendly Care worksheets,
 358t–360t, 362t–365t
 age/sex warnings, 241f
 anticholinergic, 196–198, 196t–197t
 approaches to, 88f
 assessment of 4Ms in, 164t, 240–242
 care plans and, 164t, 237
 categories of, 64–69
 costs of, 64

delirium and, 97
deprescribing, 87, 164t, 383t–384t
for depression, 103–104
description of, 4
documentation of, 230–232
essential measures, 287f
falls and, 110, 122
measures, 191t–192t
nonadherence, 64, 104
personal action plans, 89
plans of care and, 162t
questions to be asked about, 89
reconciliation methods, 230–232, 231f
reviews of, 90, 241f, 370t, 372t–374t,
 380t
risks-benefits analysis, 70
targeted, 187t–188t, 196t–197t
Medi-Span, 241f
Megestrol, 79t
Mental health, older adults and, 93–104
Mentation, 93–108
 Age-Friendly Care worksheets,
 358t–360t, 362t–365t
 assessment of, 106, 232–233, 242–243
 description of, 4
 falls and, 110–111, 122
 measures for, 105t
Meperidine, 80t
Meprobamate, 77t
Metoclopramide, 79t
Mineral oil, 79t
Mini-Cog screening tool, 242, 248f
MinuteClinic, USA, 34–36
Mistakes, information about, 270
Mobility, 109–143
 Age-Friendly Care worksheets,
 358t–360t, 362t–365t
 assessment of, 163t, 164t, 235–236,
 244–245, 377t, 385t
 business case for safety in, 130
 care plans in, 123, 165t
 case studies, 123–128, 132–136
 daily goals, 135f
 description of, 4
 EHRs and, 115–118
 falls and, 111
 goal tracking, 245f
 measures of, 136t

screening, 189t–190t, 195t–196t, 371t, 381t
support, 244f–245f
urgency of culture change, 128–131
Mobilization, decision tree for, 134f
MOLST. *See* Medical Orders for Life-Sustaining Treatment (MOLST)
Monoamine oxidase inhibitors (MAOIs), 104
Months Backward Test, 53–54
Motivational Interviewing Network for Trainers (MINT), 345
Multidisciplinary care teams, 18t
Multilex, 241f
Multiple chronic conditions (MCCs), 254
Multiple sclerosis, 30–31
Muscle relaxants, 197t
"MyMobility Plan," 236

N
Narratives, effective, 283–284
National Health Service (NHS), 27
National Standards for Culturally and Linguistically Appropriate Services (CLAS) guidelines, 45–46
Nervous system agents, 84t–86t
Nonpharmacologic Delirium Prevention, 101
Non-steroidal anti-inflammatory drugs (NSAIDs), 81t
Nothing by mouth status (NPO), 234
Nurses
care team roles of, 150t
communication scores, 24
navigators, 17, 47
training for, 289
What Matters conversations with, 47
Nurses Improving Care for Healthysystem Elders (NICHE), 101
Nursing homes, 42t, 153t, 268–269
Nutrition assessment tools, 261t

O
Observability of change, 276
Observation
4M workflow and, 156
real-time, 157–158

Older adults. *See also* Age; Aging populations
4Ms for, 161t–162t
care measures, 157–160
care plans for, 16–18
care team roles of, 149t
collaboration in care management for, 2–3
cultural preferences, 147t
education on 4Ms, 154
EHR function in care of, 225–251
health literacy levels, 147t
health outcome goals for, 10
mental health of, 93–104
open-ended questions for, 157
patient volumes, 146–147, 146t
preferences *versus* clinical advice, 17
prescription risks for, 64–69
risk stratification of, 222
scale-up for improving care for, 277–280, 277t
What Matters to, 9–39
Online tools, What Matters, 341–343
Open-ended questions, 24
Opioids, targeted, 198t
Orientation of patients, 162t, 375t
Outcome measures, 172t
ambulatory/primary care, 184t–185t
campaign success and, 285
care concordance with What Matters, 338–339
collaboRATE tool, 410t
delirium and, 179t–180t, 410t
dementia and, 94–95
emergency department, 172t, 410t
HCAHPS, 177t–178t
hospital care settings, 176t–177t, 179t–180t
lengths of stay, 172t, 410t
readmissions as, 172t, 176t, 410t
surveys of, 172t
Outcomes
comorbidities and, 254
depression and, 94
What Matters process and, 18t

P
Pain, delirium and, 97
Pain medications, 80t–82t

Parkinson's disease, 86t
Participation, PFCC goals for, 27–28
Patient advisors, 32
Patient and Family Advisory Councils
    (PFACs), 26–27, 29–36
Patient- and family-centered care (PFCC),
    26–27, 27–28
Patient-centered medical homes (PCMHs),
    259–262
Patient Councils, 34
Patient education, 16–17, 154, 258t. *See
    also* Health literacy levels
Patient-facing portals, 15
Patient Health Questionnaire-2 (PHQ-2),
    103, 242
Patient Priorities Care, 342
Patients
    engagement of, 131, 261t
    experience scores, 24
    goals of, 16–17, 49
    life context, 48–50
    participation in decision-making, 27
    post-discharge surveys of, 23
    preferences of, 45, 49, 147t
    preferences versus clinical advice, 17
    priorities of, 48–49
    self-reporting of What Matters, 47
    transitions of care and, 256t
Patient safety rounds, 33
Patient volumes, 158–159
PatientWisdom, 345
Peer-coaching webinars, 268–269
Personal Action Plans, 89
Personal adaptive equipment, 234
Person-Centered Health and Care
    Programme, 342
Pharmacists, roles of, 150t
Physical records, documentation of, 13t–14t
Physical therapists, roles of, 150t
Physician Orders for Life-Sustaining
    Treatment (POLST), 230
Picker Institute Europe, 27
Plan-Do-Study-Act (PSDA) tools, 154–156
    4M care sustained using, 160–165,
        160f
    Age-Friendly Care Systems and,
        401–407
    change campaigns and, 278

    multiple cycles, 407
    sequence of improvement, 279f
    testing changes, 280
Plans of care. *See* Care plans
Policies, public health systems and, 311
POLST. *See* Physician Orders for Life-
    Sustaining Treatment (POLST)
Polypharmacy, 2, 63, 90, 122, 261t
Population health, public health and, 312
Post-discharge patient surveys, 23
Potentially inappropriate medications
    (PIMs), 69–70
PowerNote, 230f
Preferences. *See* Patients
PREPARE for Your Care, 51, 345
Preventive care, 214–215
Primary care settings
    4Ms in, 155f, 163t–164t
    care concordance with What Matters,
        339
    collaboRATE scores, 184t–185t
    cost savings in, 207
    dementia screening in, 193t
    depression screening in, 194t–195t
    EHR use in, 238
    measures, 172t, 175t, 182t–183t,
        190t–191t, 191t–192t, 287f, 399t
    Mobility screening in, 195t–196t
    observations in, 158t
    PDSA cycles in, 404–406
    process measure overviews, 185t
    PSDA tools in, 407
    rate of ED visits, 181t–182t
    What Matters documentation, 337
Process-flow diagrams, 154
Process improvement measures, 173–181
Project Implicit assessments, 45, 342
Proton-pump inhibitors, 80t
Providence St. Joseph Health, Oregon
    Region
    case study, 301–302, 301f
    Mobility programs, 132
    testing of the 4M approach, 5–6
    What Matters conversations, 57–59
Psychotherapy for depression, 103–104
Public health systems, 310–311
    Age-Friendly Health Systems and,
        309–323, 319f

description of, 310–311
foundational capabilities of, 311–312
key roles of, 313–318
silos in, 319–320

Q

Quality improvement. *See also* Plan-Do-
    Study-Act (PSDA) tools
adoption of, 272
CMS surveys, 205–206
cost benefits of, 204–206
to improve documentation, 20
organizing for acceleration of, 272f

R

Race/ethnicity
    data stratification by, 284f
    data stratified by, 173
    life expectancy and, 296–297, 296f
    patient preferences, 147t
    stratification by, 410
Readmissions
    cost of, 254
    hospital outcome measure using, 176t
    Medicare beneficiary rates, 253
    outcome measures, 172t
    outcomes measures, 410t
    prevention of, 2
    reports, 245
Referrals, community resources and, 18
Reframing Aging Project, 320
Rehospitalizations. *See* Readmissions
Relationship-based care, 43
Religion, patient preferences, 147t
Reluctance, patient, 50–51
Reminiscence therapy, 96t
Resistance to change, 269–271
Resources, public health and, 312
Resources for Enhancing Alzheimer's
        Caregiver Health (REACH II), 96t
Respect, PFCC goals for, 27–28
Returns on investment (ROI), 206–207,
        208f
    Annual Wellness Visits and, 215, 215t
    calculation of, 411–424
Risk factors, ERA approach and, 113t, 116t
Robert Wood Johnson Foundation, 313
Rogers, Everett, xviii

Rush University Medical Center (RUMC),
    Chicago IL, 297–301

S

SCAN Foundation, 11
Screening Tool of Older persons'
    Prescriptions and Screening
    Tool to Alerty to Right Treatment
    (STOPP/START) criteria, 70, 104
Sedative-hypnotic drugs, 67–69
Selective serotonin reuptake inhibitors
    (SSRIs), 103–104
Self image, cognitively impaired adults
    and, 44
Self-management, environment changes
    and, 281f
Self-mobility programs, 130
Self-monitoring, assessment tools, 261t
Sensitivity analyses, 206–207
Sensory adaptive equipment, 163t
Serious Illness Conversation Guide
    (Ariadne Labs), 52, 58, 344
Shared Decision-Making National
    Resource Center, 342
Short Blessed Test, 53–54
Simulated presence therapy, 96t
Skeletal muscle relaxants, 82t
Skilled nursing facilities, 42t
Skin integrity assessment tools, 262t
Sleep, management of, 65–66
Sleep deprivation, 97, 376t
Sleep impairment, 101t, 234–235
SmartLink, created using Epic, 229f
SmartPhrase, 229f
Snoezelen, 96t
Social support assessment tools, 262t
Social workers, 17, 47, 150t
Sponsors, roles of, 149t
Stakeholders, mapping of, 273–275
Stanford Medicine Bucket List Planner,
    51, 342
Stanford School of Medicine
        Ethnogeriatrics Ethno Med
        Website, 342
State of Health Equity (SDOH), Rush,
    297–301
STEPS Forward, 343
St. Mary Mercy Livonia, Livonia, MI, 133

Stomp Out Stigma Summits, 34
Stopping Elderly Accidents, Deaths &
    Injuries (STEADI), 121
STOPP/START (Screening Tool of
    Older persons' Prescriptions and
    Screening Tool to Alerty to Right
    Treatment criteria, 70
Strategic plans, change and, 281f
St. Vincent Medical Group
    case study at, 210
    distributed leadership case study,
        289–290, 289f, 291f
    outpatient case study, 211–216
Substance abuse assessment tools, 261t
Sulfonylureas, 79t
Support resources, online tools, 341–343
Surveys
    ambulatory/primary care outcome
        measures, 184t–185t
    as an outcome measure, 172t
    concordance of care with What
        Matters, 180t–181t
    pre-visit, 51
Symptom assessment tools, 261t
Syncope, 84t

T
Tags using EHRs, 15
Tailored Activity Programs (TAP), 96t
Tannenbaum, Cara, 65, 67
Team Action Planning (TAP), 267, 293
The Conversation Project (IHI), 10, 51
Timed Up & Go (TUG) Test, 235
Tradeoffs, care planning decisions and,
    16–17
Transforming Patient Experience, 343
Transitional Care Model (TCM), 259–262,
    260t, 262
Transitions of care, 253–265
    assisted living settings, 255
    caregivers and, 256t
    communication, 256t, 262
    continuum of care and, 256t, 259–262
    effective, 255–258
    electronic health records, 236–238
    long-term services and supports and,
        255
    patient issues in, 256t

person-centered, 2
using EHR in implementation,
    236–238
Trauma, history of, 46
Tricyclic antidepressants, 104
Trinity Health, 5–6, 21
Trust for America's Health (TFAH),
    310–311, 313, 318

U
Ultra-Brief 2-Item Screener, 53–54, 99,
    101f, 233
Urinary tract issues, 86t, 116t
Utilization rates, 2, 207

V
Validation therapy, 96t
Value-stream maps, 154
Vanderbilt Medical Center, Nashville,
    TN, 32
Vision impairment, 101t
VitalTalk, 345
Vote & Vax, 313

W
Walton Rehabilitation Hospital, 30–31
Waszynski, Christine M., 217
Webinars, use of, 268–269
Wellness visits. *See also* Annual Wellness
    Visits (AWVs)
    4M workflow, 155f
    appointments for, 148
What Matters conversations, 42–61, 42t
    audio/video resources, 345
    blog posts, 343
    books, 344
    care touchpoints, 42–43
    case studies, 57–59
    conduct of, 52–57
    considerations, 43–46
    content of, 48–50
    continuation of, 57
    documentation of, 57
    examples of, 351–353
    follow-up on, 56–57
    guides, 343–344
    guiding questions, 49–50
    initiation of, 47–48

invitation to, 58
length of, 58
Mobility plans and, 122
online tools, 341–343
patient preparation for, 50–51
preparation for, 52–54
questions in, 54–56
records of, 53
settings for, 53
support resources for, 341–345
trainings, 345
What Matters process, 226–230
Act On use in, 239–240
ambulatory care settings, 378t–381t
ambulatory/primary care outcome
   measures, 184t–185t
brochures, 51
care concordance with, 20–21,
   338–339, 372t–377t, 382t–
care plans and, 164t
case studies, 29–36
Cerner used in, 239f
conversations with patients, 24
cost-effectiveness and, 205–206
description of, 4

documentation of, 12–16, 186t–187t,
   190t–191t, 227, 335–337, 369t,
   379t
Epic used in, 239f
essential measures, 287f
key actions, 368t–369t
measures, 18–21, 18t
multicultural questions, 347–349
Older Adults Toolkit, 11
PDSA cycles, 401–403
plans of care and, 162t
survey of care concordance with,
   180t–181t
use of Cerner for, 230f
What Matters SmartText, 247f
Whitby Mental Health Center (WMHC),
   Whitby, Ontario, 34
Workflows
   customization of, 294
   medical assistant/RN, 240f
   Rush case study, 300–301

Y
"You CAN" campaign, 33
Your Conversation Starter Guide, 344

Made in the USA
Thornton, CO
04/24/23 12:44:00